INFANT LOSSES,
ADULT SEARCHES

Second Edition

INFANT LOSSES, ADULT SEARCHES

A Neural and Developmental Perspective on Psychopathology and Sexual Offending

Glyn Hudson Allez

KARNAC

First published in 2009 by
Karnac Books Ltd
118 Finchley Road, London NW3 5HT

Second edition published in 2011.

British Library Cataloguing in Publication Data

A C.I.P. for this book is available from the British Library

ISBN: 978 1 85575 808 7

Edited, designed and produced by The Studio Publishing Services Ltd
www.publishingservicesuk.co.uk
e-mail: studio@publishingservicesuk.co.uk

www.karnacbooks.com

CONTENTS

ABOUT THE AUTHOR   vii

INTRODUCTION   ix

CHAPTER ONE
Introduction to attachment   1

CHAPTER TWO
Neuroscientific additions   15

CHAPTER THREE
The insecurely attached child   43

CHAPTER FOUR
Puberty and adolescence   73

CHAPTER FIVE
Adult attachment styles   103

CHAPTER SIX
Narcissistic personalities   117

CHAPTER SEVEN
Psychopathology, personality disorders, and schizophrenia   129

CHAPTER EIGHT
Relationship dynamics and co-dependent relationships   149

CHAPTER NINE
Cyclothymia and the bipolar spectrum   165

CHAPTER TEN
Sexual addiction   173

CHAPTER ELEVEN
Internet addiction and offending   183

CHAPTER TWELVE
Stalking and violence   221

CHAPTER THIRTEEN
Paraphilias and sexual offending   235

CHAPTER FOURTEEN
The neurobiological effect of psychotherapy   273

REFERENCES   305

INDEX   361

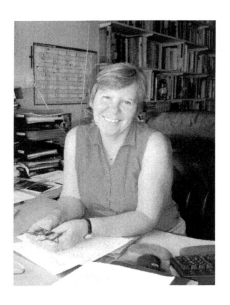

Dr Glyn Hudson Allez is a BPS Chartered Psychologist, specializing in counselling and forensic issues, and is a UKCP Registered psychosexual therapist. She has worked as a therapist for nearly thirty years, eight of which were in primary health care. She currently has a large private practice, specializing in working with sexual offenders. She has published numerous papers, theses, and book chapters, and two books: *Time Limited Therapy in a General Practice Setting* (1997, Sage), and *Sex and Sexuality: Questions and*

Answers for Counsellors and Psychotherapists (2005, Whurr). Glyn has two fellowships from the Association of Counsellors & Psycho-therapists in Primary Care (CPC) and from the British Association for Sexual & Relationship Therapy (BASRT).

Introduction

The first edition of this book was written in 2007, and, as neuro-science is such a fast-moving discipline, I was pleased when Oliver Rathbone of Karnac asked me to write a second edition. This book is a commentary on years of work with unhappy and sometimes distressed people who have managed to get themselves into situations that have made things worse for themselves rather than better. In trying to piece together my knowledge from different disciplines, I wanted to construct a heuristic that both therapists and clients alike could conceptualize and use as a road map for the client's journey to successful psychological health, which could later be evaluated through rigorous research.

An efficacious model needed to cover both physical and psychological aspects. I have always been uncomfortable with therapists who refused to offer suggestions regarding physical well-being when counselling, in terms of examining a client's lifestyle in diet and exercise, the premise being that a therapist simply reflects back what is being heard and it is not our place to advise. This seems as short-sighted as the medical practitioner who does not consider the psychological consequences of physical illnesses. I have always felt that we ignore the mind–body link at our peril.

Anxiety, panic, and depression all produce very identifiable physical responses, and if one first calms the person's fight-and-flight system that is in overdrive, it is much easier to deal with the obsessive rumination and cognitive distortions that accompany them. Similarly, if a medical practitioner is working with someone with coronary heart disease, hypertension, or diabetes, she needs to consider the psychological impact of these illnesses and how this will influence the treatment and prognosis of the patient.

I first became interested in attachment theory when I was teaching A-level psychology in the late 1980s. In those days, attachment theory was out of fashion, as feminists were attacking it as a misogynous proposal designed to keep mothers in the home. However, it did make sense to me at the time, and I could also identify my own insecure attachment from the work John Bowlby had published. Bowlby had built his theories formulated on his own experience; he had been brought up in an upper-middle-class family, and his first four years were spent with a loving nanny. When she left her job, the young Bowlby was devastated. Bowlby never forgot this infant loss, which made him search as an adult for an explanation (Bowlby, 2006). Years later, he stepped away from classic psychoanalytic theories to formulate his own developmental and cognitive theories of attachment and loss.

However, as with all theories that offer some merit or make intuitive cognitive sense, it got hijacked. I am not a political animal, but it would be remiss not to consider the changing political fortunes of Bowlby's ideas. Bowlby's original paper, based on examining forty-four juvenile thieves (Bowlby, 1944), highlighted the psychopathology and affectionless character of orphaned children. This was published in 1944, and was a gift for a government that, a year later, had a vast number of unemployed men demobbed at the end of the Second World War, whose wives had been employed in many of the occupations previously undertaken by the men who were away at war. Working mothers subsequently had nursery placements removed from them, using attachment theory as the evidence, forcing the women back into the home ("where they belonged"), leaving the jobs available for so many otherwise unemployed, discontented men.

Of course, now women had experienced a taste of living autonomously while so many men were in Europe, they were decidedly unhappy at having to stay at home looking after the children while men developed their careers and their personalities in a challenging working environment. Therefore, it created a feminist backlash, which had followed political changes from giving women the vote and equality in education, followed by the development of oral contraception, giving women the freedom of relationship choice, instead of living in fear of pregnancy and being publicly shamed. Bowlby's theories lost favour, as it was argued that they pressured women to be the sole carer of the couple's children. Equally, as women demanded to do the same work as men, men moved into women's domain, and women were happy to let them. Chamberlain described the time eloquently:

> When men took the place of women at birth and birth moved from home to hospital in the 1940s, Mother Nature was not invited to come along. In the 1950s prematurely born babies were starved for forty-eight hours for fear they might choke on "excess fluid". Men advocated cow's milk instead of mother's milk, advising women to feed their babies from bottles every four hours. Men coached mothers to let their babies cry unattended, and even opposed the use of rocking chairs! In hospitals, men promoted circumcision as if the excruciating pain and robbery of sexual parts were a matter of no importance to infants *or* parents, and men insisted on taking babies away from their mothers to house them in nurseries. In these days, fathers had no rights and were barred from attending their wives during labor and delivery; and mothers of preterm babies were barred from attending them in nursery. [Chamberlain, 1998, p. 206]

Prescott (1996) argued that a further tragedy of the rightful pursuit of gender equality has been women's misdirection to follow the male path, which meant that women were becoming more violent towards their children as power became more important than love. It is true that despite all of the organizations involved in child protection, the situation of childhood abuse is getting worse. Eight out of ten cases of child neglect are due to the biological mother (Strathearn, Gray, O'Callaghan, & Wood, 2001). However, Bowlby did talk about attachment to fathers (Bowlby, 1988), and later research focused on the importance of multiple attachments to grandparents (Schultz, 1980), nannies, and close family friends (Schaffer & Emerson, 1964). But another problem was that now mothers had excelled themselves in education, they had brains that did not respond well to being tied at home for 8–10 years (allowing two years per child if they had had up to four children to look after) at the prime time of their lives. The need for adult stimulation and intelligent conversation, which did not focus on nappies or the latest designer buggy, made some women spiral into depressive states. This low mood interfered with their relationships with their husbands and partners. Some women raged when the men came home at night after a demanding day at work if he could not conceptualize the equally demanding day she had had with the kids screaming, moaning, and playing up. Not surprisingly, statistics showed that a large proportion of divorces were occurring within two years of the birth of a child (Pacey, 2004). No wonder the birth rate started to drop rapidly.

So, women needed to go back to work to save their sanity. However, they had another problem to deal with in doing so: guilt. They may feel that they need to get away from the children, and may feel decidedly relieved, even though they have left the child sobbing with the child-minder. But how could they stop feeling guilty about it? Well, if Bowlby's theories did not focus on the mother so much, and the term could be replaced by something more politically correct, like "care-giver", then mothers need not feel quite so guilty that they are trying to meet their own needs at the same time as bringing up their children. Interestingly, the UK is swamped with language designed to change how things really are, so that people are not made to feel "bad", and although changing the terminology of attachment figures did attenuate the guilt felt by many women who left their children to go work, it could not completely take it away. Why? Because of the dynamic of the mother–child interaction; just looking into the fear and loss in the child's eyes as mother walks away taps into the mother's own sense of loss when her own mother walked away from her. Transgenerational transmission takes generations to override.

The next political hi-jack in the UK came with Thatcherism. Now, all modern young couples needed to buy their own homes, and with the spiralling costs of houses and mortgages, it was virtually impossible to do so on one salary alone. So, mothers were forced into a situation of returning to work at the end of their maternity leave, just as the children are reaching their practising period for attachments (see Chapters Two and Three), and for many of these women, there is no option if they want to stay in the homes that they chose when the couple were earning two salaries. Yes, there will be some cases where the father of the child earns less than the mother, and they make the choice for the father to become the househusband while mother works, and there may be similar arrangements made for gay couples bringing up children. Child-minding and nursery costs have escalated, though, and women are now wearing themselves out with the demands of a busy job, a home, and young children, with a considerable proportion of her salary being eaten up with child-care costs. As Perry (2001) argued, all societies reap what they have sown.

Ridgway and House (2006) pointed out that recent neuroscience research has been prolific, yet our ability to act on our knowledge has been incredibly slow. As the neuroscience literature on the development of a child's brain and its link to attachments has filtered through into public awareness, only a few researchers, such as Schore, Gerhardt, and Sunderland, have been brave enough to risk feminist flak and to highlight that what the child needs in the very early years, if he is going to develop the emotional centres of his brain into a secure attachment template, is his biological mother (Gerhardt, 2004; Schore, 1994; Sunderland, 2006). This is because of the child's genetic pre-birth programming to search for biological mother from the moment of birth in order for him to maintain his personal survival needs. The child will form multiple attachments as he grows, but it is the biological mother that the child "plugs" into to develop his neural emotional centres (see Chapter Three). It is the biological mother that the child searches for during the practising period for feedback on his autonomous adventures, as, up until this stage, the child does not have a concept of being separate from mother, and it is not until this stage that the child learns that he has a separate self. So, this feedback from mother, mediated through her eyes (Chapter Two), needs to occur when the child needs it; it will not necessarily happen during the time that mum picks up the child from the child-minder, rushes home, cooks tea, and then gives the child a quick bath and a quick story before bedtime.

Adopted children can learn to develop a secure and confident working model of life (see Chapter Three), but they will have already constructed a LOSS circuit, which, with happy and loving adoptive parents, may lie dormant throughout the childhood. But one day, a loss may trigger that circuit which had been myelinated (Chapter Two) from the earlier years, and will raise huge emotional insecurities in the person. This is why we, as therapists, see so many people who were adopted as children, and why so many adoptees get to the stage where they want to search for their biological origins.

Play is one aspect that the modern generation of children are losing out on. First, children are not allowed out of the house to play, for fear of a paedophile behind every bush. This is not to undermine the very real distress that parents feel when their children fall victim to predators. But, as Matravers (2003) vehemently argued, the incidence of children murdered by sexual predators has not increased in real terms since the 1970s, yet the media overemphasize its prevalence by high profile reporting, encouraging the outpouring of grief and rage in the general public, which the government endorses by endless knee-jerk policies. The consequence is that parents are fearful of letting their children out of their sight for a minute, and, thus, children cannot use their SEEKING system to search the local environment for themselves, or build their own play structures (Chapter Two). Second, the use of technological equipment such as videos, DVDs, televisions, computers, mobile phones, etc., reduces the incidence of rough and tumble play between children, which is vital for social bonding. Panskepp (1998) argues that this lack of physical play in young children is responsible for the vast increase in attention deficit and hyperactivity disorders (ADHD) found in modern Western societies. Adolescents are choosing mobile texting, Facebook, and MSN, messaging each other in preference to meeting and spending time in each other's company. It will eventually mean that their relationships will only be able to be conducted if some form of communication machine mediates them.

It is impossible to read this book without considering one's own parenting, as well as one's own way of being a parent. And the issues of blame and responsibility emerge. However, blame is an unhelpful construct here. I agree with Zeanah (1996) that the pejorative labelling of parents is unhelpful and counter to prevailing clinical practice. Therefore, I discourage the blaming of parents when working with clients for the following reason. Our parents, even if they were toxic and abusive towards us, are the product of their own parenting, and transgenerational transmission is covertly pervasive. Fonagy and colleagues found that the attachment style of the mother during her pregnancy predicted the attachment style of the child at one year old (Fonagy, Steele, & Steele, 1991). A one-year-old child assessed as insecurely attached demonstrates more interactive disturbances with their mothers and with their teachers than securely attached children (Sroufe, 1983b; Waters, Wippman, & Sroufe, 1979). People are not taught to be parents. They muddle on, doing what they can, based on what had happened to them. Using this framework, sometimes they make changes, determined that similar events never happen to their own children, and sometimes they repeat what happened to them without remembering. Some people, even though they have tried to change their future based on their knowledge of the past, have found themselves subconsciously repeating it anyway. But knowledge is power. I mourn for not having this knowledge when I was bringing up my own children; however, I am determined that they will understand the processes and make more informed decisions when considering my grandchildren. Similarly, with clients with young children or planning to have children, the more they know, the more informed choices they can make as to their futures, and the futures of their children, in preventing transgenerational transmission.

There is one more political implication of this material that needs to be alluded to, and that is the implications for our immigration policies. In the UK we have been generous in encouraging and protecting people from war-torn or less advantaged countries of the world. People who seek asylum in the UK are given housing, benefits or work, education, protection for a better way of life, and then we leave them to get on with it. What we do not give them is any form of psychological support. Immigrants and asylum-seekers who have broken attachments from their countries and families of origin, who have witnessed war atrocities or trauma, who have been the victims of violence or rape, who have been sold into sexual slavery at an early age, or who have experienced family persecution on the basis of their race, culture, or class, will have predominantly unresolved and disorganized attachment styles, and will, as a consequence, bring their maladaptive coping strategies with them into our country. Longitudinal studies have shown that the male children of women who were pregnant during the German blockade of Holland during the Second World War, whose mothers were severely malnourished during their first and second trimesters of pregnancy, have two and a half times the rate of antisocial personality disorder than other men (Neugebauer, Hoek, & Susser, 1999). Persecution, discrimination, migration, and involuntary social transplantation are all known risk factors for psychological disturbance (Brisch, 1999). Without psychological support, victims will still be manifesting extreme emotions with an insecure template, producing emotions of FEAR and RAGE, directed towards their rescuers (see the Karpman triangle in Chapter Seven), the birth-people of the UK. These damaged and vulnerable incoming individuals will create their own societies within our society, because that is what makes them feel safe. But, without healing the rifts of their own childhood trauma, and without receiving help with their post-trauma stress, they will be unable to provide the right environment for their children born in the UK. As Siegel (2003) pointed out, lack of resolution of trauma or grief in a parent creates paradoxical, unsolvable, and problematic situations for their children. Cozolino (2006) eloquently tells the story of Joaquin, an American-born man of an Eastern European family of origin, who had the persecution of his family hidden from him, yet he still behaviourally acted it out. That is why we find that it is not necessarily the immigrants to the UK who get drawn into terrorist activities, but their British-born children, who, torn between a clash of two cultures in which they live, act out the unresolved trauma of their parents that they, too, have inherited, and are subsequently vulnerable to predatory terrorists who will offer them security and hope through extreme dogma and inflexible rules.

The last few chapters of this book focus specifically on offending, but, although I discuss treatment options, particularly for men who have committed sexual offences, I have not discussed the prison regime. Matravers (2003) has argued that society's popular preoccupation with predatory paedophiles makes current policy misdirected. Of course, society's desire for natural justice means that offenders have to be punished. They need to face the consequences of their behaviour through being taken away from all that they know and love. But does it achieve this? For many men, it is being outside of the institutional structure of prison that is the scary place; having to function in a world that values material success, beauty, and prowess; a world where they possess neither the skills nor the confidence to function appropriately. So, for some men, prison becomes their safe base, and recidivism is occurring not because the offender is essentially bad and incapable of living a moral life, but because he needs to get back to the institutional setting where he can live cheaply and without the stress of having to make decisions, pay rent or council tax, and can quietly avoid relationships.

And what a wasted opportunity prison is. Instead of encouraging each inmate to embark on some form of therapeutic attachment to work through the demons of their history, people languish in cells, alienated from themselves and society, forming dysfunctional sexual attachment groups between themselves. Then society is outraged when, on release, these men do not function according to society's mores. Outcome literature shows us that what prevents an abused child becoming an adult abuser is an ongoing attachment relationship with someone through childhood (Kaufman & Zigler, 1987). If an offender has to serve several years in prison, what a golden opportunity to provide a therapeutic attachment figure in the prison system to enable that offender to work through the trauma of his history, to build up a trusting relationship, and then to launch the person back into society with the confidence of living life differently. As Davenport and Fisher (2007) argue, how is it that the childhood trauma of offenders apparently evaporates in the way society treats them once they reach the age of eighteen? At what point in their lives does the child victim change into being the adult perpetrator? At what point do we stop treating the victim with compassion and start treating the perpetrator with disgust and outrage? How does the child victim know not to repeat or adapt what was done to him, if we provide no interventions or support between the two scenarios? Adams (2003) argued that the most compassionate thing we can do for sex offenders and for their future victims is to compel them to address their own childhood trauma histories as a major part of sex offender therapy. We must stop treating the symptoms of our sick society with quick (four-year election-during) fixes and start addressing the real reasons why people offend. Professionals in the mental health world in the UK have an international reputation (thanks to the National Institute for Clinical Excellence (NICE)) of wanting cheap, quick fixes. When will they start considering the long-term human cost of crime? They expect the complex damage of decades or even generations to be healed with 6–12 sessions of cognitive–behavioural therapy (CBT), because that is the only therapy that responds well in outcome research, while ignoring the finding that the wrong psychotherapy for the wrong person can cause harm (Lilienfeld, 2007). When will politicians acknowledge the false economy of discounting individual therapy for fiscal reasons, preferring the cheap option of group therapy for some prisoners in some prisons?

I have started this book by talking about the effect that having children has on women, whereas much of the book will be illustrated by the effect of child-rearing practices on men. This is because many of the presenting issues that are discussed in this book, which I have specialized in working with as a therapist, are predominantly issues for men. As Hazan pointed out, it is men who benefit the most from an attachment relationship, and men who suffer the most ill effects when attachment is disrupted (Hazan, 2003, p. 52). But women do have paraphilias, they do stalk, and they do offend against children, but the incidence in all of these behaviours is much lower for women than for men. Where there is a difference between how men and women respond in certain situations, I have elaborated it in the respective chapters. Where there has been no difference, I have alternated the pronoun between he and she for ease of writing and to show no preference.

I decided to present just one case study throughout the book, to elaborate the situations that I discuss, at the beginning and at the end of each chapter. The story of Gordon highlights the developmental perspective taken, and, in particular, transgenerational transmission. It shows how Gordon's parents' families of origin influence their own attachment styles, and that determines how Gordon is treated as a child. Gordon responds similarly to his own son, Conner, who is at risk of behaving in a similar way to his own children, unless he can develop sufficient earned security through his own attachments and determination.

Attachment styles and working models in the brain formulate templates of how a person expects life to work out, and the consequent behaviour reinforces these expectancies in self-fulfilling ways. However, experience can change these working models. A secure child can become insecure following a trauma or attachment insult at a critical period of right-brain development, either in childhood or in adolescence. Similarly, a secure adult can become insecure following an attachment injury (see Chapter Eight) within a loving relationship. Equally, insecure adults can develop emotional security and earn or learn secure attachment, given sufficient mindfulness and emotional regulation. So, the developmental progress of attachments is not a theory of determinism; it is a theory of adaptation to one's life history.

Gordon is a compilation of many men that I have seen over the years. If someone feels that they identify themselves in Gordon or Rachel as they read, then this is coincidental. The description of Gordon's birth in Chapter One introduces us to him and to the work of John Bowlby. Chapters Two and Three elaborate the understanding of neuroscientific research in relation to attachment theory and how an insecure attachment template can be developed in a child's brain and the damage that can be caused by abusive parenting or traumatic events. Chapters Four and Five take Gordon through puberty, adolescence, and into being a man with an insecure attachment template. Narcissistic style is not usually part of attachment literature, but, in my view, is a manifestation from the practising period, is covered in Chapter Six, and is considered again as part of a personality disorder in Chapter Seven. Chapters Eight and Nine introduce Gordon's partner, Rachel, to help us understand the process of co-dependent relationships, domestic violence, and bipolar disorder. Gordon has always been a heavy user of pornography, and Chapters Ten and Eleven show how he becomes addicted to sex and to pornography on the Internet as his relationship to Rachel is breaking down. By Chapter Twelve, Gordon's insecurity is extreme, as Rachel and their son Conner are removed from him and he starts to harass and to stalk. In mourning his loss from his family, by Chapter Thirteen (unlucky for some), Gordon has become so addicted to sex, the Internet, and to extreme pornography as a means of soothing himself that he loses cognizance of his own behaviour and ends up being arrested and labelled as a sexual offender. Therapeutic methods are discussed intermittently throughout this book, which finishes in Chapter Fourteen with a discussion about the neurophysiology of therapy, the mind–body link and right-brain soothing. Gordon is placed into a situation where he can create some change for himself if he is willing to stick with it and through it. We are left unsure of his outcome, mirroring the uncertainties that we all face in life in changing our attachment templates.

What is different about this edition compared to the earlier one? As well as including more up-to-date research, listening to the feedback from readers, I have included new sections into this book. Specifically, in Chapter Two, I have elaborated more on neuropeptides and the relationship between mother and infant at birth. In Chapter Three, I have included more on the consequences of trauma and a section on childhood sexual abuse. In Chapter Four, I have elaborated more on adolescent processes. Chapter Eleven includes an elaboration of the addictive process, and Chapter Thirteen clarifies the differences between the psychopathological and legal aspects of paedophilia. Finally, Chapter Fourteen includes more of my way of working, including my method of assessment of individuals, couples, and offenders, and more on right-brain soothing. I hope I have heard everyone's request.

My particular thanks must go to Brian Allez for his patient work in constructing the diagrams for this text from a less than patient innovator.

For my parents Florrie and Bill Cooper
Despite their insecure attachments, they have celebrated
sixty-eight years of marriage (and still counting)

From them came my infant losses and adult searches

CHAPTER ONE

Introduction to attachment

He listens to the regular, pulsating beat of her heart, the gurgling of her bowels, and the swirl of blood and fluids all around him. His movements are slow and undefined as he bounces within the amniotic fluid. He can manage to get his hand into his mouth to suck on tiny fingers. It feels warm and comforting. He feels safe.

Suddenly, her body swirls and falls. He hears her voice let out a scream and he bounces on the top and then the bottom of his uterine walls as she falls to the floor, his arms flailing out to clutch at something. A sudden blow impacts into her stomach. He flinches from the pain of the blow, his little heart pounds faster with a surge of adrenaline and cortisol. He hears another scream of pain. His hands reach out to bang on the sides of the placenta, and fire surges through his system from the umbilical chord. Terror is surging through his body. He can hear another voice, deeper, less clear, screaming close as she tries to get up, but again she falls to the floor. He kicks out with his feet and his arms in the fluid. "Remember me! Remember me! Will I survive?"

The screaming has stopped, but there are new sounds now. Sirens wailing, strange voices making comforting noises, but sounding uncertain. His body still feels on fire, and the walls of his shelter keep becoming taught, compressing, pushing him further down into her body. She is screaming again. He can feel her fear. Her fear is his fear.

He is tired now. He has been struggling, fighting, and scared for so long. His energy has all gone. He feels he is slipping away. Another scream, and a strange sensation on his head; painfully clamped; feeling cold and dry. Huge hands clasp his head as he is pulled into the cold. He struggles weakly; he does not want to go. He would rather stay where it is safe and warm. He feels a constriction at his throat, getting tighter as he starts to leave her. There is pressure in his head and neck, and the cold burns on his skin. Fingers push against his throat; something hard and cold pressing against it. A snap, and he feels his throat released. Now he has the sensation of moving through a cold, dry space, hands rubbing his chest, a hard tube pushed down his throat. Leave me alone! He retches his first breath and lets out a wail of fear. Voices mention that he is too small and his skin is yellow. He is wrapped tightly in dry cloth that feels harsh on his delicate skin and he is lowered into a box. The box is warm, but echoes, with strange buzzing noises, and the lid bangs when it shuts, making him start. He keeps wailing, hoping she will hear his plea. Where is she? Why can't he go back where he was?

He wakes from a slumber. A hand emerges through the side of the box and fingers gently slide against the side of his face. The smell is familiar. He knows it is her. He hears her voice, comforting and clearer. He tries to orientate his face to where the sound is coming from. She loosens the wrapping binding around him and his little arm jerks out, trying to grab on to the familiar sound.

"Hello, Gordon," he hears her voice say. "Welcome to the world. Happy birthday." Again he waves his arm in the direction of the voice, trying to reach the sound. He feels her touch his fingers. He grabs on to her, and grips his fist tightly around her finger. He feels the warmth from her hand trace up his arm into his heart; it makes his heart beat stronger and warmth surges through his body. He feels safe. He is reconnected.

What is attachment?

Attachment is defined as "the affectional bond or tie that an infant forms between himself and his mother figure" (Ainsworth, Blehar, Waters, & Wall, 1978, p. 302). It is a process that starts at birth as the infant begins making emotional connection to his parents, starting with the biological mother (I will use the term "biological mother", as opposed to "care-giver" in this context, and an explanation for this decision is given in Chapter Four), and then later to other familiar figures, including the father, grandparents, and other members of the extended family and close friends (Schaffer & Emerson, 1964). This attachment process of providing a secure base for a child is vital to the survival of the species because it facilitates the emotional pairing between mother and child, which, in turn, leads to the protection of the infant during his most vulnerable years.

Over the years during infancy, childhood, and adolescence, confidence is built in the slowly developing child with the aid of attachment figures. A child learns confidence from the attachment figures, that they will be available to him whenever desired, and will provide loving, supportive, and predictable caring. In learning this, the child builds up a mental template, or inner working model, in his mind, providing the expectancy that things usually work out for the best, and when times do become difficult, the child knows a place or a safe haven (the mother) to return to in order to be soothed and supported. When adult, such a child will be much less prone to feelings of intense or chronic fear through the development of this expectancy and confidence, and will have learnt to manage the extremes of his emotions.

Slade described the functions of attachment as:

1. A child being born with the predisposition to become attached.
2. The child organizing her behaviour and thinking to maintain the attachment that is key to her physiological and psychological survival.
3. The maintenance of this attachment may be at the cost of her own functioning.
4. Distortions in thinking and feeling stem from early disturbances in attachments and the parent's inability to meet the child's emotional needs. [Slade, 1999, p. 576]

Attachment is vital in developing a strong sense of self in the child and an empathetic understanding of others. Should this attachment bond be interrupted, Bowlby proposed that it would induce interpersonal anger in the child as a form of protest behaviour, the function of which is directed at regaining contact with the attachment figure (Bowlby, 1951). For an infant who has not yet developed language or logic, an absent or unpredictable mother is interpreted as a threat to life from separation or abandonment, producing extreme emotional responses in the child of terror, grief, and rage.

Bowlby (1973) held that the predictions that a child makes of how attachment figures are likely to behave towards her are reasonable extrapolations from the way adults have behaved in the past, and that this insecurity continues into her adult behavioural repertoire. Thus, the child's mental template is a working model, providing a prediction of how people are going to behave towards her. This then facilitates how the person will later behave, using that predictive expectation, and will influence her thoughts, feelings, and expectations in future relationships. Bowlby proposed that if the secure base and safe haven were not available for the child, she would develop an insecure attachment that would manifest in all later childhood, adolescent, and adult attachment relationships. Bowlby further held that the distortions in thinking and feeling that occurred as a result of insecure attachments underpinned many dysfunctional relationships and much individual psychopathology.

Ainsworth and her colleagues subsequently developed Bowlby's theories and used the attachment process as the basis of a research methodology, "The Strange Situation" (Ainsworth, Blehar, Waters, & Wall, 1978), in watching how toddlers responded when their mothers left a room where the child was playing when a stranger was present (producing fear and uncertainty). How the child responded when the stranger tried to interact with the child, and how the toddler responded when mother returned, demonstrated the child's attachment style. The Ainsworth studies demonstrated three categories of response: the securely attached (type B), the avoidant insecurely attached (type A), and the resistant insecurely attached (type C) child. In these early studies, it was thought that about 70% of children were securely attached; that is, mother provided the safe haven for the child, who was comforted after mother's absence. However, about 20% of infants were avoidant, and failed to enjoy the reunion with mother, wanting to be near her but not wanting to be held by her. A further 10% were resistant to her, showing ambivalence in wanting to be picked up and then immediately wanting to be put down, or the child would turn his back on mother as she was attempting to comfort him. These attachment styles are universal and have been demonstrated across cultures (van IJzendoorn & Sagi, 1999). More recently, Holmes (1996) suggested that, in average populations, 20% of children are avoidant, 17% are ambivalent, and one in twenty (5%) are disorganized. With the addition of a preoccupied style, this proposes that half of children are now insecurely attached, and one might hypothesize that this increase is linked to the increase of mothers returning to work before the child reaches two years old. This hypothesis is discussed further in the following chapters.

Schore (1994) has emphasized that there is a critical window of opportunity for a child to develop secure attachments. He called this time the practising period, which occurs when the infant is between twelve and twenty-four months old. At this time, the infant starts to develop a sense of autonomy, and separateness from his mother as he begins to pull himself up on his feet and toddle away. During exploration away from the mother's embrace, the child constantly looks back to watch mother's facial expression, waiting for feedback on what is safe and what is acceptable. This is an exciting yet scary time for the child as he learns that he is no longer a part of mother, but a separate entity. Sometimes, as he explores, the fear will become too much, and he will want to rush back to the safety of mother's arms. Mother's warm welcome and caring expression amplifies the positive arousal and excitement of exploration, encouraging it to be repeated. When infants have a mother who is encouraging yet responsive, sensitive, and attuned to the child, the child will develop a secure attachment. The mother will have an awareness of her child's inner experience, and will sense when he is attuned or misattuned. Misattunement is not a negative experience, and research has demonstrated that a healthy attachment can develop with only 32% attunement (Sunderland, 2006), so a mother does not have to be perfect. On the contrary, misattunement is vital for the healthy growth of resilience to stress in the child, for it is only through misattunement that the child learns appropriate rapprochement in the reunion with mother, repair of the extreme emotions that misattunement elicits, and the ability to self-soothe or to search for mother or another for soothing. This resilience in the face of stress is an important indicator of a secure attachment (Greenspan, 1981). Thus, as Sroufe and colleagues emphasized, from the social dependency of the child in early years comes the self-reliance and resilience found in adulthood (Sroufe, Egeland, Carlson, & Collins, 2005).

All infants start off being egocentric, focusing purely on their own needs for survival. However, this narcissism and omnipotence depletes when the secure attachment process builds and empathy is introduced, as he develops an understanding of another's emotions and needs in relation to his own. A securely attached infant learns to feel, understand, and regulate the extremes of his emotions appropriately. By monitoring facial expressions from his mother, he will learn to correlate facial expressions with the felt emotion, the beginning of emotional intelligence (Goleman, 1995). In this way, as he learns the nuances of non-verbal emotional communication, he will develop the capacity for understanding the states of minds of others; the development of empathy. Human beings are the only animals with the white visible around their eyes, providing feedback for the observer as to where the person is looking, imparting information regarding possible intentions. Thus, by viewing the facial expressions of others around him, using feedback from his mother, the child will make an approximation of how others may be feeling, which is the beginning of social intercourse. In developing empathy, he will learn compassion, prosocial values, and morality, which will protect the child from antisocial behaviour and alienation. He will become socially outgoing and confident, will be willing to explore his environment in a confident way, and will be less fearful of risk while being mindful of the needs of others. Indeed, preschool children who are securely attached to their mothers use this information to develop stronger and closer friendship bonds when they do go to school. Children who were securely attached at age three showed more open emotional communication and better language ability with their mothers and with their peers at age four and a half (McElwain, Booth LaForce, Lansford, Wu, & Dyer, 2008). The interpretations that children make in their relationships with their family form the working model for their ability to get along with their friends.

Birth trauma and premature babies

Ridgway and House (2006) argue that the bonding of an infant to his mother occurs both pre-conceptually and throughout the pregnancy, as the infant and mother unite through shared senses. Birth is traumatic for the infant *per se*, but becomes even more so when the child is evicted from the uterus too early, or gets dragged into the world via Caesarean section. The medicalization of the birth process has had the beneficial effect of protecting both mothers and infants from the dangers of separation during delivery. Maternal and infant mortality has been greatly reduced, and premature infants of increasingly younger gestation are surviving with the aid of incubation and Special Care Baby Units (SCBU). However, this medicalization has a negative aspect, too, in that priority is given to this process: the attachment of machines on the baby's head pre-birth can interfere with the mother's natural birthing position. The invasion of strangers' (nurses, midwives, and doctors) interventions on an infant's body to provoke breathing or to pull the baby out with forceps, the surgical removal of the child from the womb before he feels ready or able during Caesarean section, or the removal of the child from the mother, sometimes (for premature babies) for months, into the isolation and artificial environment of an incubator. On one level, modern-day birthing techniques acknowledge the importance of reconnecting the infant with the biological mother by placing the newly born infant across mother's stomach or chest in skin-to-skin contact. But when there is a medical emergency, this need for infant–mother contact is understandably swept aside to deal with the ongoing threat to life. When the emergency is over, the assumption seems to be made that all is well, as no external physical damage can be detected. But this trauma is one that the infant remembers and stores in preverbal somatic and emotional memories, and the longer the period between the separation and physical reunion between mother and baby, the greater the potential for attachment and bonding ties to be broken. Verny and Kelly (1981) suggest that when premature babies become adults, they always have this sense of feeling rushed or hurried, and never fully catching up with others.

Of course, paediatric nurses and doctors do know this, and encourage parents to spend time with infants in SCBU. The medicalization process, however, has to be prioritized to protect the infant's mortality, yet it does so at the cost of the mother being available *when the infant wants it*, and not just when it is convenient for the medical staff or mother to provide it. The type of touch is important, too. To a premature baby, the dry, mechanical environment of an incubator will feel alien because she is pre-programmed to spend the last trimester in the wet, hot, noisy, safe environment *in utero*. Mother reaching out and touching the tiny baby's hand through the incubator's side, or lifting her on to her lap awkwardly so as not to detach the wiring from the machines, is not the kind of touch that the infant is pre-programmed to feel. Baby wants to feel real skin-to-skin contact, hearing the familiar rhythm of her heart, feeling her heat, hearing her voice, smelling her smell, and feeling completely surrounded by her in a protective embrace. To the baby, they are still a single unit, as she has no sense of being separate, so mother's absence will feel like a missing limb. Some SCBU workers, therefore, encourage the "kangarooing" of the infant, which is placing the infant inside the clothing of the parent, as a way of helping with reconnection. These babies gain more weight and have less physical and somatosensory complications than babies who do not experience this (Strathearn, 2003).

Feher (1980) argued that the correlation between birth problems and later behavioural difficulties cannot be ignored. She found that babies born with the aid of instruments grow up with a need to lean on others and have difficulty in using their own initiative. Premature babies tend to be clinging, resist change, and avoid responsibility. Babies born in a breech position over-react to their environment and can be aggressive, expecting to be pulled through difficult life situations, and babies born by Caesarean section tend to need a lot of help to achieve their goals and tend to blame others for not giving support if they fail to achieve. Verny and Kelly (1981) agreed, and proposed that these individuals need a lot of physical contact, which might be due to sensual loss of vaginal birth, producing intense feelings of both extreme pleasure and excruciating pain, both the forerunners of adult sexuality.

However, there is always an interactive dynamic between infant and mother at this vulnerable early stage. Strathearn and colleagues found that there is a significant difference in how mothers respond to their babies depending on whether their deliveries were vaginal or through Caesarean section (Strathearn, 2003). In addition, birth difficulties do present a risk factor for child protection services. Fifteen per cent of premature babies are reported to child protection services, twice as many as babies born at full-term, and some have been reported ten or fifteen times each (Strathearn, 2003). Also, medical risk factors such as low birth weight, male gender, and young maternal age are independently associated with maltreatment of the child. We need to remember that a lot of pre-term babies are born into socially deprived areas. However, Verny and Kelly (1981) also blame the isolation of premature babies in incubators for weeks or months after birth and the devastating psychological effects this has on the mother, making her more likely to physically abuse the child later.

Research is ambivalent regarding the incidence of insecure attachments in premature infants, with some investigators saying that the incidence is no different than with babies born at full-term (Goldberg, Corter, Lojkasek, & Minde, 1990), whereas others argue that the incidence of insecure attachments is increased in premature babies (Sajaniemi et al., 2001). However, a retrospective study of a large number of men found a correlation between birth complications, maternal rejection, and violent behaviour in adulthood (Raine, Brennan, & Mednick, 1994). Similarly, a prospective longitudinal study found a correlation between birth complications, disadvantaged family backgrounds, and risk for violent crime when adult (Piquero & Tibbetts, 1999). Although these studies do not propose that birth complications cause violence or crime, it is one factor on the pathway to adult offending behaviour discussed throughout this book. Clearly, the incubator will get in the way of the natural bond between mother and child, and, as is discussed in the next chapter, the infant will not "understand" the disconnection from his mother as he is only working on the developing pre-programmed emotional circuits, and will, therefore, develop a LOSS circuitry based on feelings of the threat of abandonment and fear for survival.

Children in day care

The need for predictable and responsive parenting poses the question regarding young children in day care, given that contemporary Western society has such a large proportion of working mothers. "Is this harmful to small children?" is the question asked by anxious and guilt-ridden working mothers. Bowlby originally argued that it is not until a child reaches the age of three and a half years that he can manage a half to a whole day away from his mother without experiencing separation anxiety (Bowlby, 1988). More recently, Rauh and colleagues found that, without exception, when a child changed from a secure attachment measured in the first year of the infant's life to an insecure attachment style measured in the second year, it was because the child experienced an abrupt introduction into day care at about twelve months old (Rauh, Ziegenhain, Müller, & Wignroks, 2000). Belsky (2006) similarly found that children who spent early, extensive, and continuous time in day care were more likely to show later behavioural problems, such as aggressiveness and disobedience. This acting out suggests that these children are feeling insecure. Sagi and colleagues reported that poor quality of day care with a high infant–adult ratio increased the likelihood of the children becoming insecurely attached (Sagi, Koren-Karie, Gini, Ziv, & Joels, 2002). With the best will in the world, working mothers do provide their children with unpredictable parenting. A child under two years old has not achieved the cognitive ability to understand that when mother leaves for work in the morning, she will return at night. Therefore, these children respond from a base of fear of potential abandonment. However, what is also clear is that the best buffer to protect children from this is the sensitivity of the mother in managing the transition of the child into day care (Scharfe, 2003). Richard Bowlby emphasized that children can bond with secondary attachments to nannies or grandparents, but there is a danger of an attachment injury should the nanny leave the family, as happened to his famous father. He also warned against the tendency of some parents to repeatedly swap child carers to prevent a bond developing, or to choose a nursery where the child–carer ratio is such that it prohibits babies from developing such a bond (Bowlby, 2007).

Contemporary thinking about attachment has moved on from seeing it as merely a psychological construction of what happens between an infant and parents into a developmental template of behavioural activity (Sroufe, 1977). Sroufe and his colleagues have focused upon the attachment behaviour patterns that occur, particularly in the first five years of life (Sroufe, 1983a; Sroufe, Egeland, Carlson, & Collins, 2005). In synthesizing the framework of Bowlby's internal working models (Bowlby, 1988), Sroufe's understanding of behavioural patterns, and contemporary understanding of how the brain works, a process of neural templates can be considered, providing a physiological underpinning for the psychological and cognitive expectancies of inner working models. It can be argued that these schematic memory processes are hardwired by neural connections, a full discussion of which occurs in the next chapter.

Gordon's review

Gordon's conception was unplanned, which already places him at a higher risk of early mortality, which, within the first twenty-eight days is two and half times greater than for infants where the pregnancy was planned (Roe & Drivas, 1993).

His parents had been together, in an intense and highly sexually charged relationship, for only five months when he was conceived. They had met in a local pub, and after only a few meetings became inseparable. They had not planned to conceive a child, but they had not thought to use contraception either. They had just not thought about it, as they were so preoccupied with each other.

Gordon's father, Joe, was an unemployed builder's labourer, who, at twenty-two, was five years older than his partner. Much of his unemployment benefit was spent in the pub, where he would meet many friends and feel in good company. He could not be bothered to get a job now, however, as, in previous employment, he found it difficult to take orders from people whom he did not respect. Joe lived at home with his parents, who also drank heavily. Rows were common in Joe's household, and his parents were often violent towards one another.

Gordon's mother, Jenny, at seventeen, had only recently left school and was working in an insurance office. She lived with her single-parent mother, who was very involved in community work and local women's projects, and, therefore, could give her daughter little time. Jenny did not know her father. Jenny was captivated by Joe's handsome face and infectious laugh. Being more serious than Joe, Jenny felt that she could help Joe make something more of himself. She had never felt so loved before, and even though Joe could be unnecessarily jealous, she excused it as an example of just how much he loved her.

When Gordon was at nineteen weeks gestation, and Jenny's pregnancy became obvious to the outside observer, Joe and Jenny realized that they needed to do something about a pregnancy they had so far been overlooking and avoided discussing. They discussed termination; Joe was in favour, Jenny was scared, but anyway they realized they were probably too late to make the arrangements. A mother's attitude towards her baby can be transmitted to her baby *in utero*, and some babies give up the will to live, hence one of the reasons for the higher mortality rate in unplanned pregnancies (Chamberlain, 1998). Gordon, however, was determined to survive.

Joe got himself a job. Jenny applied for a council flat, and, three weeks before Gordon was born, they moved into the flat together. The stress of the pregnancy, and their respective parents' negative responses to their partners, took its toll on Joe and Jenny's relationship. Joe's parents viewed Jenny as a "stuck-up cow" who was "up 'er own arse", whereas Jenny's mum viewed Joe as a "ne'er-do-well", and worried about his ability to support Jenny and her child. She also felt that Joe was very much like Jenny's father, who had disappeared from both of their lives when Jenny was an infant. The tension from their families of origin, and the fear of the impending obligation, had an impact on their relationship, and Joe and Jenny replaced the intensity of sex with the intensity of arguments, which eventually led to Joe starting to hit Jenny, as the only way he knew to end the disputes.

Unconsciously, each has introduced into their relationship behaviour they have learnt from their family of origin: Joe's parents mocked him when he got a job, and they taunted him about Jenny being in control. The shame and frustration of parental criticism led Joe to lash out at Jenny to assert his dominant position. Jenny's mother expressed her doubts about Joe, making Jenny critical of Joe's attempts to change as being too little and not well meant, provoking his angry and violent assaults. The more Jenny tried to rescue Joe from his drinking and lack of work ethic, the more he persecuted her (Karpman, 1968). Her shame and humiliation led her to hide the violence and pretend to the outside world that everything was well between her and Joe.

What are the implications of this pre-birth and post-birth domestic violence for Gordon? From the twenty-fourth week of gestation, Gordon is listening to his mother all the time (Verny & Kelly, 1981). As Jenny cries over the rows with her mother and the fights with Joe, her adrenaline and cortisol levels increase substantially. Jenny's fear of Joe's unpredictable violent outbursts becomes a chronic stressor. Gordon is, therefore, experiencing a stressful environment *in utero*, through his mother's distress. Her experience of intense stressful events and domestic violence will also be Gordon's stressful events. Her increase in adrenaline and cortisol will have the effect of pumping too much cortisol around his tiny body before he has developed the ability to cope with it (Schore, 1994). Research has demonstrated that distressed and depressed pregnant mothers sensitize their infants to later exposure to stress by increasing the child's level of cortisol. This is predictive of high levels of cortisol in pre-school age children, who subsequently exhibit greater mental health problems (Essex, Klein, Cho, & Kalin, 2002). These children develop a predisposition to stress, and often start life with hypervigilance and extreme reactions to stressful events. As he develops, Gordon may demonstrate heightened stress reactions to events that others may cope with and take in their stride. This predisposition underpins a constant state of semi-arousal, alertness, vigilance, and anxiety reactions. The dendrites of his hippocampus in his tiny developing brain will shrivel (Siegel, 1999), impairing his ability to remember events, whereas his amygdala and the pathways to his sympathetic arousal system will be overdeveloped and hypersensitive (Atkinson, 2005) (see the next chapter for a fuller explanation of this). Gordon may show an inability to learn sufficiently at school, as the absorption of education requires the child to be relaxed and receptive, but the hypervigilance gets in the way. The inability to learn sufficiently may lead to learning and behavioural difficulties, as children often act out their fear with disruptive and sometimes aggressive behaviour. They will show inattentiveness, hyperactivity, and conduct concerns as they constantly test the boundaries of authority searching for a safe place (Sroufe, 1979).

Thus, even as Gordon arrives in the world, his future potential has already been impaired.

CHAPTER TWO

Neuroscientific additions

Gordon awoke with a start to the sound of a loud, angry voice in another room. He felt cold, hungry, and alone. The darkness of the room swirled around him in strange frightening shapes. Where is she? He wailed out his loneliness in a long screeching cry. Will she return?

"Can't you shut that fucking brat up?" the distant angry voice demands.

The door opens and light pours into the room, circling her head as mother comes bustling in, wearing floppy slippers and a loose dressing gown. She lifts Gordon out of the cot and holds him close. His wails lessen slightly, but he continues to cry.

"Come on, Gordy. Don't do this to me, lovey. You know what he's like when he's had a few drinks."

Jenny sat in a nearby chair and plonked Gordon on her lap, pushing a cold rubber bottle teat on top of his vibrating tongue. He looked up to her face, searching for her eyes. But her face was turned away from him, her cheeks pale, and her mouth drawn down. Gordon coughed out the cold liquid as it started to invade his airway. Jenny sat him up to pat his back. In her distraction she did not realize how hard the pats were, making Gordon cough and cry even more. She stood up and swung Gordon up on to her shoulder, pacing up and down while bouncing him on her hand. Gordon dribbled milk down her back, but quietened a little. He wants to feel connected. He wants to feel safe. But he does not feel safe like this. He could feel her agitation shaking through his body. He could taste her fear.

"Get back in 'ere, woman!" the distant angry voice demands.

Jenny swung Gordon down on to his back, lowering him rapidly into the cot; Gordon's arms flail, trying to catch something in the air to stop him falling. As she scurried away, closing the door behind her, Gordon's fear-filled wail floods the darkness.

The architecture of the brain

It is not the remit of this book to provide a definitive description of the brain. However, in order to understand the discussion that follows, it is necessary to provide an outline of the brain's construction. Those readers who are familiar with this physiology can skip to the next section.

The central nervous system comprises the brain and spinal cord, and, together with the peripheral nervous system, it activates our behaviour. Part of the peripheral nervous system is the autonomic nervous system, which has two activating processes: the up-regulating sympathetic nervous system (often called the "flight and fight" system), and the down-regulating parasympathetic nervous system (often called the "rest and digest" system). These two systems mostly work antagonistically to one another, so when the sympathetic is switched on, internal processes like digestion and self-system analysis are switched off. However, together they maintain balance, or homeostasis, within the body's activating systems.

The brain has a tripartite nested construction (Figure 1), sometimes considered hierarchical in evolutionary terms (MacLean, 1990), although contemporary thinking now disputes this (LeDoux, 2002). The central part of the brain, without which we would inevitably die, is the brain stem, responsible for our vital functions such as heart rate and respiration (Figure 1). Wrapped around this inner core is the limbic system, sometimes called the midbrain, where much of the hormonal and emotional processing takes place. On the top is the cortex, which is where most of our more

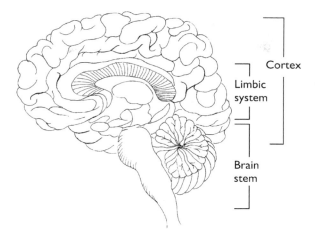

Figure 1.   The tripartite brain.

sophisticated intellectual processing takes place, as well as our motor functions.

On the surface of the cortex are sulci, depressions or fissures in the surface of the brain that surround the gyri, creating the characteristic appearance of the cauliflower-like structure readily identified as the brain. Large furrows (sulci) divide the brain into lobe fissures, identified as performing specific functions. This cortical structure is divided into two halves, the left and the right hemispheres which cross at the corpus callosum; thus the right hemisphere controls the left side of the body, and the left hemisphere activates the right side of the body. These two sides are not identical in shape. The left hemisphere has an expansion in the lower parietal lobe, around the speech areas, and the right hemisphere has an expansion on the prefrontal temporal lobe, where the attachment areas are. These expanded areas are perhaps enlarged by the demand our usage puts on them. The two hemispheres are connected in the middle by a large band of fibres called the corpus callosum, which facilitates communication between the two cortices.

Brain matter consists of billions of nerve cells called neurones, which may be microscopic in size, or over three feet long as they travel from the brain down the spinal column. In addition, there are glia, cells that support the neurones and strengthen synaptic connections (Fields, 2004). A neurone has a cell body with its own heart or nucleus, and a tail called an axon, ending in finger-like protrusions called dendrites (Figure 2). Human brains potentially have several trillion dendrite connections (Damasio, 2003) providing the potential to create millions of different neural pathways. Axons are generally considered to be output channels, whereas dendrites are input channels (LeDoux, 2002), and each of these connect to form pathways, very much like a connection of roads in a road map. A single neurone may have only a few dendrites, or it may have thousands. This allows for the vast variation in potential connections, and, thus, the vast potential behavioural templates or personality traits of each individual. The complex architectural structure of axons and neurones creates what is perceived as the grey matter in the brain.

A child is born with an activated sympathetic nervous system and sparse neural connections, but by the time she reaches age six, she may have twice as many neurones as an adult. The neurones are fired by an electrical spike, or charge, which runs from the cell body down the axon to the dendrites. As neurones do not actually touch one another, the dendrite releases a chemical called a neurotransmitter, providing a fluid through which the electrical spike can pass the gap between neurones, called the synaptic gap (Figure 3).

These neurotransmitters are "key coded", in that they can only pass on to the next neurone if they have the right chemical structure that will fit the receptor on the cell wall of the receiving neurone. If they do, the electrical charge can pass through the

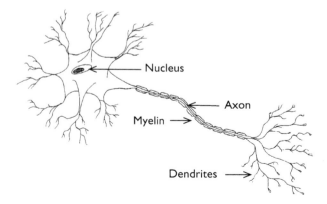

Figure 2.   The structure of a neurone.

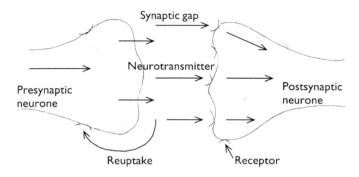

Figure 3.   The synaptic gap, or cleft, between neurones.

synaptic gap, and a pathway is created. If it is the wrong shape for the receptor lock, the neurotransmitter will be deflected and will eventually be reabsorbed back into the original firing neurone, called reuptake. This is a form of recycling of peptides that keeps the brain maintaining its balance, or homeostasis. Some neuro-transmitters are designed to facilitate the firing, or excitation, of the nearby neurone, whereas others are designed to inhibit its firing, thus creating the structure of behavioural neural pathways.

Once an infant has had a neural pathway activated, the neural axon gets covered with a fatty sheath, called myelin, which estab-lishes and protects that pathway to facilitate reuse and to speed up the process. The thick mass of myelinated neurones makes what is perceived as the white matter in the brain, and more white matter is found in the left hemisphere than in the right. Every move that we make, every thought, sense, emotion, perception, or idea involves the firing, or excitation, of neural pathways from one neu-rone to another, which is then activated, or maybe inhibited, by neural peptides, amines, and hormones. The easy use of prepre-pared pathways allows individuals to learn routines of behaviour that make life quick and easy for us. However, equally, these routines may do us a disservice if we outgrow their usefulness.

Split brain research

As mentioned above, the brain has two halves, a left side and a right side. Controversy abounds as to whether these two halves are designed to undertake specific, different functions, and whether they are two halves of a whole, or two separate systems that look similar but perform different tasks. Hemispheric lateralization of the brain means that the two sides of the brain undertake different functions. The right brain develops earliest in infancy, while the verbal left brain does not start to develop until the latter part of the second year. Both can express emotions from the limbic system, but the right brain is likely to access the expression of non-verbal emotions and bodily responses, whereas the left brain will store verbally mediated mood states. The right side is dominant from birth until about three years old, when the left side assumes dominance in preparation for speech and learning, and it is this early dominance of the right brain that underpins our discussion regarding attachments.

The seminal work of Roger Sperry, for which he won the Nobel Prize in 1983, was crucial in our understanding of the dual processing of the two hemispheres of the brain (Nebes & Sperry, 1971; Sperry, 1982). Sperry's work contributed to the understanding of the true extent of the lateralization of the brain as not two halves of a whole unit, but, rather, two separate brains with different functions (Friedman & Poulson, 1981) and different levels of consciousness (Harrington, 1985), only one of which is dominant at any one time. Lateralization of the brain suggests that the left cortex is responsible for language, logic, mathematics, and other "executive" functions, whereas the right brain is more concerned with preprogrammed emotions, spatial awareness, novelty, colours, and arts and crafts. But there is a duality of function in the two hemispheres. For example, although the majority of emotions are stored in the early developing right brain, more social emotions are evaluated in the left hemisphere, as are positive emotions like joy, happiness, and interest, and shows greater activation in manic states (Migliorelli et al., 1993). The right brain tends to be more responsive to the neurotransmitter dopamine and its pathways for more specific negative emotions like fear, distress, depression (Bench, Frackowiak, & Dolan, 1995), anxiety, and disgust, particularly in midbrain areas of the amygdala and cingulate, and parts of the frontal lobe called the ventromedial prefrontal cortex (Figure 4). The left brain has more noradrenaline pathways and moderates or inhibits negative emotions and behaviour found in the right brain (Ross,

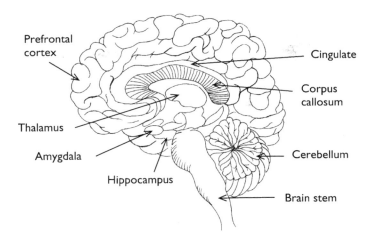

Figure 4. The right hemisphere.

Homan, & Buck, 1994). Again, although most of the language centres are in the left hemisphere, there are language centres within the right, for example, one's own name is processed here, as are single words like "no" and "good", intense emotional expressions, and swear words.

There is a tendency to describe an individual according to the dominance of the side of the brain. Those who are right brain dominant are considered to be artists, actors, musicians, playwrights, and generally creative, colourful figures of society, whereas those who are left brain dominant tend to be those attached to executive, logical, and mathematical forms of work. Interestingly, there are few gender differences in the structure of the brain, other than a female's brain tending to be smaller, but it has been found that men and women with a left hemisphere dominant brain have a thinner corpus callosum, and so have less cross-talk between their two hemispheres (Morton & Rafto, 2006). The corpus callosum of a woman's brain tends to be thicker than that of a man's, allowing greater hemispheric co-ordination and integration, which may account for the tendency of women to use both hemispheres in speech, whereas men tend to only use the left side (Shaywitz et al., 1995).

Solms and Turnbull were fairly derisory about hemispheric lateralization theories, arguing that there is no clear empirical support for the ideas, and that their clinical work suggests otherwise (Solms & Turnbull, 2002). However, other contemporary thinking suggests that the previously held non-dominant role of the right hemisphere has been largely undervalued and misunderstood (Watt, 1990), and it is now considered that the right brain plays a huge role in social processing. Ramachandran, also a clinician, pointed out the contrasting cognitive style of each hemisphere, suggesting that the left is goal-directed and likes coherent plans of action, whereas the right monitors to search for discrepancies (Ramachandran, 1994). Schiffer and colleagues also conducted clinical studies that confirmed their view that the two hemispheres manifest separate, autonomous, mental functioning systems with different psychological properties (Schiffer, 2000), and with each hemisphere producing different physiological responses to visual stimulation (Wittling, 1995). McGilchrist (2009) posed the question: Why would nature evolve two brain hemispheres unless there was a specific reason for it? He argues that they can be rivalrous, like squabbling siblings, each with their own take on the world. He notes that the larger and more asymmetrical the cortices are becoming, the smaller the corpus callosum between them, rather than the other way round. Does this imply that the larger and more independent each hemisphere becomes, the less cross-talk is needed, the more each half would wish for independence? The difference in function for the two hemispheres for McGilchrist is that of attention. The left brain attends inwardly, being a coherent self-referencing system of narrow, focused attention with its own agenda to manipulate and use the world, presumably originally designed to feed and provide for itself, whereas the right brain broadly looks out into a wider view of the world to see what is there, to analyse others, and to prepare in the event of danger. The requirement of two opposing attention mechanisms, one narrow and focused on the self and the other broad and open to the world, in McGilchrist's view accounts for the necessity of the two separate systems.

I tend to agree with McGilchrist, and take the view that the left hemisphere is thought to interpret our experiences of life by our linguistic interpretation of events that formulate in our conscious awareness by labelling, categorizing, and elucidation of events (Gazzaniga, 1995). However, that explanation occurs based on the emotional response received from the right hemisphere as to how it is interpreted as it scans the world. Thus, one could say that it is the left hemisphere that makes the implicit (unconscious) processes in the right hemisphere explicit or conscious. Therefore, it provides a script, or an interpretation, of the emotion experienced via the other side. Those individuals with a smaller corpus callosum will have less cross-talk, thus less verbal access to emotions and what they might mean, creating automatic mind–body processes responding to perceptions of threat via the hypothalamus–pituitary–adrenal pathway called HPA axis without sufficient analysis of the triggering situation. More of this will be discussed in the next chapter.

Infant neural development

An infant's brain commences its development in the last trimester of pregnancy, and continues through various growth spurts, first on one side and then on the other, throughout childhood. At birth, an infant's brain weighs about 400 grams, and in the first year of life it increases to 1000 grams, so the early development is of rapid expansion.

At birth, the infant has anywhere between 15–85% more neurones than an adult brain, and requires twice as much energy, even though the thought (cognitive) processes are not yet available. The infant's brain is relatively smooth and round, without the cerebral convolutions, which appear at about five months and take at least into the first year after birth to fully develop. The baby has only preprogrammed emotional neural circuits, designed, in evolutionary terms, to protect the vulnerable infant from harm and to enhance the potential for survival. Panskepp (1998) described these seven emotional operating systems, or emotional circuits, as follows:

SEEKING: Involves active arousal, curiosity, excitement, engagement, and the desire to explore "from nuts to knowledge" (Panskepp, 1998, p. 145). Its purpose is to motivate the child to interact with the world, thus becoming proactive in his own development.

CARE: This is the warmth and tenderness when with attachment figures, and developing social empathic concern. The purpose is safety in numbers.

PLAY: To play with others is to feel joy and laughter in interaction, encouraging the social bonding process and dominance hierarchy. It produces opiates, which facilitate the development of pleasure centres.

FEAR: This is the flight and freeze mechanism of the sympathetic nervous system, designed to escape from imminent danger.

PANIC: This is separation anxiety: fear of separation from important others, and includes loneliness and sadness. It precipitates separation distress vocalisations, and behavioural movements back to the important other, whose absence may place the child's life under threat.

RAGE: Again attached to the sympathetic nervous system producing the 'fight' response. This is a self-protection mechanism.

LUST: Sexual arousal and satisfaction motivates reproduction of the species.

These preprogrammed emotional templates all produce peptides, creating physiological changes in the body that motivate the infant to behave in particular ways, so that her survival needs are met. There is no volume control on the extent of these emotions; that comes later with the development of the left prefrontal cortex, which has a substantial growth spurt around two years of age, and then again at age five (Solms & Turnbull, 2002). Currently, these are on or off raw emotions, which are activated via the amygdala. The amygdala and the hippocampus of the limbic system are the only parts of the infant's limbic system online at birth (Schore, 1994). The SEEKING system uses the amygdala as an orientating one, designed to search for safety (i.e., search for the mother) and protect against threat or harm. It focuses with the warmth of the CARE and PLAY systems when interacting with the mother. In mother's absence, the amygdala triggers PANIC and has a direct line to trigger the sympathetic nervous system's response of fight (RAGE), flight or freeze (FEAR), via the HPA axis.

Following birth, the first desire of the infant is to use the SEEKING circuit to find CARE at mother's breast, using his strong sense of smell and taste. An infant placed upon a mother's stomach will "worm" his way up to mother's breast using the olfactory sense. (This preprogrammed search for biological mother is considered to have evolved from survival of the species. It would not protect the life of an infant to have an "any mother will do" approach, because

when food is scarce or when danger is threatening, only a biological mother is likely to risk her own life to protect or feed the infant.)
Indeed, the sense of smell is the only sense that is not mediated by
the thalamus; hence its immediate impact. Sucking of the breast
releases the neuropeptide oxytocin through the pituitary and hypothalamus "affiliation" pathways, producing a feeling of calm and
connectedness. Oxytocin is also thought to stimulate the brain's
dopamine "reward" pathways through the ventral striatum, a
reward region at the cross-roads of the oxytocin and dopamine
pathways (Skuse & Gallagher, 2009), and on to the medial prefrontal cortex. Both these pathways appear to be strongly influenced by our early maternal care. Oxytocin produces feelings of
increased trust, reduces anxiety, improves recognition of faces,
decreases FEAR responses and increases eye-gaze, which commonly occurs when the infant is at mother's breast. Breast-feeding,
therefore, has a protective factor in the mother–infant bonding
process, as it releases oxytocin and dopamine in the brain of both
mother and, subsequently, infant, reducing stress and anxiety, and
facilitating the attachment process.

Within minutes of birth, the infant will see, hear, and move to
the rhythm of his mother's familiar voice (Ridgway & House, 2006).
After finding the breast, the next desire of the infant is to focus
on mother's face, and for about forty minutes there is a period
of intense calm as mother and baby gaze at one another, exciting
the warmth of the CARE circuit. This biologically preprogrammed
process ensures survival and neural development, which is
triggered by the amygdala and facilitated by arousal and curiosity
from the SEEKING circuit. The child has already been in communication with his mother *in utero* through a neuro-hormonal
dialogue (Borysenko & Borysenko, 1994), and this ability of an
infant to decode the emotional state of the mother is vital in the
development of the attachment relationship (Brazelton & Cramer,
1990). A child is, therefore, not a passive recipient waiting for
mother to attend and provide what he needs, but an active,
demanding entity, searching for what he genetically knows he
needs.

Chamberlain (1998) pointed out that newborn babies are all
eyes (SEEKING), their amygdalae scanning their environment with
their eyes moving about every half second, even when they are in

the dark. Babies are able to focus from birth at close distances, representative of the distance they needed to focus when *in utero*. This focus on mother's face is the learning of attentional processes, which the child will use throughout his life. The more mother activates this attention, encouraging the child to focus, the greater the investment in how that child will learn in later years. Noticeably, infants watch their mothers intensely in brief tranches and then look away; even at this early stage, staring is considered socially unacceptable. Feuerstein called it "mediated-focusing" (Sharron & Coulter, 1994). As mother and child focus on each other in eye-to-eye communication, most commonly while nursing, the infant develops a schema, or template, for mother's face, based on the infant's *in utero* knowledge of mother's smell and the sound of her voice (Lancker, 2006). The mother's facial expressions are mimicked by the infant within an hour of birth (Meltzoff & Moore, 1995), probably by using mirror neurones (Rizzolatti, Fadiga, Fougassi, & Gallese, 1999), and are remembered with his emotional states. Even at this early stage, if mother closes her eyes to prohibit eye contact, the baby looks puzzled, distressed, and then looks away (Papousek & Papousek, 1979). Reciprocally, mother's dopamine pathways respond to her own baby's face, which will not occur with other babies (Strathearn, 2003). This use of the eyes in such early stages, facilitating the SEEKING circuit, is so fundamental to the infant that the retina will double its size and reach full adult size by the time the infant is one year old (Chamberlain, 1998).

According to Prescott (1996), this early bonding between mother and child is based on trust, affection and love using the vestibular–cerebellar sensory system. The somaesthetic (touch) sensory system provides the foundation for affection, and the olfactory (smell) sensory system provides the foundation for intimacy. In normal development, these emotional–sensory systems are combined in rich patterns of complex sensory stimulation, which results in the development of basic trust. In addition to regulating their baby's external temperature, mother regulates the baby's hormone and enzyme production, as described above, and their respiration and heart rate. Babies of mothers with low heart rates tend to sleep for longer periods, fall asleep faster, and cry less. Chamberlain (1998) calls this "private tutoring in the womb".

As the child feels nourished and safe, that is, good CARE, he will also SEEK to PLAY, encouraged by the production of the neuropeptides oxytocin and prolactin. PLAY, which comes on line at the end of the second month, has been shown to emerge after a warm and supportive base has been established, as fear or hunger will eliminate it (Panskepp, 1998). PLAY is not a frivolous circuit, but is a vital aspect of child survival, as a child alone will die. As Ridgway and House (2006) point out, a child can live without eyesight (insecurely) or hearing, but he cannot live without touch; such children fail to thrive, a condition called *maramus* (wasting away).

PLAY promotes laughter, which can be infectious, and encourages humans to bond together. Teasing and tickling are important aspects of PLAY. A child cannot tease or tickle himself; he needs social interaction. Thus, PLAY encourages social connectedness and social bonding, and the development of this circuit may enhance our social intelligence. Indeed, Charlton (2000) pointed out how vital it is for humans to learn the strategic social intelligence found in all mammals with a large prefrontal cortex. Thus, using internal working models of social relationships, together with a theory of mind and empathic responding, a child can learn to predict and manipulate the social behaviour of others and of himself in reference to them.

PLAY produces excitement in the production of endogenous opiates, but the child also needs quiet, down time to prevent the development of hyperactivity. Thus, tiredness from PLAY encourages the child to SEEK CARE again (Figure 5).

If mother is missing for a time, the PANIC circuit will be triggered. The panic circuit initiates endogenous opiate and oxytocin withdrawal; separation anxiety promotes physical pain. Physical pain initiates stress hormones of adrenaline and cortisol. The child will vocalize this distress in crying and search the environment (SEEKING) using his senses and motor actions available at the time to find his mother to re-establish contact and CARE. Reunion with her calms the distress, as her CARE releases oxytocin that dissolves the cortisol; reunited, they link back into the CARE circuit.

The child stores this information in the hippocampus, imprinting snapshots in visual memory schemata (Stuss & Alexander, 1999), with its attached emotional tag (body feeling), in the right

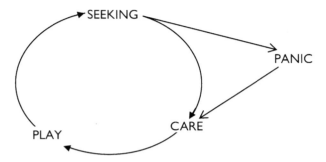

Figure 5.   The nurturing emotional template: secure attachment.

hemisphere of the brain. These schemata formulate very important "flashbulb memories" (Brown & Kulik, 1977) of the infant's inter-action with his mother, which are often vivid and enduring (Neisser & Fivush, 1994). They will be remembered in the body and in the senses, but have no verbal labels. These imprinting experiences form rapid learning processes, providing the memories and default pathways that form the basis for later attachment development.

From about eight weeks old (Yamada et al., 2000), the growth development of the visual neurones in the infant's brain allows him to be able to distinguish mother's face from other faces (Morton & Johnson, 1991). He will be using the amygdala to visualize the face, the hippocampus to store the memory, and the cingulate cortex for the emotional processing. The communication between mother and infant is mediated via their retinae (Hess, 1975) in eye-to-eye conversation (Buck, 1994), which makes both mother's and infant's right hemisphere available to one another. Thus, in this syncho-rhythmic state, entitled by Trevarthen as protoconversation (Trevar-then & Aitken, 1994), the child is able to access his mother's feeling state in a direct way. Parenthetically, the right brain can appraise facial expressions in under 100 milliseconds, yet to become con-sciously aware of that appraisal (left brain) requires five times longer.

Thus, the visual pathways are vital to the healthy development of the CARE and PLAY emotional circuits. The infant communi-cates and plays with mother, limbic system to limbic system (Buck, 1994; Trevarthen & Aitken, 1994), as their eyes lock together to become a single unit, like an electrical plug going into a socket, the child absorbing mother's emotion as if it were his own, and attaching these emotions to the developing database of visual images, sounds, and senses. As mother nurses, her brain produces oxytocin and vasopressin, neuropeptides released by the hypothalamus and pituitary gland, which facilitate bonding and nursing behaviours. As these make her feel warm, safe, and comfortable, simultaneously her baby will produce oxytocin too. Oxytocin is known to have anti-stress effects by reducing the levels of cortisol (Petersson, Hulting, & Uvnas-Moberg, 1999), creating feelings of calm. Similarly, as mother and child PLAY together, mother's brain will produce endogenous opiates, or endorphins, and the baby's brain will produce these, too. Interestingly, most secure mothers nurse their babies initially on the left side of the body, which tucks the baby's right eye into her breast, leaving the left eye available (left eye is activated by the right brain). This nursing position allows access from mother's right brain to the infant's right brain via the child's left ear and eye (Harris, Almergi, & Kirsch, 2000).

An infant's brain development is, therefore, extremely sensitive to the cues in his visual, aural, and somatic environment, so much so that he can soon develop an awareness of an incongruence between the emotion mother is experiencing and the expression on her face (Gergely & Watson, 1996). As the infant's brain develops, other parts of the emotional system start to be activated, in particular the ventromedial region of the prefrontal lobe. This region develops as the child learns complex social emotions and the development of sympathetic and empathetic responses (Damasio, 2003). The infant will also continue emotional development during sleep states, especially during REM (rapid eye movement) sleep, when most of the dreaming occurs (Koukkou & Lehmann, 1983). Later, the left brain accesses the non-verbal memories in the right brain and processes them in the form of dreams. This may account for the symbolic nature of dreams and the ability to problem solve during the sleeping state.

These early, or "primitive", emotional circuits of SEEKING, CARE, PLAY, PANIC, FEAR, RAGE, described by Panskepp, provide the physiological responses, emotional feelings, and behavioural consequences for an infant with as yet no verbal thought processes to moderate them. It is using these circuits, together with the genetic predispositions of the infant and experiential environmental circumstances, that lead the child to develop new, more sophisticated emotional circuits, sometimes called emotional operating systems (Panskepp, 2004).

Here, a metaphor might more readily explain how the system seems to work. Imagine that you are going down a country road that is familiar to you, when unexpectedly the road ahead is blocked. You are at a junction, so take a turn to the side, hoping to bypass the blockage, and come to a field of long grass. As you travel through the field, the grass is flattened, making a pathway through to the other side. It might take several diversions on the route before you can get back to where you want to be, leaving a flattened trail of your route. In this metaphor, the country road is the preprogrammed circuit; say of SEEKING to get CARE. However, the route is blocked by the unexpected absence of the mother. The turning into the field is the brain's potential to find new ways to the same place, and the billions of blades of grass represent the billions of neural connections yet unused. By making a pathway through, the grass is flattened, or the neurones are myelinated, creating a new pathway, or emotional circuit (Hebb, 1949). Next time your route is blocked, you are more likely to use that same pathway, facilitated by the myelin sheath.

As discussed, the inability to obtain the desired CARE triggers the PANIC circuit, provoking separation anxiety and distress vocalizations with the behavioural desire to SEEK the mother for CARE. Her absence, however, may trigger the FEAR or RAGE expressions of separation anxiety, until the CARE from the mother is re-established. This trigger of the PANIC system is physically extremely painful, as it produces opiate and oxytocin withdrawal in the brain, which is experienced as physical pain. However, after a time of intense expression of separation anxiety, the child dysregulates the separation vocalizations and changes into a parasympathetic activation of withdrawal, which Solms and Turnbull (2002) suggest is very similar to that seen in adult depression. This is a new learning for the infant, which will create a new emotional circuit that we could call LOSS (Figure 6). LOSS is a terrifying circuit for an infant, as it is underpinned by rejection and abandonment, which ultimately means death.

Going back to the grass field metaphor, it is a new pathway through the grass field from which the infant would prefer to

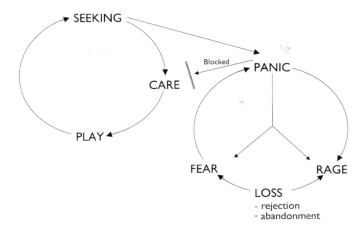

Figure 6.   The development of the LOSS circuit.

escape. This circuit, which is associated to the loss of the mother, may comprise the hurt and pain of rejection, the emptiness and hollowness of abandonment, and the terror (in survival terms) of immanent death without her. In future, the trigger of the PANIC system will automatically take the child through this pathway to the LOSS circuit, until it becomes a well-used, earth-trodden pathway through the grass. Rowe (1991) argues that whenever a child experiences the conflict of not being able to get what he wants, he will experience this subjectively as a loss. Venga (2005) elaborates "loss likely to convey . . . a reduction in one's survival chances, feelings of insecurity and ultimately it poses a threat to the stability and existence of the self" (p. 95).

Attached to the LOSS circuit are snapshot memories that create a default of expectation that mothers, care-givers, or attachment figures are unavailable, unpredictable, or absent, which has both physical and psychological sequelae. Figure 6 shows a model of how the circuitry could work, with expectation of the LOSS circuit becoming a default pathway. The implications of this circuit for the insecurely attached will be discussed in the next chapter.

The SEEKING system using the amygdala in the limbic system of the brain in these early stages of the child's life, provides the proactive life force of the child to focus on her own survival and development, and is the gateway to the development of the emotions. Neurotransmitters, released in the synaptic gap between neurones, facilitate the development of emotions to create behavioural pathways. In particular, increased levels of the neurotransmitter dopamine precipitate arousal in the brain, and enhance the metabolism and growth spurt of the individual neurones, particularly in the prefrontal cortex. However, Allan Schore proposed that in addition, serotonin, particularly in the front orbital part of the cortex, plays a vital part in the first few months of life in regulating sleep, body heat, and appetite (Schore, 1994). This may account for the regressive repertoire that becomes manifest during phases of depression, where a depletion of serotonin has been identified.

The development of the circuits of the infant's brain progresses sequentially from inside to out, like the web of a spider, commencing with the amygdala, cingulate, insula to orbitofrontal cortex (Schore, 2003a). As this occurs, a competitive process ensues in the development of the cortex whereby axons on the circuits that are used become myelinated (i.e., get covered with a fatty protective sheath) and form default pathways, whereas those neurones that are not used have no such protection, therefore later atrophy and die. As the brain constructs its default pathways, there are critical windows of development where certain events need to occur at specific times to create a fully functional brain. It has to adapt to certain situations at certain stages of development, which may not be a necessary function at a later stage. This process of change and adaptability allows for more complex systems to be incorporated into the developmental repertoire. However, as Scott (1979) pointed out, "there can be no reorganization without disorganization" (p. 233). Thus, during this process the infant is in a very fragile state, and even small stressors can throw the infant completely off balance.

As previously mentioned, for the first three years of life, only the right hemisphere is being developed (Chiron et al., 1997), as the infant's left hemisphere does not start to develop until the child reaches about two and a half years, and has achieved about seventy words in vocabulary (Schore, 2003c). Within this right brain, the infant's behavioural templates are using the raw, unmodified, and unregulated preprogrammed emotional circuits, which are being adapted and added to with new circuits over time by interactions with the parents, attachment figures such as grandparents, and with the world. During critical periods of brain maturation, these neural circuits with behavioural templates develop and form the default pathways of childhood and later adult emotion-driven behaviour.

Up until the age of three, children may spontaneously remember and talk about their birth, as their consciousness is attached to the right brain limbic system memories (Verny & Kelly, 1981). Then, as the development moves over to the left hemisphere, the birth memory becomes unconscious, as with the other preverbal memories. These limbic system memories have no sense of time or of knowing the difference between the past and the present. They are just "here and now" responses, which is why memories triggered from the unconscious can have such a profound affect on the adult.

The development of new emotional pathways wane when the right brain is not having a growth spurt, so that new neural development is based on the enrichment of established pathways. Thus, the adage that "neurones that fire together are wired together" (LeDoux, 2002) is especially poignant during the development of neural pathways at critical periods in the child's life during right brain growth. These neural pathways formulate implicit automatic behavioural templates that remain entrenched until they are made more explicit through self-awareness. Later, the development of appropriate attachments allows the orbitofrontal cortex, via the hippocampus, to provide higher levels of coding and analysis of emotional situations. This is the long processing route providing the "volume control" of emotional expression, instead of operating directly from the fear centre of the amygdala to the periaqueductal grey matter, the short-cut route which LeDoux called the "quick and dirty" route (LeDoux, 1996) with "sloppy generalisation" (Goleman, 1995) (Figure 7).

It can be seen, therefore, that although genetic material provides the development of the child's personality via the DNA, a considerable proportion (some say 50–50 (Panskepp, 1998), others say 83% environment (Dobbing & Sands, 1973)) is open to adaptation and change through life experience. During this maturation process, different areas of the brain mature at different rates and at different critical periods in the child's life. The areas of the brain that have the most growth are also the areas that are the most sensitive to external stimulation. The later maturing areas of the cortex are

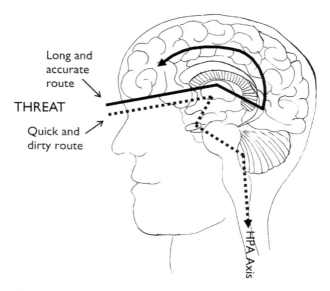

Figure 7. Two routes for the analysis of FEAR.

particularly sensitive to post natal influences (Schore, 1994), especially the orbitofrontal system, called the thinking part of the
emotional brain (Goleman, 1995), one of the few areas of the brain
that is privy to all of the signals of activity in the mind and body at
any given time (Damasio, 1994). Girls' brains tend to develop
earlier than boys' brains (Gregory, 1975), and this may underpin
why girls and boys respond differently to early childhood experiences.

The development of infant attachment

In synthesizing neuroscience and psychological research, Allan
Schore has contributed enormously to the nature–nurture debate
in understanding child development. We are now clear that it is
not an either/or process of genes or environment, but an interaction between the two: "Attachment is thus the outcome of the
child's genetically encoded biological (temperamental) predisposition and the particular caregiver environment" (Schore, 2003b,
p. 73).

Indeed, Thomas and colleagues argued that the infant brain is actually designed to be modified by its environment (Thomas et al., 1997), to be shaped and honed like a sculptor's stone.

As discussed in the previous chapter, the function of attachment is predominantly to search for pleasure and safety, using the CARE circuit. On achieving this, the child develops confidence within his sense of security to explore (SEEKING) novel aspects of the physical and social world (PLAY) (see Figure 1, p. 17). These attachment processes occur in the developing infant during a critical window of opportunity for the child's developing brain. It first appears at around seven months, can be reliably observed at one year, and continues up to his second birthday. The process then ceases, as maturation of other parts of the brain take over.

This attachment has been described as a process of psychobiological attunement (Field, 1985) to develop stable or secure attachments, which are vital for the infant's continuing neurobiological development. They are mediated through the child's developing emotional limbic system via the eye contact with the mother. The infant learns to explore the world, feeling for the first time that he is separate from the mother. Excited in his exploration of a new environment, he is simultaneously looking back to mother's face for feedback on the emotional content of his exploration. When mother's eyes are full of warmth and support, and sensitive to the child's needs, the child will be willing to explore further while still feeling safe. Even the child's innate fear of snakes and spiders will not be triggered in this exploration without his mother's expression of fear to reinforce it (Hinde, 1989). Thus, attachments are about automatic imprinted expectative templates within the child to the behaviour and emotional feedback from the mother, using the SEEKING, CARE, and PLAY circuits, with the emotional tags that develop alongside these templates.

Schore described the critical period of attachment development as the "practicing period", which related to Mahler's description of the practising and rapprochement stage of infant development (Mahler, Pine, & Bergman, 1975). Both Schore and Mahler view the latter half of the first year up to the end of the second year as the *psychological* birth of the infant; the development of the self. First, the child learns to feel that he is a separate entity from the mother, and then he learns a sense of feeling about himself through the eyes of the mother. Using the newly developed empathic response and emotional feedback of how mother responds to him provides the underpinning to how he will feel about himself. Because all the emotional responses are visceral, vas Dias (2000) maintained that the experience of the self is, therefore, through emotional states. During this time, when there are high levels of pleasure expressed by mother during CARE and PLAY, these are mirrored and reflected by the infant, which, in turn, is developing the infant's neural pathways between the thinking cortex and the emotional limbic system. Contentment and pleasure becomes a default pathway, with the memory laid down in the right, non-verbal hemisphere of the brain.

It is considered that emotional memories, hyperactivity, hyperarousal, and exploratory experience are being laid down by the age of fifteen months. The maturation of these pathways is directly influenced by the infant–mother interaction. If the infant gets the appropriate feedback and support from the biological mother during the critical time, that infant will develop a secure and autonomous emotional attachment template. The affectionate memories produced by attachment situations will construct the default pathway to warmth and security (CARE) and what Schore calls "practicing period elation" (Schore, 1994). Sometimes the attunement between mother and child may not be perfect if she is preoccupied with something else or not constantly available. This will trigger the PANIC state in the child, who has yet to learn the concept of time (see Figure 1, p. 17). This misattunement is almost as important for the child to experience as the attunement, because the good repair, or rapprochement, of that misattunement is an important learning for the child. He has to learn not to trigger the FEAR or RAGE states, and to learn that comfort is predictable and close by. In this way, the child constructs concepts of the self in relation to others, and, when using this frame of reference, he starts building the inner working models of how to behave under certain conditions. This is what Fonagy (2001) called the development of the reflective self.

Paternal attachments

And what about dad? Attachment to father is very important and is considered to commence using the CARE and PLAY circuits from about 10–12 months old, after the child develops a sense of self in being separate from biological mother. Even though, in the early period, the child's relationship and interaction with father may be significant, the protoconversation between mother and child remains his primary focus for the development of his own emotional midbrain and prefrontal cortex. However, dads often become equally engrossed in the protoconversation, cooing, staring, and talking to the baby. Dad becomes particularly significant in using the PLAY circuit, as it is through the interaction with the father that the child learns social bonding and dominance hierarchy, which will later be applied to playing with others of his own age. Source, or episodic, memory does not come online until the child reaches the age of seven, so, prior to that, children get their source information predominantly from their parents (Crittenden, 2007). Thus, the bias of the parent's information becomes the bias of the child.

In the early stages of attachment development, the child will be watching the mother's eye contact and behaviour with the child's father, which will determine how the child will respond to father in those initial stages. If the mother's response to father is warm and loving, the child will mimic those feelings to the father. If the mother's response to father is angry or critical, then the child will become more fearful of interaction with father (Main & Weston, 1981). So if mother is feeling tired, angry, or resentful at times with her partner because he goes off to work while she is staying home with the baby, and this is communicated to him in front of the child, the child will absorb all the nuances of the non-verbal interaction like a sponge, which may impede the child feeling relaxed and secure in father's care. Thus, paternal attachment is contingent on attuned care-giving by the mother (Herzog, 2001).

By about eighteen months of age, the child will have developed both a maternal attachment and a paternal attachment template (Abelin, 1971; Schaffer & Emerson, 1964). However, it is thought that the neural circuitry for these two attachments is essentially different. The maternal attachment, which develops during the child's practising period, uses the ventral system and creates a pathway between the hypothalamus and the orbitofrontal cortex (Figure 8). The paternal attachment, which seems to develop during the rapprochement period (Mahler, Pine, & Bergman, 1975), uses

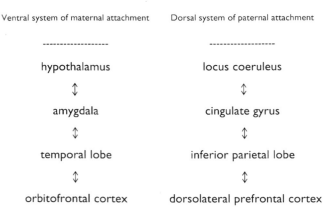

Figure 8.   The neural pathways of attachment circuitry.

the dorsal system from the locus coeruleus to the dorsolateral prefrontal cortex.

These two systems produce different psychopathology in an unattached child: difficulties in maternal attachment produce inappropriate social behaviours, impulsiveness, self-indulgent attitudes, explosiveness, increased motor activity, and sexual disinhibition in the developing child. Difficulties in paternal attachment produce lack of overt emotion, depression, and reduced spontaneity of behaviour in the developing child. As paternal attachment enhances socialization, this also becomes impaired in the absence of the father. Schore (2003d) suggests that the absence of both maternal and paternal attachments would be a potent matrix for inefficient control of aggression.

Peter Blos pointed out that experiences and memories of early protection and love from a father gives the infant a lifelong internalized sense of safety (Blos, 1984). It also helps male children particularly to learn to deal with their emotions of anger and aggression in ways that are more appropriate. The production of testosterone suppresses crying (which is why boys and men cry less than women), as will the child reaching out to father for contact comfort and relief from separation anxiety. Reciprocally, dad's brain is producing oxytocin, which contributes to his attachment and nurturing paternal behaviour (Panskepp, 1998).

In a recent study, Hagan and Kuebli (2007) found tentative evidence that it is principally fathers, as opposed to mothers, who are responsible for treating girls and boys differently, which may contribute to the child's early behavioural differences. They found that fathers with daughters tended to protect their daughters in a difficult co-ordination situation more than they did their sons, whereas they found no difference in how mothers treated their young daughters or sons. This again suggests the importance of fathers as gender socializing agents.

Theoretical underpinning

Our knowledge and understanding, from neurophysiological studies, of how an infant's brain matures and develops has provided physiological underpinning for many developmental theories proposed in the psychotherapy literature. For example, Freud proposed a theory of unconscious processes (Freud, 1901b) that arguably can be considered to be the saved visual memories of a young child, stored in the right hemisphere of the brain before the child developed words to describe them. Schore described the three levels of unconsciousness: the deep unconscious, the unconscious, and the preconscious, which mirror the developmental progression of the infant brain. Thus, the deep unconscious develops in the amygdala, then the cingulate holds the unconscious, and, finally, the orbitofrontal–limbic core with the preconscious, nested within each other like a set of Russian dolls (Schore, 2003a, p. 272).

It was Bowlby (1973) who initially described the development of attachment as the child's need to find a secure base, which was developed through a process of imprinting, as discussed in the last chapter, and now physiological evidence has been found to validate it. Similarly, Winnicott (1960) held that there is no such thing as an infant, only a mother and infant together in a symbiotic unit. From birth, the infant develops a way of relating to the mother to gain security and comfort, and their subsequent behaviour will depend on the success or otherwise of doing so (Feeney & Noller, 1996). The "good-enough mother" (Winnicott, 1971) is one who can help her infant regulate the stress of social interactions, sensitive to the needs of the child, which operate automatically outside of conscious awareness.

The attachment system is vital for the development of a healthy sexual repertoire. The delight that an infant feels when interacting through the senses with the mother formulates the template in which the later adult relates, first with one another, and later in intimate friendships and sexual relationships. Indeed, one could argue that this process of joy, coupled with curiosity and interest (Izard, 1991) underpins the survival of the species, and if this connection were not enjoyable, then the species would not reproduce.

In conclusion, neurophysiology using PET, CT, and MRI scanning of the brain has taught us such a lot about how the human brain functions, and our knowledge is expanding rapidly on a daily basis. New technologies, like diffusion tensor imaging (DTI) make neural pathways so much clearer in their identification. This new approach tracks water diffusion along nerve fibres, exposing the micro-architecture of the brain. It shows crisp outlines in red and yellow of white matter tracts running through and between the left and right hemispheres. DTI promises to open up new avenues of research into the brain's circuitry and also, later, to provide a powerful diagnostic tool.

Neuropsychology has taught us that environmental experiences form part of the child's autobiographical memory, laid down as chunks of emotionally pleasant or emotionally aversive experiences stored in the right brain. A person has access to these via the body and the senses rather than words, sometimes described as subconscious or implicit memories. It is these memories that can trigger the preprogrammed and newly developed emotional circuits, which form the implicit working templates that help the child make predictions about the world, and how to behave within it. The next chapter discusses how infants respond when their implicit working template of attachment is unpredictable and insecure.

Gordon's review

Gordon is already finding it difficult to find a secure base. Using his SEEKING system, he searched for his mother in the dark of the night wanting CARE. She came to him, but her presence did not instil a sense of security for him. He searched for her eyes to make a connection, but they were averted. This made Gordon feel afraid. Jenny always nursed Gordon on her right side rather than the left, as she needed to keep her own security system open in case of threats from Joe. Thus, Gordon's right brain seldom has unfettered access to his mother's right brain.

Jenny left Gordon to cry for long periods, which felt even longer for an infant with no sense of time, and no sense of object constancy or permanence to tell him that she is going to return. This triggered his PANIC system, and his cries of pain vacillate between his FEAR and RAGE circuits.

Jenny's night-time caring is brusque and does not soothe Gordon, as she is fearful for herself and how Joe will respond as she attends to the baby. Joe was always jealous of the time and attention she gave to the baby, so she tried to minimize how much time she gave to the child when his father was around. On the night described above, Joe had been to the pub, so Jenny knew he was likely to be highly volatile. Joe wanted feeding and he wanted sex. Jenny wanted Gordon to settle and keep quiet, so that Joe would not be wound up, as Joe had no patience with the child's crying. Gordon, however, felt that had been left too quickly without feeling soothed or supported, triggering the pain of PANIC and the terror of FEAR. Jenny, in turn, has started to build up a template of Gordon as a "difficult" child who always wakes, cries, and is demanding, and who can make her life with Joe difficult. Gordon's right brain is building the template of unpredictable parenting, a mother who can meet his needs at some times and not at others. He never feels safe, as she always feels nervous. His father never picks him up or touches him at all. Joe excuses this to Jenny as his fear that the baby is too small and he fears that he will hurt him, but really Joe has no interest in Gordon at all, and Gordon senses that. These insecurities may put Gordon's very life under threat, so he has to learn new ways of getting his vital needs met. He will need to develop behavioural ways to cope with the unpredictability and insecurity of his mother being available for him at some times and not others. He will watch for the nuances of non-verbal communication more intently, watching for her to relax when his father is not around, and being more vigilant and aroused when his father is present. He will become more vocal and demanding in his father's absence, and maintain a quiet closeness to his mother when his father is present. Gordon is developing the rudiments of manipulative behaviour and an insecure attachment.

CHAPTER THREE

The insecurely attached child

G ordon has just had his first birthday. He pulls himself un-
steadily to his feet by holding on to the coffee table strewn
with celebrity magazines and used coffee mugs. His little
legs wobble inside his red dungarees, padded inside with a dispos-
able nappy overdue for changing. He turns to look at his mother.
Jenny is slouched forward in a grubby chair nearby, with her
elbows on her knees, her unkempt brown hair lank around her face.
She draws deeply on her cigarette as she stares into space. A television is flickering with a magazine programme in the corner of the
room, but she is not watching it. Gordon tries to attract her attention by calling "mamma", but can only vocalize "ah, ah". Jenny still
does not respond to him, but takes another long pull on her cigarette. Gordon edges sideways along the table to get closer to her
and stretches across to balance himself on her knee. He calls out
again, louder this time, searching for eye contact and emotional
feedback. Jenny looks down at Gordon, but seems to look through
him, her pale face wet with tears. He sees a cut across her eyebrow,
framing a blackened eye. He reaches out a chubby hand to stroke
the injury in tender caring. But mother snaps awake, pushing the
potential touch roughly away. She pulls herself to her feet; with one

hand holding up her swollen belly, and the other pushing the hair from her face, with the cigarette singeing a few loose ends, she strides out of the room. The abruptness of her move swings Gordon around, and his knees collapse under him. He drops down on to to his sodden nappy, and his face reddens with shock and disappointment. He screams out his pain as he watches her leave the room.

The role of the amygdala

To recap from the previous chapter, an infant's memories and emotional experiences are laid down in the right hemisphere of the brain as snapshots of flashbulb memories for the first three years of life (Chiron et al., 1997), as the left brain has not commenced its developmental growth. Only the amygdala and hippocampus of the limbic system is activated at birth, which provides an interface between visual and auditory stimuli via the thalamus to trigger the FEAR and RAGE circuits, and a means to remember the stimuli (Adolphs, Tranel, & Damasio, 1998; Dolan et al., 1996). The amygdala also provides the interface for the "SEEKING system" (Panskepp, 1998), which induces curiosity, interest, and expectancy, which is fired by the dopamine pathways (D_2) of the brain. This orientation process, motivated by arousal and curiosity, searches for mother's face to make the symbiotic connection using the CARE and PLAY circuits (see Figure 1, p. 17). This is vital for the survival of the child, so it is a preprogrammed "primitive" pathway. The amygdala (Greek for almond, from its shape) is also connected to the hypothalamus–pituitary–adrenal pathway, called the HPA axis. This pathway evokes the sympathetic nervous system process of fight (RAGE), fright or freeze (FEAR) (Damasio, 2003). So, one of the amygdala's fundamental functions is always to be on the alert for threat, using the visual pathways (Teasdale et al., 1999), although infants typically trigger their FEAR circuits in response to loud noises, strange objects, physical pain, and loss of physical support (emotional pain) (Panskepp, 1998).

In adults, the hippocampus of the midbrain stores the memory for events, but the amygdala stores emotional memories at the deepest unconscious level. These can be activated via two routes:

from the sensory thalamus or through the thinking cortex. The route from the thalamus is the route laid down in infancy before thought processes are developed. It is a high-speed response to threat triggered by visual threats, loud noises, harsh tones, aversive smells, or hurting body senses. Sometimes called "the quick and dirty route" (LeDoux, 1996), this is the instantaneous fear response that is still triggered in adulthood when something catches your attention out of the corner of your eye, or a sudden loud noise, or when someone turns up when you had not heard their arrival, making you "jump". This evolutionary response protects the developing human from danger, and can be seen in fMRI scanning as increased amygdala activation (Straube, Glauer, Dilger, Mentzel, & Miltner, 2006). In evolutionary terms, the speed of jumping away from a spider or a scorpion is more important than waiting to cognitively analyse whether the creature is dangerous or not.

The alternative route to processing threat via the insula is the slower route, which shows less amygdala activity as it develops in the left hemisphere as thought processes and self-talk, and becomes activated after the age of three years. When children are frightened by something (PANIC), they run to their parents for comfort and support (CARE) and, using physical comfort and left hemisphere language, the parents assure the child with an alternative frame of reference: "Don't be scared. It is only a garden spider and it can't hurt you." This is the development of the communication between the right and left hemispheres via the corpus callosum. The left brain language circuits develop the ability to reduce the strength of the emotional fear response in the right hemisphere by giving it an account, or a script, of what the emotion is in response to. As the child matures, this will happen through her own self-talk, which allows her to say to herself, "Hang on a minute, what am I really scared of?" to mediate, or inhibit, the fear response. This is usually, but not always, a more accurate perception of the stimulating event, which is why LeDoux (2002) called this the "long and accurate route". This slower route is mediated via the prefrontal cortex, which is the crossroads (Atkinson, 2005) between the midbrain emotional limbic system and the higher cortical cognitive systems. Here, the motorway interchange occurs and divides between the quick emotional and slow cognitive systems, and is also the place for the regulation of emotional intensity.

However, potential perceptual threats may still be distorted by expectations and cognitions, forming well-defined fear circuits in the right hemisphere. Also in the right brain are the catecholamine arousal systems for emotion and stress, which are mediated via the neurotransmitter dopamine. If there has been an increase of corticosteroids as the result of constant stress during infancy, this permanently reduces post natal brain growth, and impairs the adaptive function of emotion. Pre-learnt fear, intense stress, or threats associated with pain or danger may overcome the language inhibition from the left brain, preventing the reduction (or inhibition) of the firing of amygdala cells. This may make them respond too readily to events or threats that are ostensibly meaningless, and hardwire the PANIC and FEAR circuits. This process is thought to underpin the elicitation of repetitive fears and anxieties, as does the elevation of adrenaline and cortisol in the blood, which can precipitate panic attacks via the HPA axis. We return to these two routes to the amygdala later.

Insecurely attached infants

Much was learned from the study of Romanian orphans. As a result of severe economic decline, 65,000 children had been placed in state-run orphanages; 85% of these children had been less than one month old when they were abandoned. Chugani and colleagues (2001) found after positron emission tomography (PET) scanning of children's brains that large portions of the prefrontal lobe were missing in the institutionalized children who had missed the critical stage for the development of attachments. In addition, it was found that the orphans who were in cots near a doorway entrance had greater neural matter than those at the far ends of dormitories, where there was little through traffic of care staff. These children also had decreased metabolism in the orbital frontal gyrus, the amygdala, and the hippocampus, and showed neurocognitive deficits in language processing and memory. They exhibited behavioural problems such as self-stimulating behaviours, and had attentional and social deficits. Some of these children did improve on adoption, but deficits that were in the children when they were four years old were still there when they were six years old.

Thus, the concept of critical periods of neural development suggests that the development of the brain is not just experience dependent, but also experience expectant (Glaser, 2003). The developing brain wants to grab as much stimulation as it can get in order to enhance itself, using the SEEKING system. As the cortical regions of a toddler's brain start activating, a pathway develops between the left and the right brain. The communication is between the anterior cingulate in the limbic system in the right hemisphere and orbitofrontal cortex in the left (Gerhardt, 2004). It is this link between our emotional centre and our cognitive account of the emotion that facilitates the development of emotional intelligence (Goleman, 1995) in the securely attached child.

Kobak and Mandelbaum (2003) highlight that, for the infant, the perceived threats to the availability of the mother fall into several categories: relationship disruptions, parental helplessness, parental anger or rejection (p. 151). If the toddler's memories and experiences of interaction with the mother during the critical period of attachment were of unpredictable, unavailable, or aversive mothering, then the circuits of PANIC, FEAR, or RAGE will be triggered and the child will express separation protest. During the practising period, the child is in an egocentric and vulnerable state, and will search for the contact in mother's eyes for emotional support and feedback. If he turns to mother for comfort and support, and she is emotionally unavailable, preoccupied, depressed, busy, at work, etc., then the PANIC circuit of separation anxiety is triggered and the child experiences a sense of fear of rejection that his needs will not be met. He will feel alone (FEAR), as he has no concept of her returning at a later stage; she is just not there; he has been abandoned. This can precipitate the new neural circuitry of the experience of LOSS, as discussed in the last chapter (see Figure 2, p. 18).

There may be two common responses within the child to this LOSS circuit. The first may be an increase in adrenaline and cortisol which leads into a sympathetic nervous system response of flight or fight with FEAR or RAGE. The triggering of the circuits from PANIC into FEAR and/or RAGE into LOSS can result in a circular domino effect that may precipitate increasing PANIC into spirally heightened distress signals of screaming, crying, and wailing. As the child learns that CARE is no longer available, and the LOSS circuit is triggered on a regular basis, a new insecure circuit is developed (Figure 9).

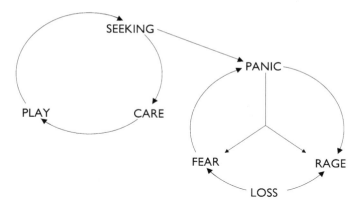

Figure 9.   An insecure attachment template created between PANIC and LOSS.

As the child metaphorically runs around the insecure circuit, there is extreme sympathetic arousal with increased heart rate and high levels of adrenaline and cortisol produced, which interferes with the child's hippocampal development. Under these conditions, a child will often struggle to be free of the care and support of another carer, throwing himself horizontally into a flat, "play dead" posture as he desperately tries to connect with his mother. Even when mother does return, because of the extremely high levels of arousal within the child, he may take some time to calm down. This event will later be memorized as a somatic fear attached to the LOSS circuit. From viewing thousands of infants in strange situation scenarios, Crittenden held that there are two places on the child's body that he will focus on to try to calm down his excessive arousal: the mouth and the genitals. These areas have many nerve endings to promote soothing. So, by pushing fingers or a dummy into his mouth, or by the slow, rhythmic rubbing of the genital area, arousal is reduced (Crittenden, 2007).

The second, alternative response to LOSS may be a decrease in opioids and a parasympathetic nervous system response of freeze, with FEAR triggering feelings of grief, despair, and shame (Hofer, 1994). In a similar way, the domino effect may work in reverse, with the parasympathetic system spiralling downward into the depression and lethargy of LOSS, triggered by further PANIC from threat of survival. The behavioural consequence will be a parasympathetic floppiness, aversion of the gaze with eyes to the ground, and a lethargic and apathetic demeanour, as one may associate with grief. Again, the child may focus on her mouth or her genitals, and the adult consequence of this is often learned helplessness (Miczek, Thompson, & Tornatzky, 1990). Both these aforementioned res-ponse systems are designed to protect the child from the feelings of rejection and abandonment that is felt when the LOSS circuit is triggered.

As Damasio has pointed out, the brain was constructed to be able to predict from past experiences and develop working models based on these predictions. But the brain always looks externally for its rationale. It cannot predict the neural or chemical signals that cause body states; it has to wait for the body to report back on what has transpired (Damasio, 1994, p. 158). Thus, the neural pathways that develop in the insecurely attached child are the expectancies, or inner working models, that attachment care-givers, and later attachment partners, are unavailable, unpredictable, or absent. Paradoxically, both response systems may promote negative mater-nal responses, and sometimes separation responses occur as the result of the child's desperate attempt to regulate the extreme emotion felt in LOSS. Interestingly, studies have shown that the mothers of badly behaved infants, that is infants who already have activated LOSS circuits, tend to believe that their child's "bad" behaviour is intentional and has to do with the nature of the child rather than the child's circumstances or insecurities. Wilson, Gardener, Burton, and Leung (2006) found that the mothers of the worst behaved children tended to think their children behaved badly on purpose and would do so regardless of the circumstances. Yet, really, infants and young children do not intentionally want to be "bad". They just want to have their needs met and to stop feel-ing the extremes of their emotional circuits.

You can see in Figure 9 how some of the emotional circuitry is bypassed when children are insecurely attached and operating on their insecure circuit. Their preprogrammed CARE circuit is under-developed, as they have insufficient connection with their mother. The PLAY circuit may be completely bypassed, reducing the vital social interaction with others, and the SEEKING circuit is reduced, as it is too busy searching for CARE rather than using the system for greater learning. A frightened child will not play in a relaxed way, nor will she reach her potential through learning. She may be restless and disruptive at school, be impulsive with poor concentration, or be an inattentive daydreamer. Her cognition will be dominated by the SEEKING areas of her brain via the amygdala, focusing on the facial expressions and hand gestures of the teacher and the teacher's non-verbal behaviour, as that is more self-protective than the teacher's verbal information (Perry, 2001). Her FEAR and PANIC circuits will be overdeveloped, and the newly developed LOSS circuit will be triggered every time she behaves in a way designed to elicit a rapprochement with her teacher that proves unsuccessful. This produces an inner working model of expectancies that influence behaviour in self-fulfilling cycles. As Rich eloquently pointed out, "the rejecting child is rejected by others, the shy child becomes invisible, the needy child avoided, and the angry child angers others" (Rich, 2006, p. 266). In elaborating on Feuerstein's method of teaching children from deprived or disadvantaged backgrounds, Sharron and Coulter (1994) noted his view that once this belief of incompetency is set in a child, it is extremely difficult to reverse.

As discussed in Chapter One, Ainsworth's strange situation test and other tests used for older children (Main & Cassidy, 1988) identified different behavioural patterns for insecure children, which have been elaborated to the following styles: preoccupied, avoidant, ambivalent, and later, disorganized (type D) was added. We will, therefore, discuss these different behavioural patterns in turn.

Preoccupied attachment style

Infants who have long periods away from their mothers, or whose mothers are absent or have died, tend to develop a preoccupied attachment style, where they are constantly searching for their attachment figure. Their emotional and behavioural sequelae result in a very needy, greedy style, constantly wanting attention and reassurance. This results from the overdevelopment of the FEAR and PANIC circuits in the search for CARE, which triggers the HPA axis via the amygdala. The child's arousal centres will be heightened; she will be anxious, nervous, fretful, needy, and will want reassurance and attention from being picked up and held. The constant demands and inability to settle because of her increased arousal may have the self-fulfilling response from the mother of less attention and allowing the child to cry for longer periods, as mother gets desensitized to the child's distress vocalizations. This will trigger the child into the LOSS circuit, and then back into PANIC. This neediness is manifest in children by being very hypersensitive with attention deficits and hyperactivity.

In adults, the preoccupied style manifests many forms of sympathetic nervous system-driven anxious behaviour, including generalized anxiety states and obsessive rumination, preoccupied jealousy, and an inability to be alone, obsessive–compulsive behaviour, and compulsive eating disorders. The symptoms of obsessive–compulsive disorder (OCD) are unwanted, uncontrollable, repetitious (preoccupied) thoughts that result in compulsive actions. Preoccupied adults identify with a victim position, so become very resistant to any ideas that they may be able to control their own destiny (Shorey & Snyder, 2006). In fMRI scanning of people with this behavioural style (using an MRI scanner to determine the functions of the brain), a brain circuit connecting part of the frontal cortex with the basal ganglia in the brain stem, a region involved in the co-ordination of movements, is shown to be highly active. Here, the importance of activity and exercise might help to calm the person down (see Chapter Fourteen). In extreme circumstances, adults with a preoccupied attachment style can exhibit behaviour similar to those with histrionic and borderline personality disorders (Bartholomew, Henderson, & Dutton, 2001). See Chapter Seven for a fuller discussion of this.

Avoidant attachment style

Infants with brusque or rejecting parents are likely to develop avoidant attachment styles. Such parents are likely to dismiss, deny, or minimize the child's overtures for attachment, sometimes in a cruel or derogatory way (Clulow, 2001). For this infant's brain, the short route to the amygdala monitoring threat is always open, as is the SEEKING system, searching for some sign that the parent will pay attention and provide warmth, and him not wanting to miss it should it come. The visual pathways will be very strong as the child monitors the faces of those closest to him, searching for the nuances of the threat of volatility. This leads to an undeveloped CARE circuit, as the warmth and security is too unpredictable, with an overdeveloped PANIC circuit triggering a constant state of hyper-arousal and hypervigilance, triggering the RAGE side of the inse-cure circuit (Figure 10). This may not necessarily be overt RAGE, but a person with an avoidant style is more likely to develop a passive–aggressive stance, as he is unlikely to risk the threat of more rejection or criticism by showing overt anger.

Should a parent express critical or ambivalent vocalizations to the child at the practising stage, then the self-representation that the child develops during this developmental period may be negative and linked to the production of feelings of shame. In addition, the FEAR and RAGE circuits may become intertwined with the avoid-ance, making the child feel depressed, sullen, and unco-operative, with passive–aggressive behavioural responses. Interestingly, although the child is showing an outward low-key presentation to the mother, internally, the child's heart rate and galvanic skin responses are very high, demonstrating a discrepancy between internal and external emotional states (Fisher & Crandell, 2001). Parenthetically, as the child becomes adult, this down-regulation of outward emotional expression with high internal physiological stress will lead to the manifestation of somatic illnesses. In addition, he may adopt strategies that idealize his parents and his upbring-ing, as a defence against the painful reality.

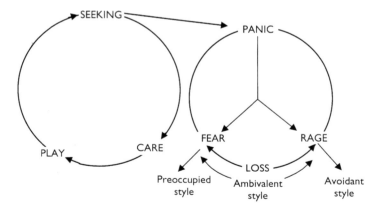

Figure 10. The insecure attachment template, showing different behavioural styles. The preoccupied style overuses the FEAR side, the avoidant overuses the RAGE side, while the ambivalent swings between the two.

A mother who is addicted to recreational drugs or alcohol tends to be unable to respond to the needs of her child. The addiction seems to usurp the attachment circuitry, bypassing the oxytocin systems while exaggerating the dopamine reward systems feeding the addiction. Strathearn and colleagues found that mothers with addictions tended to be more harsh and threatening to their infants, more overly involved, more authoritarian, and more neglectful than other mothers. They would often demonstrate role reversal, encouraging the child to take care of the parent, and they were less tolerant of the child's needs (Strathearn, 2003). In this situation, the child may start actively avoiding his mother, particularly by avoiding her eye contact, so expectations for love and security are never fulfilled. This may occur in the first few weeks or months, long before the attachment style is considered to have developed. Keeping a distance using the avoidance strategy protects the child from being further hurt by mother's emotional absence and serves the self-protective function of avoiding LOSS, with the potential for rejection or abandonment. Avoidant children show no interest in adults who are trying to attract their attention, and show little interest in maintaining any form of contact, losing the ability to interpret emotional signals (Crittenden, 1995). Thus, mother may blame the child by suggesting that the child is unlovable and that the child chooses to be rejecting of her. Consequently, a general aversion to physical contact builds up between them, and mother will avoid the infant's approach and keep her head above that of the child to avoid the eye contact. Kalin (1993) found that avoidance of eye contact produces freeze responses in children, which produces increased levels of cortisol, mobilizing the body for a stress response. Here, the paradox of a hyperactive stress system in a frozen, paralysed body will inevitably result in psychosomatic reactions, and a later predisposition for addictions as the child becomes an adult and tries to fill the emotional empty spaces.

Children with an avoidant style often have a hyper-developed sense of shame. Schore sees shame as the regulating and socializing emotional circuit in attachment, which is associated with unfulfilled expectations. It is not usually observed in the infant until about fourteen months old, when the parasympathetic system becomes activated (Siegel, 1999). It is linked to the shift from sympathetic to parasympathetic autonomic processes, and produces low arousal, facial flushing, reduction of heart rate, and a drooped, eyes-averted, head-down posture in the child. If the mother sees and acknowledges this posture with warmth and sensitivity, the child will learn to moderate and socialize the sense of shame. The ability to learn to experience shame helps the child to learn empathy and social awareness. Once activated, shame does not have to be the result of an external presence, but may be internalized as "the eye of the self gazing inward" (Morrison, 1983). Schore believed that an unregulated sense of shame might underpin social phobia, which is an avoidant style caused and maintained by a perception of another's negative appraisal, and the constant monitoring of the self in comparison to the ideal self and to others. Shame is a preverbal, right-brain emotion developing before a child has access to language, in contrast with guilt, which is a left-brain, cognitive, sophisticated emotion, which Sroufe (1979) believed a child developed at around thirty-six months old.

Children manifesting an avoidant style will be unco-operative, and will often avoid playing with other children, preferentially heading for solitary electronic games and computers that will not threaten them in the same way as interpersonal contact. An avoidant child can also be a bully (Main, 1995). In identifying with aggressors, he will attack others (RAGE) seen as equally needy and vulnerable as he feels inside. As he has learnt that he rarely has his desire for closeness with his mother met, when mother is present, he will stay close enough to her to get some protection, but not so close as to provoke her rejection. He feels ashamed of his desire for closeness, and then ashamed because he feels ashamed, which feeds into his low self-esteem. When mother is absent, the child will feel his anger, but will stop expressing it when mother returns, although physiologically he will still be experiencing heightened sympathetic arousal (RAGE) inside.

Adults manifesting an avoidant style will often be social isolates and IT specialists; the loneliness of the long-distance runner. When mothers who have an avoidant style are shown pictures of happy faces, they show brain activation in their dorsolateral prefrontal cortex, that is, a cognitive response (Strathearn, 2003). Comparatively, if secure mothers see similar faces, they get emotional reward responses via their ventral striatum dopamine pathways, and they get more oxytocin activation in the hypothalamus and pituitary regions (Strathearn, Fonagy, Amico, & Montague, 2009). Avoidant insecure mothers, alternatively, have less activation of their reward-based pathways, and demonstrate less eye gaze and less maternal sensitivity. They also tend to be predisposed to more parasympathetic disorders, like recurring depression and chronic fatigue. In more extreme examples, they can develop severe paranoia, avoidant personality disorder, and anorexic-type eating disorders (see Chapter Seven).

Ambivalent attachment style

Infants with inconsistent parents, who may be over-involved with the child on some occasions and dismissive at others, tend to develop an ambivalent attachment style. Such parents may have been confused by their own attachment figures in a muddled, angry, or fearful way (Clulow, 2001). Unpredictability is extremely stressful for an infant, who has yet to learn the concept of object permanency; that the mother still exists despite her absence. An ambivalent child senses the inability of the mother to be consistent, so clings on to any nurturance to get as much as he can in a short space of time, but then, as soon as contact is established, may switch to pushing mother away, turning his back on her, or avoiding her. This behaviour may develop due to chronic stressors within the mother occurring during the practising period and therefore absorbed by the child. Stress over a long period of time alters the developing neuro-modulators and impairs adaptive function. Such a child may, therefore, slip between sympathetic and parasympathetic arousal states that may manifest in ambivalent behavioural states, the behavioural sequelae being to vacillate between FEAR and RAGE: approach or avoid. These children may be labelled as having difficult temperaments, with intense expressions of emotion, which are unbound-aried and impulsive. As children, their behaviour becomes inconsistent, sometimes being hypermanic, at other times being absorbed and cut off. They constantly test parental discipline boundaries, as the inconsistent parenting may mean inconsistent rules, and they have not learnt a cognitive strategy that allows them to deal with the inconsistency (Crittenden, 1995).

As adults, a person with an ambivalent style may be described as moody and unpredictable. She may develop binge eating disorders, vacillating between the FEAR-based compulsive eating and then flipping to the RAGE-based purge and vomit. More damaged people with an ambivalent style may even move into cyclothymic or bipolar spectrum states (Chapter Nine).

Disorganized attachment style

The disorganized / disorientated attachment style has such a high prevalence among children who have been sexually, emotionally, or physically abused (82% compared to 19% in a control sample (Carlson, Cicchetti, Barnett, & Braunwald 1989)), that it has become synonymous with traumatic childhoods and threatening parental behaviour (Hesse, Main, Abrams, & Rifkin, 2003) and has been strongly linked to disruptive behaviour in later childhood (Lyons-Ruth, Alpern, & Repacholi, 1993). Sometimes called a type D pattern, it is marked by the overuse of the FEAR circuit, producing fear, freeze, and dissociative behaviours in the child. The child responds with a variety of symptoms:

- hypervigilance;
- hyperactivity;
- decreased stress flexibility with a low window of tolerance;
- stereotypical automaton motor movements;
- trance-like states: freezing;
- attention deficit;
- speech disorders;
- cognitive deficits;
- lack of empathy;
- failure to thrive.

This produces a fragmented sense of self in the child, who lives life without feeling a participant within it. Thus, the circuitry shown in Figure 10 would be fragmented and disconnected, rather than a continuous template. This attachment style is more commonly encountered when infants have experienced some form of trauma or abuse during their practising period (Lyons-Ruth & Jacobvitz, 1999), or when the mother has a history of abuse or some unresolved loss in her history (Main & Hesse, 1990). This child becomes hyper-vigilant for the nuances of non-verbal behaviour, being highly sensitive to the anger and disgust in what Peto called "mother's terrifying eyes" (Peto, 1969), burning into the child's memory in a flash-bulb image branded on to the child's concept of self. As a consequence, the child formulates a concept of what Klein called "bad-me" (Klein, 1957). Watt suggested that this produces a neural template or circuit of BAD-ME, which will consist of a snap-shot visual image of mother's face (especially her angry eyes), a soundbite of mum's angry or critical voice, and a somatic memory of the felt fear or terror attached to an emotional tag of shame (Watt, 1990). Despite his fear of mother, he will still seek comfort from her, sometimes to his own detriment. Regardless of the child's fear and need to avoid danger, he may double and redouble his efforts to feel safe with mother, "trying to be good" (Herman, 1992, p. 100) with the one person who is supposed to protect him. This is what Main (1995) called "fright without solution". In a self-fulfilling cycle, often the "trying to be good" routine provokes further rage from the abusive mother, who perceives the child as weak and sycophan-tic. Liotti suggested that then the child's self fragments into incom-patible working models of self as a victim of an abusing parent, self as persecutor of an out-of-control parent, and self as a rescuer of a vulnerable parent (Liotti, 1993). This fragmented sense of self becomes a classic aspect of the adult presentation, as is discussed further in Chapter Five.

The BAD-ME circuit will be fused with the LOSS circuit, so the rejection and abandonment feeling is perceived by the child as his own fault. This template will then be internalized into the child, meaning that he learns that he is not worthy of comfort, warmth, or attention, and reinforcing his own feelings of shame and worth-lessness. In addition, the sight of an angry or fearful human face triggers the pathway to the amygdala, setting off internal FEAR responses even in safe situations, triggering repetitive dissociative states. For some children, they feel they are so "bad" that the only way to make the situation better is to take their own life. Although there may be a tendency to dismiss very young children's attempts at self harm as accidents, Rosenthal argued that children as young as two and a half years old had deliberately attempted to take their own lives (Rosenthal & Rosenthal, 1984). These children showed a general loss of interest, had morbid ideas, depression, and greater impulsivity, hyperactivity, and running away behaviour

compared to children with behavioural disorders. They also showed significantly less pain and crying after injury. These children
were unwanted, abused, or neglected by their parents.

Alternatively, there may be a situation where the child's
memory of an abusive or traumatic event, that is, the episodic
memory in the hippocampus, is different from, or even contradicts,
the semantic memory in the prefrontal cortex from what the child
has been told by others had happened. If others insist that their
version of events is true, it creates confusion in the child's own
sense of reality, leading to fears of insanity, which can, perversely,
trigger mental ill-health. This often underpins the enlargement of
the need for secrecy, as highlighting the contradiction would make
it appear that the child was creating unnecessary conflict. Byng-
Hall suggested that it might be this process that is the manifestation
of the family ethos of keeping secrets (Byng-Hall, 1999).

Domestic violence and other forms of child abuse

Davies and Cummings (1995) argued that violence between parents
creates an insecure attachment within the child, as it leads to the
child's anticipation of unpredictable and unavailable mothering. It
is estimated that 80–90% of children brought up in homes where
violence occurs are aware of this, either at an implicit or explicit
level (Jaffe, Wolfe, & Wilson, 1990). For children who are brought
up in abusive environments, the need to maintain constant vigilance triggers hyperactivity in the child's HPA axis. The chronic
stress releases excess cortisol, a powerful steroid, into the child's
brain, enlarging the brain stem and increasing the activity in the
amygdala, while shrivelling the hippocampal dendrites and, thus,
reducing the size of the hippocampus (Atkinson, 2005) and the corpus callosum (Teicher, 2000). These physiological changes within
the memory and learning structures of the brain no doubt account
for many of the functional difficulties that occur with people who
later present with stress-related syndromes, including trauma and
post traumatic stress disorder (Perry, 2001).

As stress triggers activation of the amygdala, cortisol is released
from the adrenal cortex, which travels to the brain and binds to the
receptors of the hippocampus, weakening the dendrites. The

hippocampus is the part of the brain involved in the storage of explicit memories, and does not mature until around three years of age; hence we remember very little before then. As the hippocampus has atrophied, the ability to retain new information is consequently reduced and the episodic memory for the actual abusive events may be lost. In fact, because the hippocampus has the ability for neurogenesis, i.e., the development of new neurones, until around thirty years of age, trauma-related damage in early childhood may well be masked (DeBellis, 2002). The physiological consequence of early childhood abuse subsequently could make the child perpetually hyperaroused (sometimes misdiagnosed as some form of hyperactivity, or conduct disorder) and hypervigilant (Perry, Pollard, Blakley, Baker, & Vigilante, 1995). The domino effect of this comes from the need for an abused child to maintain alertness, which will interfere with the creation of pathways in the prefrontal cortex, the "long and accurate route" (LeDoux, 1996), which the left brain would use to moderate the amygdala from triggering the stress response in the HPA axis. Teicher (2002) found in a clinical study of psychiatric patients with a history of abuse that their right brains were overdeveloped (presumably from hyperactive emotion), their left brains were underdeveloped (presumably from insufficient cognitive processing), and their corpus callosum, facilitating communication between the two sides, was also underdeveloped. So, by inhibiting the learning and thinking processes, the abusive situations directly inhibit the development of the child's brain, and directly reduces brain volume (DeBellis et al., 1999). As Stein and Kendall (2004) pointed out, it is an overdeveloped stress system in an underdeveloped thinking cortex.

Thus, abuse actually changes the structure of a child's brain, making the amygdala over-excited while the hippocampus loses inhibitory control (Vyas, Mitra, Shankaranaryana Rao, & Chattarji, 2002). It may be that this also enlarges the anterior cingulate, which makes people fearful and worry more (Gundel et al., 2004). We also know that a mother who is a victim of domestic violence will initially nurse her infant at her right breast, covering the left eye with her right breast, thus impeding the mother-and-child symbiotic right-brain-to-right-brain communication (Schore, 2003a). This could be seen as this mother's implicit need to protect her baby, both from a threatening environment and from some of the transference of negativity between herself and another adult, e.g. the father. But again, this is impairing the development of the child's brain.

Sheline and colleagues have shown that in women who had suffered major bouts of depression, the hippocampus was 15% smaller than controls, and the longer the woman had been depressed, the smaller the size of her hippocampus (Sheline, Gado, & Kraemer, 2003). This may account for why so many women with proven histories of childhood sexual abuse have no conscious memory of what has happened. Recent research has suggested that, under these conditions, the abusive somatic memory is stored in the amygdala, so the memory may be remembered in the body without any verbal explanation or account of the event (Bremner & Narayan, 1998).

Schore (2003b) proposed that domestic violence and abusive childhood experiences leads to severe right brain attachment pathology, and when the child becomes an adult, will predispose him to respond to stressors that some might consider trivial, as if it were a threat to survival (Scaer, 2001). The vulnerability to trauma and retraumatization evokes a predisposition in later life to domestic violence (Lyons-Ruth & Jacobvitz, 1999), addiction disorders (DeBellis, 2002), and puts the person at high risk of post traumatic stress disorder (Gordon, 2002). Similarly, LeDoux suggested that these physiological changes may account for the memory disturbances that people experience during stress-related episodes, depression, or post traumatic stress disorder (LeDoux, 2002).

The hyperactivity of the fight and flight system will also lower the body's immune system, making the child and subsequent adult more prone to physiological infections. In fact, a major study conducted by Felitti and colleagues in San Diego on adverse childhood experiences demonstrated that abused children were up to twelve times more likely to develop alcoholism, depression, drug abuse, or to attempt suicide. They are more likely to smoke, to have numerous sexual partners, and are more likely to acquire a sexually transmitted disease. They are also twice as likely to get heart disease, cancer, diabetes, and strokes (Felitti et al., 1998). As Herman (1992) argued, trauma destroys the child/adult's fundamental assumptions about the world and how safe it is, and raises existential questions as to whether it is worth continuing to live in an unsafe environment.

Childhood sexual abuse

For children who experienced sexual abuse, the LUST circuit, which should lie dormant until the pre-pubescent right brain growth spurt around the ages of five to nine, is prematurely activated before the child has developed sufficient emotional intelligence to deal with it. This may account for why some children, when being sexually abused within a loving family, actively initiate the sexual activity after instigation. They may also choose not to tell a parent when abuse occurs within the family, as they may already perceive that the other, non-abusive parent is unresponsive to meet their needs. Thus, as Finkelhor elaborated, such a child will manifest four specific symptoms:

- traumatic sexualization leading to dissociation;
- stigmatization leading to low self-esteem and suicidal ideation;
- feelings of powerlessness;
- feelings of betrayal leading to depression and somatic symptoms (Finkelhor, 1986).

As seen in Figure 11, the LUST circuit will either attach to the secure circuit for those in a securely attached adult relationship, introducing sexual activity into the dynamic of SEEKING, CARE, and PLAY, which is a very intimate and bonding experience, or it will attach into the insecure circuit, vacillating between PANIC and LOSS, thus merging LUST (sex) with strong feelings of FEAR and RAGE. In addition, when sexual activity occurs with a child, the memories of the abusive acts are often connected with exhortations of secrecy and sometimes with threats to herself or those she loves. So the child merges the LUST circuit with BAD-ME, and feels responsible for the behaviour and responsible for any negative consequences that manifest from it, such as the break-up of the family upon disclosure. More is discussed about the LUST circuit in the next chapter.

With the neural changes that occur in the amygdala and hippocampus, physical and sexual abuse in infancy can promote emotional and somatic responses later in life. As outlined above, the somatic memories may be stored in the right brain without words to describe them, which may be re-enacted later in adulthood at an

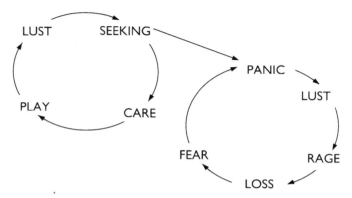

Figure 11. Introduction of the LUST circuit. When a girl reaches six or seven, and a boy reaches eight or nine, the LUST circuit comes online in preparation for puberty. For children who are insecurely attached, the sexual template gets merged into a LOSS ↔ PANIC template.

implicit, or unconscious, level. Flashbacks in specific situations seem to emerge from the very rapid right brain memory retrieval of visual images perceived by the amygdala as threatening (Braeutigam, Bailey, & Swithenby, 2001), triggering the FEAR or BAD-ME circuits. The experience of trauma is even greater if the abuse occurred in familiar surroundings that should be safe, such as in the home. Van der Kolk and colleagues suggested that in these traumatic situations, it is the body that keeps the score as the experiences emerge in somatization (van der Kolk, Perry, & Herman, 1991).

Despite these physiological stress and fear processes, abused children stay strongly protective of their abusive care-givers (Crittenden, 1995), as the threat of an abusive care-giver is not as bad as no care-giver at all, which may threaten life. Hesse and colleagues pointed out that attachment processes drive an infant frightened by her parent away from, but also towards, the abusive parent, creating an unsolvable experience that can lead to disorganization and disorientation of the child (Hesse, Main, Abrams, & Rifkin, 2003). In addition, some abused children fear the response of other adults should they disclose what has happened to them. They fear their abuser being prosecuted and the family being torn apart. They fear the abuser being sent to prison, and they feel partly or wholly responsible (Bagley, Wood, & Young, 1994). As Bartholomew and colleagues pointed out, the fact that a child's attachment figure is abusive does not reduce the intensity of the child's desire for attachment, does not allay her anxiety at separation, nor does it reduce her inconsolable grief if the child protection services move in and force a separation (Bartholomew, Henderson, & Dutton, 2001). As a consequence, many adults continue to protect their abusive parents, defend them against threats of prosection, and continue to submit to their sexual demands, even in adulthood (Herman, 1992).

One aspect of this presenting syndrome that needs to be considered, which manifests frequently in the therapy room, is that of an adult who, as a child, experienced frequent, painful, or intrusive medical interventions, especially of a gynaecological or proctological nature. It is assumed that because the invasive procedures were conducted by medical practitioners with the intention of making a sick child well, the child will respond in a positive way. But the neural template the child develops as a consequence is similar to that of a child experiencing abuse: she feels bad, she feels out of control, humiliated, dominated, and hurt, and may also learn dissociation as a way of protecting herself from the process. Thus, the child will display all the adult symptomology of someone who experienced childhood sexual abuse.

Dissociation

Infants and young children are not capable of fighting or fleeing when they are scared, so a common defence response in those who have had chronic abusive experiences is dissociation (Boardman & Davies, 2009; Carlson, 1998). This may be a state of depersonalization, trance-like fugue states, altered identity states, or may even manifest as dissociative identity disorder (Hesse, Main, Abrams, & Rifkin, 2003). Dissociation is a state commonly missed by health care professionals, thus the child (later adult) may not receive the help and support they require when they need it (Boardman & Davies, 2009), even though, as Putnam (2003) argues, dissociation is a strong predictor of suicidality, violent behaviour, and multiple psychopathological conditions. And even when it has been diagnosed, it is remarkably difficult to treat. As Lifton (1973) suggested, it is a form of paralysis of the mind.

Ogawa and colleagues have found that the most significant predictor of an adolescent experiencing dissociation at the age of nineteen is the classification of a disorganized attachment style at age two, irrespective of any intervening trauma (Ogawa, Sroufe, Weinfield, Carlson, & Egeland, 1997). Also, more recently, Neufeld Bailey, Moran, and Penderson (2007) demonstrated empirical support for the link between a person who dissociates and their unresolved attachment style. Usually, in the child's brain, the trigger of the PANIC circuit elicits SEEKING CARE; in FEAR, it triggers fight or flight. However, if a child is placed in an irresolvable dilemma where the danger may be the person one seeks care from, it produces an internal conflict of behavioural drives. The FEAR and PANIC with lack of CARE triggers the HPA axis into a freeze response from a sense of helplessness and hopelessness (Vianna, Graeff, Brandao, & Landeira-Fernandez, 2001). The child will stare with a glazed look, become numb with terror, speech will cease, and she will become compliant and avoidant, as pain-numbing endogenous opioids trigger the parasympathetic nervous system into a freeze. Freeze has an evolutionary function, as it mimics the "playing dead" process of animals when they get into a situation from which they cannot escape; what Putnam (1995) called "escape when there is no escape". This dissociation is a passive state that has elevated levels of endogenous enkephalins that reduce pain, trigger immobility, and inhibit cries for help (Kalin, 1993). It is a separation of mind and body, which may be the psychodynamic concept of splitting, and enables the child to absent herself from inescapable physical or emotional pain. Children exposed to chronic violence may report a variety of dissociative experiences, such as floating under the ceiling, watching themselves from a distance like watching a film, or fantasizing about being a superhero, whereas very young children might develop catatonic immobility. Interestingly, Perry (2001) reports a gender difference in how children respond to violence. Girls are more likely to adopt the dissociative (freeze) stance described above and become anxious and dysphoric, whereas boys are more likely to display the fight and flight responses and become impulsive, hyperactive, and aggressive themselves.

It may be very functional for a vulnerable infant as a survival mechanism, but, as a default pathway for later adult behaviour, dissociation becomes very maladaptive, as the individual becomes split off from her real emotions. In addition, it has been found that individuals who tend to dissociate at the time of a traumatic event are more likely to develop subsequent symptoms of post traumatic stress disorder (PTSD) (Krystal, Bennett, Bremner, Southwick, & Charney, 1995). Circularly, people with a history of PTSD are susceptible to freeze responses and retraumatization following events unrelated to the previous traumatic life event (Kolb, 1987). People with PTSD find it very difficult to be relaxed, but always have heightened arousal and vigilance. This increased arousal persists through sleep as well as waking hours. They take longer to fall asleep, are more sensitive to noise and bright lights, are more likely to wake, and instead of habituating to unpleasant stimuli, keep responding with heightened arousal or panic (Herman, 1992). The HPA axis in people predisposed to PTSD has heightened elevated levels of adrenaline and cortisol that provide a hair-trigger response to the slightest event.

Adopted children

Although much neural development occurs post natally, an infant is not born *tabula rasa*. She is born with memories based on senses experienced *in utero*. The knowledge of mother's voice, taste, and smell provide information in the SEEKING circuit for reconnection with biological mother that begins instantly from birth. If the child is subsequently taken away from biological mother and cared for by another carer, even a warm, responsive, and loving other, the infant still knows that this person is not the one whom she had been preprogrammed to find in SEEKING. As a consequence, the infant will trigger PANIC, then FEAR/RAGE, and then develop the LOSS circuit as her first newly developed emotion. This emotional circuit will produce feelings of rejection and abandonment, laid down in the preverbal right hemisphere, and the child will develop a working model of herself as unwanted and undeserving of love, with an expectancy that the adoptive parents will also eventually reject and abandon her. The child may develop an earned secure attachment style (Siegel, 2003) with very sensitive and loving adoptive parents, providing that loss has been resolved (Levy & Orlans, 2000), and she may then grow into a happy and secure child (Chisholm, 2000). Alternatively, she may develop a secure attachment style until something triggers an attachment injury (see Chapter Eight), such as the death of the adoptive mother, which then triggers the hitherto dormant LOSS circuit.

However, a child who has not resolved her loss of her biological mother will maintain her allegiance to the birth mother, and she may find that her LOSS circuit keeps triggering, and that she behaves with the assumption that people will reject or abandon her. She may become hostile to the adoptive mother, provoking physical punishment or rejection to confirm her negative expectations. She may triangulate the parents, by being hostile with one and loving with the other, and may become very manipulative and abusive towards siblings, especially if they are biological siblings (Levy & Orlans, 2003).

Veríssimo and Salvaterra (2006) investigated whether the age of children when they were adopted predicted attachment security. They found that although girls were more likely to become securely attached than boys, there was no relationship between the age of adoption and the security of the child. Therefore, they concluded that it was not having the adoption occurring immediately after birth that contributed to the development of security in the child, but the security and, thus, the sensitivity and co-operativeness of the adoptive parent. An issue experienced between the adopted child–mother dyad is that they have no real shared experience of the child's history. So, although the adopted mother may have an understanding of what happened previously in the child's life, the new parent is unable to provide the source material to frame it for him. This will feel like a cut-off for the child, and elaborates the LOSS circuit.

The infant's brain development is dynamic. It is not a passive recipient of experience as it comes along, but is actively capturing what it can and adapting to the environment in which it finds itself. However, aversive experiences in infancy can have permanent detrimental effects, even if the children are subsequently removed and adopted into better environments (O'Connor, Bredenkamp, Rutter, & English and Romanian Adoptees (ERA) Study Team,

1999). Wismer Fries and colleagues looked at the development of the neuropeptides oxytocin and vasopressin in four-year-old orphans from Russian or Romanian orphanages where they experienced little human contact, in comparison with attached children (Wismer Fries, Ziegler, Kurian, Jacoris, & Pollak, 2005). The orphans had less vasopressin, a hormone thought to be specifically involved in recognizing familiar people, and no comparative rise in oxytocin when they played with their adoptive mothers. As discussed in Chapter Two, oxytocin is thought to play a role in the soothing process of security and protection that one experiences when feeling securely attached. The researchers' observations are consistent with reports that children reared in institutionalized settings (even for the short duration of one and a half years, as in this study) continue to demonstrate social problems even after settling into a loving adopted family environment. The lack of oxytocin production in adopted children suggests that playing with an adoptive mother does not have the same physiological effect as playing with a biological mother; thus, the infants are less likely to be soothed during emotional dysregulation when the PANIC circuits are triggered. In addition, the adoptive children who are unable to produce oxytocin for themselves will also be unable to precipitate the production of oxytocin in the brains of their own children, thus facilitating transgenerational transmission.

Perry (2002, p, 89) agreed that children who were in an institution prior to their adoption, particularly in their first three years of life, may show disruptions to neural development that can lead to compromised functioning throughout life, even if they are adopted into loving and caring environments thereafter. Inattentive, chaotic, or ignorant care-giving of an abandoned child can produce pervasive development delay (O'Connor, Bredenkamp, Rutter, & English and Romanian Adoptees (ERA) Study Team, 1999). They may show particularly intense behavioural dyscontrol, manifesting in aggression, violence, and destructiveness towards themselves and to others (Ames, 1997). Dennis investigated institutionalized children raised in a Lebanese orphanage. If they stayed in the institutional environment until the time they reached adolescence, their IQ reached only 50; if they were adopted between the ages of two and six years, their IQ would increase to 80; and if they were adopted before they were two years of age, their IQ would reach the normal population average of 100 (Dennis, 1973). However, it has also been found that children reared in institutional environments that were stimulating and developmentally sensitive would have normal intelligence, but still have disordered attachments (Tizard & Hodges, 1978).

Levy and Orlans highlighted that adopted children with compromised attachment are more likely to come to the attention of the mental health, social service, and criminal justice systems. They are twice as likely to display psychological symptoms in later life, five times more likely to be referred for psychological treatment, and ten times more likely to be diagnosed with attention deficit hyperactivity disorder (ADHD), demonstrating problems with attention, hyperactivity, and impulsivity, than their non-adopted peers (Levy & Orlans, 2003, p. 177). Similarly, Rutter noticed that there was a surprisingly higher incidence of children on the autistic spectrum in children adopted from Romanian orphanages than one would expect to find, suggesting links between deprivation and autism which challenges our current understanding of the disorder (Rutter, 2000; Rutter et al., 1999).

Children who have experienced extreme abuse or deprivation may develop a reactive attachment disorder (ICD10: F94.1) or a disinhibited attachment disorder (ICD10: F94.2). In the former, the disorder is one of non-attachment, where the child never had the opportunity to develop at least one attachment with a reliable caregiver throughout the child's life. In the latter, the disorder is one of indiscriminate attachments where the child is over-familiar with strangers and will accept anyone as a care-giver. Zeanah is unhappy with these categories, however, as he argues that the categories are not based on empirical developmental research. He points out that although all disordered attachments are insecure, not all insecure attachments are disordered (Zeanah, 1996). He prefers a system that conceptualizes disordered attachment in relation to the child's ability to use the mother as a secure base, and proposed three secure-base distortions:

- a child who is excessively clingy and extremely inhibited (preoccupied);
- a child who moves away too easily without checking back even in times of danger (avoidant);

- a child who inverts the parent–child role and excessively worries about the mother (disorganized).

Zeanah, Mammen, and Lieberman (1993) suggest that these attachment problems become later psychiatric disorders when the behaviours create persistent distress or disability for the child.

Similarly unhappy with current classifications, Federici (1999) proposed a concept of a "neuropsychologically-based attachment disorder" for these children as opposed to the more widely held "reactive attachment disorder". This proposal demonstrates the importance of secure attachment behaviour during the critical time of right brain development, without which the subsequent damage becomes extremely difficult to change.

More than 85% of children removed from their parents for abuse or neglect have disturbances in attachment (Perry, 2002) and are at increased risk of aggressive and violent behaviours when adult. Neglect also has an effect on the size of the child's brain and can affect brain growth. Only neglect (not abuse) is an independent predictor of cognitive decline in the child and a significant reduction in brain circumference (Strathearn, 2003). Breast-feeding is a protective factor against a child being neglected, and although some adoptive mothers achieve this, many do not. Mothers who do not breast-feed are 2.5 times more likely to maltreat their children, and four times more likely to neglect them. However, breast-feeding is not a protective factor against physical or emotional abuse (Strathearn, 2003). Such neglect can have long-term consequences for the child becoming adult. The physiological changes of hypoarousal and low cortisol levels are consistently found in people with antisocial personality disorder (Virkkunen, 1985).

Fraiberg and colleagues have emphasized the importance of working on the acknowledgement of loss for adoptees in the therapy room (Fraiberg, Adelson, & Shapiro, 1975), either when working with adoptive children or adoptive parents. Describing the process as "ghosts in the nursery", they suggest that, for the adoptive mothers, these women may not have been able to grieve for their loss of their ability to have their own children. As attachment is a dynamic between mother and child, this can interfere with a woman's capacity to attach with foster-, step-, or adopted children, and may unconsciously place upon the child expectations and fantasies about the children she wanted to have. In addition, the adopted child will vociferously communicate his devastated feelings of loss of his biological mother at times, which may undermine the adoptive mother's confidence. Verrier (1993) opined that no matter how loving the adoptive parents are, and no matter how much the biological mother wanted to keep her child, the infant experiences the separation as abandonment, and she described this as the primal wound. This is why most adults who were adopted as children end up searching for their biological origins at some stage in their lives: infant losses; adult searches.

Transgenerational transmission

As we have discussed the various forms of attachment style, it becomes clear that how sensitive the mother is when she responds to her child will determine how the child will cope with other relationships in a social situation. And how the mother responds to her child may be very dependent on how her mother responded to her, and so back through the generations. Similarly, a mother who was abused may find her unresolved trauma can be triggered by the behaviour of her child, which can lead to re-enactment of the original trauma.

So, can we predict from the mother's behaviour how the child is going to turn out? Main and colleagues found a relationship between the attachment style of the mother and the subsequent attachment style of her child. Mothers who had a dismissing (avoidant) style had children who became avoidant, and mothers who were preoccupied had resistant children (Main, Kaplan, & Cassidy, 1985). By assessing the attachment style of the mother before the child had been born, and then making a comparison of the child's behaviour with this prediction in prospective studies, the stability of transmission of attachment across generations has been confirmed, not just across two generations, but across three generations from grandmother, to mother, to child (Benoit & Parker, 1994).

No one can change their parental history. Most people believe that parenting comes naturally, but it is, in fact, behaviour learnt from our family of origin, and our parents learnt it from theirs.

Most parents do not intend to give their children difficult, danger-ous, or aversive outcomes. But the intention and the outcome may be very different. Insecure attachments are not problematic *per se*. They are reasonable strategies that a child develops to cope with the danger she feels and is facing with her parents. Even for those chil-dren who have had very aversive upbringings, they can change their emotional experience of it and their response to it in adult-hood once they become aware (mindful) of what is happening and what they are doing. They can then consider new ways of parent-ing their own children, rather than repeating the errors of their parents, providing no further damage occurs at critical times on the pathway to parenthood. The next chapter will review two more critical stages in the development of a child's brain: puberty and adolescence.

Gordon's review

Gordon is a year old, and his mother is already pregnant with her next child. The violence between Jenny and Joe has escalated, and Jenny has sunk into a depressed state. Developmentally, Gordon has reached the practising period for the commencement of his attachment circuitry. As he starts pulling himself up on to the furni-ture to make his first adventurous steps into autonomy, he is devel-oping a sense of his own self as separate from his mother. He searches for his mother's support and approval in his adventures, but he finds he cannot get eye contact or positive reinforcement for his daring departure to the coffee table and back. He tries unsuc-cessfully to attract her attention vocally, but she is hurt, depressed, and unable to feel warmth for her son's milestone. Gordon is trying to show his new sense of separateness from his mother. He is trying to show caring for her bruised face, touching her wound, as she would do for him. But mother's shame and humiliation at Joe's violence towards her makes her reject the intimate act of her child, and she brusquely leaves the room. Gordon is learning that inti-macy is a risk, and if you try to be warm and tender, you may end up being hurt and rejected. He must learn to keep close to her in case caring is available, but not so close that he gets hurt or rejected. Gordon is starting to develop an avoidant attachment style.

CHAPTER FOUR

Puberty and adolescence

Gordon slipped out of the school gates at lunchtime, after telling his teacher that he was going home for lunch. His eyes did not flinch from the teacher's gaze as he lied, but the shame of confessing that he had no packed lunch or money for a school dinner was greater. He is now nearly seven years old. His father disappeared from his life when he was five, and they have not met since. His mum cried a lot at first, but then she got herself a job, and then a new boyfriend. Since she started working full-time a few months ago, Gordon was no longer allowed to have free school dinners. Mum said she had not got enough money to buy dinner for him; however, she often forgets to pack him a lunch. She drops him off at the school gates at 8.15 in the morning to go to work and gets home at 6.30 at night. A key has been placed under a flowerpot at the side of the house so that he can let himself into the house after school. Sometimes she forgets to leave that, too, and he has to wander outside in the garden or in the streets until she gets home. Often Gordon goes back home at lunchtime, lets himself into the house, and stays there. He gets so hungry; he searches the kitchen for bread, biscuits, or crisps. Sometimes he gets into trouble at school for stealing other children's chocolate bars or pocket money. It's not fair, he thinks, that they have good things and he doesn't!

Today, Gordon does not go straight home, but wanders to the park along from the school. There is a fenced section for the children to play on the swings. Inside, a woman is placing a small child into a pushchair, watched by a man seated on the nearby bench. Gordon sits on a swing sullenly, kicking at the ground to make the swing move, and watches as the woman leaves. The man has a friendly face and smiles, but then looks away. After a few minutes the man looks back and calls, "Do you want a push?"

Gordon nods warily. He has been told not to talk to strange men as they might be bad men, but this man does not seem bad. He looks ordinary. The man pushes the swing for a while, quite high, but not scarily so. Gordon feels elated. His dad had never pushed him on a swing.

"I'm tired now," the man says. "You've worn me out! What a tough little man you are! I'm going to have to sit down for a while." The man goes back to the park bench, and when the swing slowly comes to a stop, Gordon slides off and sits next to him. The man reaches down into a haversack on the floor, pulls out a bag of crisps, and starts eating them. Gordon's stomach growls as he eyes the crisps enviously.

"Want one?" Gordon reaches in the bag and takes out the largest crisp he can see, but the man does not scold him like his mum would. The crisp tastes lovely, his favourite flavour. He smacks the salt from his lips, and the man lets out a chuckle. He has warm, kindly eyes that twinkle with his amusement.

"Here," the man says, offering Gordon the packet. "You have these. I have another pack here". He reaches into his bag and brings out another packet, and they sit side-by-side, saying little, other than introducing themselves. Gordon's packet of crisps is finished in half the time of the man's.

"Wow!" He eyed Gordon with a tilt of his head. "You miss lunch today?" Gordon nods dumbly, accompanied by another growl from his stomach.

"What's your favourite sandwich, Gordon?"

"Peanut butter. But mum doesn't buy it very often. She says it's too expensive."

"Peanut butter. Well, fancy that. I tell you what. See over there?"

He nods to some houses at the other side of the park. "I live over there, facing the park, so you'll know where you are. How about we go to my house, and I'll make you a peanut butter sandwich for lunch, and then there will still be time for you to get back to school for afternoon lessons. What d'you say?"

Gordon thinks for a moment. "Crunchy or smooth peanut butter?"

"Which is your favourite?"

"Crunchy."

"Well, crunchy it is then, and if you are very good, I'll make you a chocolate milk shake for afters."

Gordon needed no more thinking time. He leapt to his feet and was walking, hand-in-hand, with the man across the grass.

Puberty: the sexual template

The previous chapters have taken us through the right brain development during the first three years of life. These preverbal processes provide an unconscious template of behaviour based on the developed attachment style. However, these infantile unconscious processes still operate in the older child and later into adulthood (Fischer & Pipp, 1984; Krystal, 1988). At age 2½–3 years, the development of the right brain plateaus as the left brain takes over for the introduction of learning and language. Thereafter, the right brain and the left brain oscillate in turn in their further development. In the process of this development, some children develop behavioural difficulties that get progressively worse throughout their lives. One in ten children between the ages of one and fifteen develops a mental health disorder, and, although estimates vary, research suggests that 20% of children have a mental health problem, and in any given year about 10% have a mental health problem at any one time (Mental Health Foundation, 2004). This chapter will aim to elaborate more on how some mental health conditions develop through childhood.

By the age of six, the brain is around 95% of its adult size when the next important growth spurt occurs in the right brain. This development tends to be earlier for girls than for boys; six or seven for girls, with the ages of eight or nine being particularly significant for boys. This is another critical window in neural development, and includes the activation of the LUST circuit, or sexual template (Figure 12).

Crittenden (2008) points out that attachment and sex use the same systems. Both are biologically based, require proximity and closeness, both elicit feelings of affection, both require touch, both generate long-term bonds, and both are essential for the survival of the species. The only difference is genital contact. This is because the sexual system builds on the already developed attachment system, and uses the same circuitry. In attachment, genital contact may be with the self (as in soothing), whereas in sexual behaviour, genital contact is usually with another (but, of course, not always). This sexual template prepares the child for the onset of puberty at around ten years old (McClintock & Herdt, 1996), and subsequent sexual play and adolescent sexual experimentation. Interestingly, Smallbone quoted Belsky, Steinberg, and Draper (1991) in elaborating the biological bases for the development of the sexual template according to the attachment environment. Those who have a secure attachment, who experience safety in their familial relationships, tend to have late-onset puberty, delayed overt sexual behaviour, fewer relationships that involve sex, fewer children, and high parental involvement. Those with an insecure attachment, where the familial relationships are rejecting, aversive, or unpredictable,

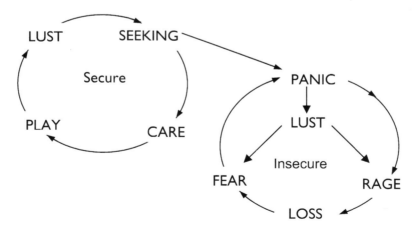

Figure 12. The addition of the sexual template, the LUST circuit, formats the attachment system in adult loving relationships.

have early-onset puberty, low levels of parental involvement in their children (Belsky, Steinberg, & Draper, 1991; Smallbone, 2006), a lower age at first intercourse (Miller, Norton, Curtis, & Hill, 1997), many short-term unstable relationships, later sexual promiscuity (Cookston, 1999), and a greater number of sexual partners throughout their lifetime. Indeed, sexual promiscuity in the adolescent has been commonly linked to suboptimal parental attachment (Walsh, 1995). How pervasive transgenerational transmission is.

This sexual template provides the internal working model of how that child will behave sexually when adult, and many people develop an awareness of their sexuality at this time. Any awareness of homosexuality, paedophilia, or transgenderism may start emerging into conscious awareness this early. As mentioned in the previous chapter, if the LUST circuit activates in a child with an insecure template (see Figure 11, p. 62), then the sexual repertoire will formulate around the PANIC and LOSS circuits, and so sex will be used to reduce the extremes of FEAR and RAGE. This template is empty of the intimacy that is found in CARE and PLAY of the secure template, which are both bypassed in the insecure template. Thus, dysfunction in the attachment template creates dysfunction in the sexual template, and vice versa. Both are designed to protect the child's life, both in the present and in the future. Attachment protects from danger, so that the child is protected in the present. Sex protects the child from isolation so that the child (species) is protected in the future.

The late John Money called this sexual template a lovemap, which he defined as an idealized and highly idiosyncratic image of a potential partner (Money, 1986). Money proposed that vandalization by sexual molestation or abuse at this stage could have critical consequences in terms of the development of later paraphilias, which he saw as having a dual existence, one in fantasy and one carried out in practice. This is similar to that discussed in the last chapter. The activation of the LUST circuit when the child is too young introduces a sexual repertoire that interferes with the normal developmental processes of sexual play and exploration.

However, it appears that the vandalization of the sexual template is not just from sexual abuse. When the right hemisphere is online, and the amygdala pathway triggering extreme and unregulated emotion is open, any severe emotionally aversive situation can have a detrimental effect. This may be physical, sexual, or emotional abuse, neglect, witnessing domestic violence, trauma from road traffic accidents, witnessing violent crime, bereavement from the loss of a parent or close grandparent, or even an acrimonious parental divorce (Neufeld Bailey, Moran, & Penderson, 2007). Indeed, being sent to boarding school at this age from a previously secure base can also have a detrimental effect. Power (2007) highlighted that a hitherto secure child may become distressed, which can make him a target for bullies, whereas avoidant children seem to be already prepared for the emotional bleakness of boarding school. As Scaer (2001) pointed out, it is not necessarily the feeling of fear or horror that can produce traumatization as much as the feeling of helplessness. Of course, the trauma resulting from assault, rape, or torture will produce the most extreme responses, as they really do represent a threat to the survival of the child, but these smaller traumatic life events, every bit as scary for the child, tend to be overlooked by adults.

An insecurely attached child will be predisposed to releasing high levels of cortisol at such times of stress, a finding that does not occur with securely attached children (Essex, Klein, Cho, & Kalin, 2002). So, for children who already have a predisposition of unregulated and extreme emotions from their insecure attachments, and a dysfunctional cortisol system from earlier life stressors, such life events may corrupt the construction of an appropriate sexual template. In addition, it is known that childhood trauma corrupts the formation of the HPA axis, predisposing the child to later addiction disorders (DeBellis, 2002).

A secure attachment template enhances the child's capacity to deal with the developmental benchmarks throughout the lifespan. Thus, a securely attached child would respond to pubescent aversive experiences differently; he would have a clearer understanding of his extreme emotions and know how to get them soothed, and it would be less likely to affect his later sexual repertoire. An insecurely attached child, however, will act up and act out, at the mercy of a tyrannical amygdala eliciting unregulated emotions, and may be demonstrating conduct disorders from a very early age. Again, environmental factors play a significant part. Eron (1987) found that childhood viewing of violence on television and DVDs was significantly associated with the level of aggression twenty-two years later. Alternatively, Heath, Kruttschnitt, and Ward (1986) found retrospectively that this was only the case when combined with the child's experiences of parental abuse. Although it is generally held that violence on television can influence a tendency for aggression in childhood, if the presence of an adult condemns the violence, the child is less likely to behave aggressively (Hicks, 1968). This research again points to the importance of the child searching for the parental feedback from situations in learning how to respond.

Sexual activity between childhood friends and siblings

Vosmer and her colleagues have highlighted that Western cultures seem extremely uncomfortable with the concept of childhood sexuality, preferring to romanticize the concept of childhood innocence (Constantine & Martinson, 1981). As such, there has been a lack of appropriate research, lest the research *per se* stimulated children into sexual knowledge and activity (Vosmer, Hackett, & Callanan, 2009). However, children do engage in sexual behaviours throughout their childhood, even before they have reached puberty. As I mentioned in Chapter Three, infants will rub their mouths and their genitals when they want to soothe themselves from high arousal states. So, even before the sexual arousal switches on, children use "sexual behaviour" as a means of providing comfort. Freud called this the phallic stage of child development, which occurs between three and six years (Freud, 1901b) (the "bums and willies" stage), thus before the sexual template actually comes on line. Prepubescent children play sexual games, such as doctors and nurses ("you show me yours and I'll show you mine"), but as their sexual template has not been activated, their play does not usually involve sexual arousal. Stimulation of the genital area as a result of climbing ropes, bouncing on tree branches, sliding along beams, or rubbing on soft fabrics may produce pleasurable feelings which the child may enjoy repeating, but will not be erotic at this stage unless interpreted as such by an older child or an adult. These behaviours are exploratory, comforting, playful, and are not hostile, aggressive, or hurtful to self or others (Bancroft, 1995).

Thus, sexual activity between childhood friends and siblings is not uncommon. They are curious about sexuality and most of the time it is harmless fun, and again can be tempered by the reaction of the parents. However, some parents are inappropriately sexually open with their children, even though they may not be actually physically abusive. This may be from sexual innuendo or overt sexual jokes in front of the child, leaving pornography around for the child to see, failing to put filters on telelvision or computer screens, or actively allowing their children to watch them having sex. Or boundaries may become blurred if a parent indulges in deep kissing with the child, encourages an older child to stay in bed with them, or uses a "hands on" method of teaching children about sexual arousal. Children who experience this form of boundary-breaking from their parents are likely to break boundaries with each other. The antithesis of this can also create difficulties, however. Parents who refuse to discuss sexual activity with young children, as if it does not happen, can create unnecessary myths around sex, considering children are surrounded by sex in our everyday society. So parents who turn the television off if a couple are getting close, or make comments about sex being "disgusting", are likely to create an atmosphere of intense curiosity, as opposed to it being a normal everyday occurrence between consenting grown-ups.

Cavanagh Johnson (2002) has defined a typology of sexual behaviour in children aged twelve and younger, ranging from normative sexual behaviour to increasingly more troubled behaviour, as follows.

- *Natural and healthy*, in which children engage in healthy, appropriate, and natural sexual experiences.
- *Sexually reactive*, in which children engage in more sexual behaviours than commonly exhibited by their peers.
- *Children engaged in extensive mutual sexual behaviours*, including children engaged in frequent and precocious sexual behaviour with a consensual peer.
- *Children who molest* includes children who coerce or force other children into sexual acts, often aggressively.

Cavanagh Johnson (*ibid.*) believed most or all of the children of the latter category have themselves been sexually or physically abused or exposed to sexually explicit materials or environments.

Boys will engage in more sexual behaviours and more often than girls (Sandnabba, Santilla, Wannäs, & Krook, 2003), and we are now seeing an increasing number of boys under the age of ten referred for therapeutic attention because of their sexual behaviour (Whittle, Bailey, & Kurtz, 2006). Too readily these children are labelled as "child sexual abusers" (Vizard, 2006) and the assumption is made that they must be acting out their own sexual abuse (Friedrich, Davies, Feher, & Wright, 2003), therefore they must be a risk to other children (Vosmer, Hackett & Callanan, 2009). A girl is less likely to be labelled as such, even though girls can be just as sexually aggressive as their male counterparts (Hutton & Whyte, 2006). Sexual activity between children becomes abusive when it involves emotional and physical abuse, using coercion by employing threats, bribes, or promises of special attention in order to maintain the secret. Under these circumstances, one can perceive an older, stronger, more powerful sibling coercing a younger, weaker sibling into sexual activity. An age gap of a minimum of five years between the two is necessary before it is usually considered abusive, although health professionals surveyed by Vosmer, Hackett, and Callanan (2009) considered a two-year discrepancy was sufficient to consider the activity abusive. Considering that two years is very small in child developmental variance, this seems to me to be very judgemental.

Sexual behaviour serves as an attachment function in providing a connection with another individual to reduce anxiety and insecurity and to increase self-esteem, so it may be that a soon-to-be adolescent sibling is rehearsing sexual activity with his or her younger siblings before taking the risk of experimenting with peers. Although sexual activity between adolescents and children can never be condoned, as children need to be protected in such situations, it does not necessarily mean that such an incident is necessarily harmful to the child (Bancroft, 1995). Potential harm involves a variety of factors, including the reaction of others to the event after it has happened, and sometimes, adult clients have presented for therapy to deal with "childhood abuse" that was normal experiential play, which has later been interpreted by someone else as abusive or exploitative when the person had confided the activity, and until such time had felt fine about it.

A child who has developed an insecure attachment template will incorporate any aversive sexual experience into his own sexual template when this comes online. As Rich (2006) highlights, such a child may become "sexually reactive", engaging in age-inappropriate sexual behaviours, which may be a re-enactment or eroticization of his own abuse. He may not consider himself a victim at all, and may willingly trade sex for attention, affection, and gifts (Lanning, 2005). This may lead to excessive sexual comments or play with his peers, or the sexual molestation of siblings or other children. He may search to find some form of security in his life, and, in doing so, he is more likely to search among his mother's belongings, especially in her absence. He may try wearing her clothes, her swimwear, or her lingerie. He will feel warm and comforted and may even get an erection. In this synchrony of events, fetishes develop at an implicit or sometimes explicit level. Any further emotional trauma at this stage, or in later adolescence, may facilitate inappropriate sexual behaviour and later paraphilias.

Adolescence

Adolescence is the time when the child makes preparation for adulthood through behavioural practice and experimentation. Until now, the parent has provided the container for the child's negative and extreme emotions (Diamond & Stern, 2003), but a post-pubertal adolescent, biologically speaking, is an adult. A secure adolescent can risk practising and asserting his autonomy with his parents without the fear of rejection and abandonment. Indeed, the more support and autonomy given to an adolescent, the less likely he is to rebel. Adolescent behaviour is not necessarily driven by pubescent hormones, but may be driven by a neurological process, which is a much longer progression.

The brain continues to develop during adolescence between the years 10–19, refining the cognitive skills of organizing, setting priorities, strategizing, and progressing from concrete to more abstract skill levels. It hones the brain functions that help plan and adapt to the social environment, and those that help to put situations into context; to retrieve memories that connect with gut reactions and learning to control impulses. During this time, the teenage brain remains more exposed, more easily wounded, and more susceptible to critical and long-lasting damage than previously thought. Neuroscientists warn that this is one of the worst times to expose a brain to drugs, alcohol, or a steady dose of violent video games.

At adolescence, the brain has reached its adult capacity, and so it starts to disorganize and reorganize itself (Spear, 2000), and has a neural growth spurt, particularly in the prefrontal cortex. Schore (2003d) maintains this is second only to the neonatal period in terms of rapid growth in response to environmental demands. At this stage, virtually all of the changes that take place in an adolescent's brain are based on experience and not genetics (Perry, 2002). Analogous of computer hardware, the adolescent brain undertakes a system analysis to determine which pathways have been myelinated and are, therefore, required for the future, and which connections remain unused and, therefore, can be considered irrelevant. Just like other cells in the body, neurones operate on a "use it or lose it" basis (LeDoux, 2002). So, a defragmentation process of neuronal pruning occurs, with a final burst of myelination of axons in key cortical areas, particularly the prefrontal cortex, at the same time removing the unused neurones and dendrites, which atrophy and die away. The timing of this again suggests a critical window for optimal development. If pubescence occurs too early, then adolescent pruning occurs quickly and may be insufficient. If pubescence occurs too late, then adolescent pruning lasts longer and may be excessive (Saugstad, 1994). Early pruning makes the brain more excitable and may contribute to cyclothymic mood swings (see Chapter Nine), whereas late pruning could lead to under-stimulation and predispose depressive states.

Teenagers and adults respond differently to the same emotional images. In a study designed to evaluate maturational changes associated with emotional responses, Killgore and colleagues utilized fMRI techniques to determine whether the adolescent brain operates in the same way as an adult brain to emotionally charged facial images (Killgore, Oki, & Yurgelun-Todd, 2001). The results showed that adults had a significant increase in dorsolateral prefrontal cortex activation during the viewing of fearful faces, whereas the adolescents showed no increase in prefrontal activation during the task. In addition, the adults showed lower activation within the amygdala relative to the adolescents, suggesting that adult maturation of the prefrontal cortex was associated with reduced amygdala activity. Younger teenagers relied entirely on their amygdalae, while older teens showed a progression towards using the frontal area. Recall that the amygdala is the threat periscope with direct access to the HPA axis that can override cognitive systems in the "quick and dirty route" (LeDoux, 1996). This suggests that teenagers, who are often criticized for behaving irrationally and spontaneously, leading them to make risky decisions, actually do not have the activated hardware online to allow them to do so. Yurgelun-Todd also found a gender difference in these studies. Teenage girls were using their prefrontal cortex bilaterally earlier than boys, who tended to use only the prefrontal cortex in the right hemisphere (Yurgelun-Todd & Killgore, 2006). This again suggests the early developmental process of girls in neural development,

These findings help us to understand why teens do not always understand the consequences of their behaviours, in particular risk-taking behaviours. Sarkar and Andreas conducted a study of risky driving behaviours of teenagers in San Diego. They found that under-twenty-fives were involved in a quarter of all crashes causing death or injury, but only made up 9% of licence holders. During the course of their study in 2007, there were seventy-two collisions involving young drivers where someone was killed or seriously injured, and on survey found that young drivers would only say they were speeding if they were driving around or above ninety miles per hour. Sixty-two per cent admitted to being in a car during which activities such as drunk driving, drag-racing, reckless driving, or other dangerous acts were taking place (Sarkar & Andreas, 2004).

The adolescent brain is at its peak of cognitive processing. It is quick, alert, and open for exploration and excitement in the transition from child to adult. So, the adolescent takes risks, becomes impulsive, tests boundaries, or rebels against the system, often just to show that he can. He might also interpret social situations differently to adults and respond with different emotions. This confirms what parents probably have known all along: adolescents do not process and think in the same way as adults do.

With adolescence, there are changes in the parts of the brain that govern the sleep–wake cycle, or circadian rhythm. Circadian rhythm refers to the biological clock that runs on an approximate twenty-five-hour cycle and appears to be reset each day by exposure to sunlight. In adolescents, the biological clock shifts, so that if teenagers were allowed to create their own sleep and wake cycle, they would go to sleep at about 1 a.m. and wake at about 10 a.m. Adolescents need between nine and ten hours of sleep each night, and the increased need for sleep seems to be a function of puberty, because hormones are released primarily at night. Many adolescents do not get the sleep they need and suffer from sleep deprivation, the correlates of which are similar to those thought to be "typical" of puberty: irritability, moodiness, changes in school performance, and changes in motivation. Perhaps the characteristics that we associate with adolescence are really a function of sleep deprivation, or a function of the enormous energy resources involved in neural pruning.

In interaction with their social environments, young people are trying to figure out who they are, what makes them unique, and where they fit in life. Identity formation is critical at this stage, and is closely linked to how they feel about themselves and what they think others expect from them. Recent studies have shown that youth in ethnic minorities who developed a strong sense of ethnic identity tend to have higher self-esteem than others (Jamil, Harper, & Fernandez, 2009), perhaps because they had a stronger earlier link through their parental attachment. The search for identity can be more complex when adolescents face the additional challenges of social injustice and discrimination; this might be especially true for LGBT (lesbian, gay, bisexual, transsexual) youth, who often start their identity development by being considered "different". Diamond and Stern (2003) point out that secure adolescents can express anger or sadness about parenting failures, which strengthen rather than weaken the attachment relationship. They argue that direct anger is a more productive and healthier coping strategy than withdrawal, self-punishment, or self-harm found in adolescents with an insecure attachment style.

Based on the confidence that a secure attachment has given him, a secure adolescent can make the important step to autonomy and separation from the family of origin. Thus, adolescence is, *per se*, a transitional practising period: to practise making autonomous life-changing decisions on the basis of the previous decade and a half of parental role models. The more attached and secure the child was in earlier years, the stronger the sense of self in the adolescent. At this stage, parental views and values eventually become less important as those of one's peers, as the need for attachment makes a transition from parents to the social group. As Moretti and Holland (2003) pointed out, it is a time of intense preoccupation with the self as they make a comparison between their own attributes and of those around them in their peer social network. Acceptance within the peer group is vital to maintain their feelings of security within it, and it may be at this stage that an adolescent who does not have a strong sense of self may move into impression management and present a false self in order to be accepted by the others (Harter, Marold, Whitesell, & Cobbs, 1996).

The right prefrontal cortex participates in the construction of autonomous beliefs about the world, intentions in life, and perspectives of others. In a recent study, Shaw and colleagues found that the superior intelligence of some children is associated with slower cortical thickening during childhood neural development, followed by a period of less pruning during adolescence (Shaw et al., 2006). They consider that IQ is related to the dynamic developmental properties of cortical maturation, which might provide an extension to the critical period for the development of high-level cognitive cortical pathways.

Securely attached adolescents will become proactive in planning their futures, responding appropriately to the excitement and challenges of their future autonomy as an adult. They will respond to aversive events in an appropriate way, turning to established support systems for help and protection. Leaving home is part of the transitional process, but may trigger attachment issues either in the adolescent or in the parent as it reactivates attachment injuries from when they themselves left their own families of origin (Kobak, Ferenz-Gillies, Everhart, & Seabrook, 1994).

For the insecurely attached adolescent, however, excessive neural pruning before the brain has developed adaptive coping strategies can lead to later amygdala-driven fear states without having the cortical inhibition from the left hemisphere to attenuate the reaction. This can feel emotionally overwhelming and disorganizing (Schore, 2003b) and can lead to dysregulated aggression. Planning for the future and delayed gratification is inconceivable to an adolescent who has had abusive trauma in his history (Perry, 2001). He becomes an automatic responder to his internal fear states, and, in subconscious re-enactment, his behaviour may promote what he most fears: parental rejection and abandonment, as he tests the boundaries at home and challenges authority figures. Even low-level stressful events can elicit huge fear responses in the young person (Corodimas, LeDoux, Gold, & Schulkin, 1994), based on the individual's early history. Memories of difficult events, which are stored in the right brain as snapshot memories, trigger the HPA axis process of sympathetic arousal, leading to fight, flight, or freeze responses. The adolescent may lash out and act out his FEAR or RAGE in vandalism, mob behaviour, binge drinking, or promiscuous sex. Or he may turn in on himself in a process of self-loathing, developing self-harming behaviours, eating disorders, or drug experimentation. Rates of mental health problems among children, as previously discussed, increase as they reach adolescence. Mental health disorders affect 10.4% of boys aged 5–10, rising to 12.8% of boys aged 11–15. Similarly, disorders affect 5.9% of girls aged 5–10, rising to 9.65% of girls aged 11–15 (Mental Health Foundation, 2004). Insecure adolescents have little emotional intelligence; they behave as insecure, fear-filled children in adult, sexually practising, life-experimenting, risk-taking bodies.

Eating disorders

You will recall from Chapter Three that infants who are highly distressed and aroused reduce their arousal by pushing their fingers, dummies, and other items into their mouths. It is, therefore, unsurprising that insecure adolescents and adults push food into their mouths to soothe their mood. The correlations between people with eating disorders and those who manifest mood disorders are consistently found to be high (Barone & Guiducci, 2009; Cole-Detke & Kobak, 1996; Cooper, 1995), and, considering that 10% of all anorexic cases will be fatal (Abrams & Stormer, 2002), the problem is a serious one. In the previous chapter, the link between the manifestation of eating disorders and insecure attachments was made. Again this is not to suggest that insecure attachments *cause* problems with food, but may predispose the adolescent, at a vulnerable time in her life, to adopt maladaptive strategies to eating.

Approximately 1% of girls aged 12–18 are anorexic and 1–3% are bulimic. As many as 20% may engage in less extreme, unhealthy dieting. Young men can develop eating disorders as well, but the numbers are much lower. Additionally, over the past thirty years, an increasing percentage of young people are diagnosed as over-weight due to a decrease in physical activity, an increasingly seden-tary life style (too much time in front of the computer and television), poor nutrition, and larger serving sizes. Barone and Guiducci (2009) found a higher incidence of unresolved trauma in their study of patients with eating disorders, with a marked tendency for them to have experienced neglect, rejection, or role reversal with their parents. In particular, the relationship with their mothers was the most problematic, with the paradox of idealization of, as well as anger with, their mothers.

The SEEKING circuit provides the desire to forage for food, and the link between the nurturance of CARE and food is clear. A well-nurtured adolescent will reach out to peers for PLAY, which, for adolescents, assumes greater importance in social bonding and social acceptability. We know that the Western media portray an inappropriately thin (size zero) ideal of beauty in catwalk models, making many normally built young girls look in the mirror and feel unhappy with what they see reflected back. Secure adolescents will have greater confidence in themselves as individuals, with the sense that beauty is only skin deep. An insecure, unconfident adolescent is more likely to be influenced by peers and by the media, rather than by parental influence with the fundamen-tal generation gap. Cole-Detke and Kobak (1996) suggested that eating disorders derive from a history of negative interactions with attachment figures and are behavioural manifestations to divert attention away from attachment-related distress. Moretti, in a series of research designs, noted that girls in mid-adolescence were particularly at risk of this psychological distress if they per-ceived a discrepancy between their own and their parental, peer, or partner standards (Moretti & Higgins, 1999). Thus, the adoption of extremely punitive eating strategies may be a consequence of the development of the insecure template, and the predominant fear of rejection from the peer group or others who are important to them.

The incidence of eating disorders for girls is higher than it is for boys, as girls want to be thinner and boys want to be bigger and stronger (Sobal, 1995), and, as we have discussed, fearful girls are more likely to attack internally rather than externally, as boys do. One can hypothesize, therefore, that this attack is a form of self-harm, to be discussed in more detail in Chapter Seven. However, although most individuals with eating disorders are adult females, a significantly high proportion of people with anorexia are boys (Manley, Rickson, & Standeven, 2000). Adolescent males, therefore, are at high risk of developing this disorder if:

- they are athletic and are focused on a lean body type;
- they are struggling with their sexual identity;
- they have been diagnosed with some form of psychopathology (see Chapter Seven);
- there is a history of eating disorders within the family (Ray, 2004).

In reference to Figure 13, those who become fixed in the FEAR side of an insecure template are more likely to adopt the needy, preoccupied attachment styles. If a person becomes preoccupied with food, then compulsive eating, particularly of comfort food, becomes a way of protecting from the PANIC of LOSS. As the female adolescent starts to gain weight, this serves the function of protecting her from the (sometimes excessive) attention of adolescent boys. She does this to defend herself from LOSS, the terrible feeling of being rejected and abandoned by her peers that she is

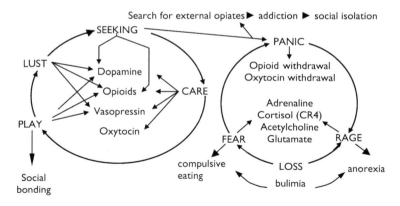

Figure 13. The insecure template is devoid of endogenous opiates that excite the pleasure centres. Thus, these individuals are more likely to turn to external means of stimulating their pleasure centres. Food, drugs, alcohol, or sex may all stimulate the missing "feel good" centres.

convinced will happen despite the attention. But, of course, the self-fulfilling side is that she *is* rejected and abandoned by her peers, who prefer the antithesis of her body shape.

The anorexic, alternatively, is fixed in the RAGE side, and is very much turning her anger inward with punitive passive–aggressive self-harm. This manifests in two behavioural consequences. First, the sense of power and control over her own body, as it releases endogenous opiates to anaesthetize and protect from the pain of hunger, which can be very addictive *per se*. Second, as the body shrinks with the loss of body weight, puberty and menstruation ceases, sexual desire is switched off, and the adolescent stays in the child-like state, perpetuating an infantile, dependent position (Orzolek-Kronner, 2002). Again, this protects her from the threat of rejection and abandonment by adolescent peers by separating herself from the demands of sexuality. And again, this has the self-fulfilling paradox of rejection and abandonment by adults who become frustrated and angry at the uncompromising self-punitive behaviour.

Persons manifesting with bulimia are those with ambivalent attachment styles, who flip between FEAR and RAGE, and, as a consequence, compulsively eat when they are fearful, searching for comfort, trying to fill the empty space of lack of emotional nurturance, and then purge and vomit when they hit the anger with themselves and self-loathing. Interestingly, this behaviour can also manifest in sexual relationships, when the person will initially become preoccupied and demanding, especially sexually, then very suddenly "purge" the partner away. This link between food and sexuality (especially female sexuality) is considered by Panskepp to be due to the vicinity of the SEEKING system, which sits astride the pituitary stalk, enabling it to orchestrate hormonal, foraging, and sexual receptivity changes (Panskepp, 1998). The differences in the neurochemistry of the secure and insecure templates will be discussed more fully in the next section.

Addictions

In the previous section, we discussed how emotionally immature individuals use the method of oral soothing, that is, eating or drinking, as a form of comfort. It is, therefore, a short step away to consider that other oral devices, like drinking alcohol, smoking cigarettes, or popping pills can serve the same purpose in an attempt to change the way one feels. It is then a further short step for the neural pathways to use alternative methods of ingestion to obtain the same feelings, either through the nose, under the skin, or directly into the veins. MacLean (1990) proposed that people develop addictions to compensate for the lack of biochemicals produced naturally through stimulating relationships, and this attachment model is consistent with this view. Figure 13 looks at the secure and insecure templates. The secure template produces endogenous opiates that facilitate the warmth and caring of a secure attachment style. The SEEKING and PLAY circuits release dopamine and endogenous opioids, producing interest and excitement. These are also produced from the CARE circuit, with the addition of oxytocin for the warmth and enjoyment of nurturing. Vasopressin is produced from LUST for sexual excitement. Indeed, Panskepp (1998) noticed that the levels of oxytocin increases threefold in some parts of the male brain with free access to sexual gratification, and as oxytocin is produced in both men and women from the CARE circuit, this suggests that an ongoing sexual relationship will motivate the man to nurture both the woman and any offspring in a long-term relationship. This is consistent with the understanding that generally men in long-term relationships need to have sex with their partner to show they care (whereas women need to feel cared for before they want to have sex).

However, the insecure template does not produce endogenous opiates. In fact, the PANIC circuit does the reverse, as it precipitates opiate and oxytocin withdrawal, which can feel like going cold turkey to an addict (Herman & Panskepp, 1978). The FEAR and RAGE circuits elicit adrenaline, cortisol (corticotrophin releasing hormone (CRH)), acetylcholine, and glutamate. This makes an adolescent hungry for his missing pleasure centres, and he is, therefore, more likely to search for external substances to replace the missing feelings, or to remove the pain of the stress hormones. Subsequently, he may turn to addictions, either to drugs, cigarettes, alcohol, food, work, shopping, sex, or religion (all of which activate the dopamine pathways) as a means of changing the way he feels.

Most commonly, the first substance tried by adolescents is alcohol. In a study by Beniart and colleagues, it was found that up to a quarter of thirteen- and fourteen-year-olds claimed to have "downed" at least five alcoholic drinks in a single session, and the figure rises to a half of all fifteen- and sixteen-year-olds. Among these, 27% reported three or more binges in the past month. By the ages of eleven or twelve, 9% of boys and 5% of girls described themselves as regular drinkers, rising to 39% of boys and 33% of girls aged fifteen to sixteen. The majority of children said their parents would think it was wrong for them to steal or use illegal drugs. However, the proportion who said their parents would object to under-age drinking declined from 91% of eleven- to twelve-year-olds to 56% of fifteen- to sixteen-year-olds (Beniart, Anderson, Lee, & Utting, 2002). This worries Tapert and Schweinsburg, whose research demonstrated that binge-drinking alcohol damages the fragile adolescent brain. It affects memory, alters sensitivity to motor impairment, and damages frontal–anterior cortical regions, producing long-lasting neurophysiological changes in the cortex and hippocampus (Tapert & Schweinsburg, 2006).

The PANIC circuit and feelings of separation distress can be soothed by external opiates such as morphine or heroin (Carden & Hofer, 1990) which interact with the *mu* receptors in the brain, again showing that maybe the addiction to external opiates replaces the missing endogenous endorphins which alleviate the pain of separation (Panskepp, 1998). The paradox of this searching for what is missing, however, is that the endogenous opiates produced from the secure template promote social bonding, whereas the external opiate substitutes promote addictions and social isolation.

The use of drugs during adolescence has some implications for the onset of later adult psychopathology. For example, McCarthy-Hoffbauer and colleagues found a risk factor for thirteen-year-old girls who abuse substances and later deliberately self-harm (McCarthy-Hoffbauer, Leach, & McKenzie, 2006) (see Chapter Seven). Similarly, Lara and colleagues pointed out that repeated administration of psychostimulants like amphetamines sensitizes the dopamine pathways and can trigger RAGE states (Lara, Pinto, Akiskal, & Akiskal, 2006), and this may account for some adolescent delinquent behaviour. Three out of every 100 teenagers experience a drug-induced psychosis, which is more common than diabetes in the young. It can be brought on by the use of drugs or from withdrawal from drugs. Amphetamines (speed) and cannabis are the most common drugs that can lead to psychosis when used heavily. For some, the symptoms disappear quickly when the effects of the drug wear off. For others, a longer-lasting mental illness, including severe paranoia, may begin with a drug-induced psychosis.

In an interesting study, Schindler and colleagues found a direct relationship between the attachment style of the individual and the type of substance used. Individuals using heroin had a fearful avoidant style and used the drug as an emotional substitute for a deficit in coping strategies. Individuals using cannabis were avoidant and used the drug to support their emotional deactivating and distancing strategies. Ecstasy users were predominantly preoccupied (Schindler, Thomasius, Petersen, & Sack, 2009). The group of non-drug-using controls was fifteen times more likely to have a secure attachment.

Cozolino (2006) points out that when people take cocaine, it inhibits the activation of the amygdala and makes people less responsive to social appraisal and, thus, reduces shame. The same response does not occur with heroin, however, and Panskepp (1998) points out that social isolation and alienation are endemic in addict populations. Similarly, Lingford-Hughes and colleagues argued that one of the reasons that people develop addictions is to reduce anxiety, pointing out that people who have social anxiety disorders, that is, those who have not developed their social bonding pathways, will be predisposed to using drugs (Lingford-Hughes, Potokar, & Nutt, 2002). In an interesting study looking at the family systems of adolescents with drug habits, Schindler and colleagues found a common theme of a triangulated family pattern, with the mother having a preoccupied style and the father having an avoidant style, making the adolescent avoidant and fearful (Schindler, Thomasius, Sack, Gemeinhardt, & Küstner, 2007). As Cozolino (2006, p. 120) succinctly pointed out, when a person depends on a drug as a substitute for love, you can never get enough.

Delinquency

There have been countless studies over the years trying to develop the predictive factors in delinquent behaviour. Sroufe and his colleagues' extensive studies at the University of Minnesota have shown that stable predictions can be made from environmental factors that will place a child at high risk of developing aggressive and delinquent behaviour (Egeland & Sroufe, 1981; Sroufe, Egeland, Carlson, & Collins, 2005). These factors are:

- chronic rejection of the child;
- parental neglect of the child / lack of supervision;
- physical abuse of the child;
- chaotic home situation with stress and uncertainty;
- domestic violence in the family.

Further, Farrington (1995) used a longitudinal nomothetic research approach (Farrington, 1995) by following boys from eight years of age into men in their thirties, and in doing so formulated a clear opinion as to the social factors that may contribute to the reasons why young men offend. Farrington (1978) found harsh parental attitude, low IQ, and separation from parents to be the best predicting factors to distinguish violent from non-violent offenders. He argued that there are very predictable events that can occur when a child is aged eight, which can account for the child's subsequent adult behaviour at age thirty-two. He further suggested that if three out of the following risk factors occurred for a child, the subsequent adult had a 75% likelihood of being convicted of a criminal offence:

- parental poverty;
- parental criminality;
- harsh physical treatment of the child;
- abusive treatment of the child;
- parental hospitalization;
- low parental education.

Farrington (*ibid.*) showed that violent delinquents averaged more criminal convictions than non-violent delinquents, and the remaining 25% with more than three of the above risk factors were malfunctioning rather than criminal. Farrington (*ibid.*) also found that there was no specific difference between the two groups when investigating transgenerational transmission. He believed it was not parental modelling or encouragement that made the difference between the two groups, but, rather, it was poor paternal supervision, so again the contribution of the father becomes significant. Moretti and colleagues showed that adolescents who had witnessed violence between their parents were more likely to become aggressive themselves. Boys who witnessed their fathers being aggressive to their mothers showed more aggression to their friends, whereas girls and boys who had witnessed their mother's aggression to their fathers showed higher levels of aggression to their romantic partners (Moretti, Obsuth, Odgers, & Reebye, 2006).

Interestingly, Shorey and Snyder (2006, p. 6) pointed out that adolescents who changed their attachment style from secure to insecure, or retained their insecure classifications, were those who had experienced one or more life event, such as the loss of a parent, parental divorce, life-threatening illness of a parent or the child, parental psychotic disorder, or physical or sexual abuse by a family member, making the adolescent more likely to act out. Indeed, Carlson (1998) found that having a disorganized, or type D, attachment style in childhood is predictive of psychopathology at age seventeen. Megargee (1966) found that offenders with strong personal control and strong inhibitions (avoidant style) are less likely to aggress. It was remarked of these young offenders that they were thought to be the least likely to be violent. However, when they were aggressive, they were so with extreme intensity. Megargee found that boys who had a record of extreme violence were shown by personality tests to be more controlled and unaggressive (sadistic?) than non-violent delinquents. Moretti and Holland (2003) described, from their research of Canadian youngsters referred to a assessment centre for disturbed adolescents, a range of anti-social or self-destructive behaviours, as well as a high incidence of psychiatric disorders, ADHD, and post traumatic stress. They identified their extremes of emotion, from rage to deep despair, and noted that the parents of these adolescents reported similar conflict with their own parents. It was also identified that more girls were classified as insecure–preoccupied, and more boys classified as avoidant.

Tarry and Emler (2007) found that teenagers with a negative attitude towards authority, such as the police or teachers, tended to report committing more antisocial behaviours such as stealing or fighting. Their moral values, such as promise-keeping and truth,

were also related to their levels of delinquent behaviour, but, interestingly, their powers of moral reasoning were not. They argued
that targeting the adolescent's attitude to authority might be a more
effective way of dealing with delinquency than focusing on their
moral reasoning. However, they warn that the adolescent's attitudes show considerable stability over time, indicating that they
were strongly held, deeply embedded in the individual's identity
and, thus, resistant to change. More recently, however, Fletcher and
Woolfe (2009) have found a robust link between schoolchildren
with attention deficit hyperactivity disorder (ADHD) and criminal
activity, such as burglary, theft, and drug dealing, as they become
older. Children with a diagnosis of ADHD were twice as likely to
commit theft late in life and 50% more likely to sell drugs than other
children. They also found a link between the type of ADHD,
whether hyperactive, inattentive, or both, and linked it to the type
of adult crime likely to be committed.

Biological factors may also be relevant. Youth and maleness
seem to be the two ubiquitous factors that are indicative of delinquent and violent behaviour. Men commit more crimes than
women. In England and Wales in 2008, 87% of violent assaults
involved male offenders (Home Office, 2008), with the peak age of
individuals offending being 16–24. So, is it androgens, such as
testosterone, that cause violence? It is known that testosterone stimulates aggressive responses, just as oestrogen and progesterone
inhibit them (Gilligan, 1996), and the levels of testosterone in males
peak in the late teens and remain high through to the middle or late
twenties, which correlates with the ages of most aggressive males.
The neurotransmitter serotonin is known to be a biological inhibitor
of violent behaviour; both homicidal and suicidal, and some men
are thought to have low levels of serotonin. Most men have higher
levels of testosterone than women, but not all men are violent.
Having said that, there is no culture in which men make up less
than 80% of violent offenders. Yet, it is known that women can be
just as violent, just as cruel, and just as aggressive as men. Dabbs
and Hargrove (1997) conducted research at a women's maximum
security prison and found that those women who demonstrated
"aggressive dominance" did have high levels of testosterone,
although they seemed to take longer to reach the threshold into
criminal violence. Women seem to have a protective factor that

builds greater resilience into their frustration, or makes them more manipulative or treacherous rather than outwardly aggressive. It may be, therefore, that rather than men being predisposed to greater aggression by higher levels of testosterone, women may be less disposed to it because of their higher levels of oxytocin. Or perhaps it is both.

Chromosomal abnormalities have been blamed, such as the male XYY genotype, which have been found in unusually high proportions in mental, penal, and high security settings. Such men are considered taller than average, with low IQ and behavioural disability, and are reported to have unusually aggressive tendencies. This was thought to be due to the supernumerary Y chromosome, although this has been disputed (Hook, 1973). However, surveys do indicate that men with this genetic makeup are more likely than other men to be inmates of prisons or mental hospitals, and it has subsequently been suggested that this is the most common chromosome abnormality in man (Walzer, Gerald, & Shah, 1978).

Given the consistent correlation between aversive environments and later aggressive, delinquent, or criminal behaviour, one wonders why, when these adolescents become adults, this aversive upbringing is discounted as an excuse. Another challenge consistently raised is: "Why is it that some people can experience the most appalling childhood abuse, yet come out unscathed as adults, whereas others end up with lives of criminality and psychopathy?" Kaufman and Zigler (1987) investigated the rate of transgenerational transmission between abused children and abusive parents. They determined that the rate was 30($\pm$ 5)%, suggesting that two-thirds are able to break the pattern. Hall and Hall (2007) discussed the reason why some people fail to report abusive situations and quoted the Bagley (1991) study, where more than half said that they could handle their childhood abuse and that it had not bothered them. Sroufe suggested that the resilience developed in childhood against adverse experience has to be learnt, and the development of psychopathy is a joint product of past experience and current circumstance. He emphasized that early aversive experiences do not directly cause later problems, but provide the working model to frame the later experience (Sroufe, Egeland, Carlson, & Collins, 2005).

If, therefore, one adds neuroscience to this hypothesis, one could suggest that should the vandalization of the child, or the traumatic experience, take place during right brain neural growth, then the damage is going to be fundamental to the vulnerable emotional circuitry and development of the expectancy templates. This may account for why many of the later adult mental health disorders, such as personality disorders and schizoid-type illnesses, manifest during adolescence and early adulthood. Should the traumatic experience occur during the left hemisphere growth spurt, however, the emotional circuitry is more protected, and the child and subsequent adult can develop a script, or rationale, of what has happened to him that can be protective from future trauma and acting out. Our technology for viewing and understanding the brain is still in its infancy, but also contemporarily developing at an exceptional pace. Schore (2003d) has proposed childhood neural and physical examinations after a child's life event to determine if physical damage has been done: for example, the lowering of heart-rate responses found in children who later develop psychopathy. One day, we will have the technology to know which cortical hemisphere was online in the child when the event took place, providing a method of prevention of future aggressive, self-destructive, or antisocial behaviour, rather than only having the retrospective process of adult psychotherapy available to us today.

Traumatic experiences that are being processed during right brain growth lay down subconscious, painful, negative emotions, which may be later reprocessed during adolescent neural organization and subsequent pruning, leaving the damaged pathways more entrenched. We have already noted that many insecure female adolescents are more likely to fixate on the FEAR side of the insecure template and attack (slash) inwardly. Adolescent girls who were abused as children are more likely to self-harm (Carmen, Reiker, & Mills, 1984) or to enter into abusive relationships. If her trust has been violated in her early years, a girl's expectancy will be that she is not entitled to care and respect, and victimization in a violent relationship will feel like the norm. Insecure adolescent males often fixate on the RAGE side and attack outwardly, and if they were abused as a boy, they are more likely to become abusive (Howard, 2000). Panskepp (1998) points out that restriction of freedom (in both the physical and emotional sense) and a mismatch between expectations and rewards can trigger the RAGE circuitry, and that we are evolutionarily prepared to externalize the causes of this anger and to blame others for the extremity of these feelings. The RAGE circuit also inhibits the SEEKING circuit, making the adolescent less likely to seek CARE in the appropriate places. One can conceptualize that a young adolescent insecure male, who cannot regulate or moderate the extremes of his emotions, lashes out and blames other people, authority, and society in general for how bad he feels. Lara and colleagues point out the similarities between the rise in anger during adolescence, anger-based impulsive disorders, and the high anger that is the core feature of bipolar spectrum disorders (Lara, Pinto, Akiskal, & Akiskal, 2006). More will be discussed on this in Chapter Nine.

In Chapter Three, we discussed how the presence of the child's father in the family could have either an aversive or a protective effect on the behavioural outcome of the child, particularly in reducing aggression and violence. Minty (1987) followed up the conviction records of 300 children in care. He found that violent adults were associated with having a father who was rejecting, neglectful, or a poor provider of care. More recently, Coley and Medeiros (2007) found that the father's involvement did appear to have a protective effect, even if they did not live with the adolescent. Teenagers who saw more of their fathers and who had more conversations him were less likely to be involved in delinquent behaviour, such as stealing and drug use.

Society plays a role in the "storm and stress" concept of adolescence, and it is noticeable that this is predominantly a Western cultural phenomenon. Teenagers are given mixed messages about preparing for adulthood and accepting personal responsibility for their behaviour. On the one hand, they are developing physically much earlier and stronger than those of a couple of generations ago. Girls from ten years may have fully developed breasts, menstruate, wear make-up, crop-tops, and short skirts similar to those celebrities they idolize. Boys at twelve could already have reached six feet in height, voices broken, and are expected (by their peers) to be sporty, computer literate and sexually functional. They are capable of having sex and conceiving children of their own. Yet, they are treated by their parents and by the law as if they are prepubescent children. If they break the law, their identities are protected; thus, they fail to learn adult responsibility for their behaviours. Insecurely attached girls are often sexually seductive, yet if a fifteen-year-old girl has sex with an older man, he is arrested and treated as if he is a paedophile; twelve months later, she is suddenly old enough to have consensual sex (but the law still deems her a child). This disproportionate response again shows the mixed messages society provides in suggesting that sexual activity is only an adult activity, and not encouraging post-pubertal adolescents to develop their own sexual repertoire in a natural, educated, and spontaneous way. In the UK, the distress demonstrated by some adolescents is a missed opportunity to nip later adult psychopathology in the bud. Our child and adolescent mental health services (CAMHS) are extremely under-resourced, second only to our geriatric services, and many isolated and distressed adolescents slip through the net. Foresight and funding in providing them with ongoing, supportive attachment figures would prevent many from acting out their difficulties during their teen years and into adulthood. The next chapter will elaborate how attachment styles manifest in the adult.

Gordon's review

Gordon, at seven years old, has reached the next critical window of the development of his right brain, and the formulation of his sexual template. Already predisposed to emotional dysregulation from his avoidant attachment style, he has been left to fend for himself a lot of the time, as he is the child of a single mother struggling to earn a living to keep them both. His mother's forgetfulness over Gordon's packed lunches fulfils Gordon's expectations that his needs cannot be met. His self-esteem is low, and he may consider that he does not really deserve to be looked after and be well fed. He may act out these expectations through his truancy, which becomes self-fulfilling "naughtiness". Such children are an accident waiting to happen when it comes to chance meetings with predatory paedophiles, who are knowledgeable in how to groom children into inappropriate behaviour in return for transient rewards of food and comfort.

Gordon did not confide to his mother his experiences with the man, as he knew what had happened was wrong, and he was unsure how his mother would react. What happened was bad enough; he did not want to be punished again. This experience had sexualized Gordon before he was naturally ready. He now takes more interest in sex when he reads about it in his mother's magazines, or when he sees it happening on the television. He has stolen some glamour magazines from the local newsagents, and he ran off into dark corners in the school breaks to paw through the centre folds. He has also tried to grope a couple of girls in his class, for which he was punished with detentions and threatened with exclusion. His behaviour has markedly deteriorated, but no one really knows why. In his bed at night, he masturbates as he revisits in his mind what has happened to him with the man on that first occasion and subsequent times when Gordon went back to see the man again. He is interested in the feelings of sexual arousal, and concomitantly revolted by how the man makes him feel. Again, Gordon accepts that closeness and physical intimacy is a risk that he should not take.

CHAPTER FIVE

Adult attachment styles

G ordon stared at himself long and hard in the bathroom mirror. He has just turned seventeen years old, his face has elongated, and his jawline is peppered with acne. He splashed some after-shave over his chin and shuddered as the spots smarted with the cologne. Mum poked her head around the bathroom door and handed him a five-pound note. "Here, Gord, go and get yourself a take-away. John and I are going to the pub." Gordon took the money silently, but his withering look is lost on the empty space at the doorway.

His mum rarely cooks for Gordon now. Her boyfriend John moved in with them three years before, and neither he nor John took to each other. In the early years there were active fights between them as they jostled for dominance in the household, his mother always taking John's side and telling Gordon he had to be reasonable and do as he was told. However, now Gordon has grown taller and broader than John, there is less conflict and more avoidance. Gordon notes that if John and mum are not "pawing each other" on the settee in front of the television, they are in the local pub. Gordon is spending more and more time alone in his room these days, playing games on the Internet with his iPod simultaneously playing rock music at full volume. If he did want company, he would wander down to the High Street and meet the crowd of youths on the street corner where they met every evening. Gordon does not have any real friends, but there were one or two he might call to meet up if he felt like it. Girls used to flirt with him when he was at school, as they seemed drawn to his aloof style, but he wasn't really interested in any of them. Girls, he believes, are too emotional and cannot be trusted.

Gordon has only one real interest: his car. He bought it from a friend's brother two years before, and it is now stored in the garage, waiting for him to pass his driving test. Over the time he has owned it, Gordon has spent hours tinkering with the engine, and replacing the standard parts with more performance-enhancing versions. He used to hang around the local car-repair garage after school, watching what the mechanics did, and asking their advice about his own car. They were impressed with his persistence, and eventually the owner offered him an apprenticeship. While Gordon was tinkering around under the bonnet of a car, he didn't have time to think about how alone he felt. He resolved that he would work hard, save hard, and one day he would buy a repair garage of his own. Then he wouldn't need anyone.

Adult attachment styles

Bowlby's original attachment hypothesis implied that children's early attachment experiences provided an inner working model in adult love relationships (Bowlby, 1988). Hazan and Shaver introduced these concepts of attachment security into romantic relationships (Hazan & Shaver, 1987), and it was their view that a secure autonomous style was found in only 60% of the population, leaving 40% of the population with an insecure style of preoccupied, avoidant, ambivalent, or disorganized attachment. Longitudinal studies have shown that infant attachment classifications show a 72% concordance with their adult attachment styles (Waters, Merrick, Treboux, Crowell, & Albersham, 2000), so there does not appear to be a significant change over time. This stability was later called the prototype hypothesis in attachment literature, and has been subsequently criticized (as has attachment theory) as being a pessimistic view of adult development, as people are forced to replay their early aversive experiences (Crowell & Treboux, 2001). However, contemporary understanding from neuroscience allows us to be more optimistic, knowing that neural development is a constant state of adaptation and change according to the existing environmental conditions, and that attachment theory *per se* is a theory of adaptation to environmental circumstances, be it positive or negative.

Heard and Lake (1997) proposed that there were the following five systems within an attachment dynamic that needed to be considered when working with adult attachment styles:

- the care-seeking system;
- the care-giving system;
- the interest-sharing system;
- the sexual system;
- the system for self-defence.

They proposed that these systems can work independently of each other, but, when push comes to shove, the self-defence system will be superior, even if it is to the person's own cost. They later collaborated with McClusky, using her research paradigm to elaborate how these preprogrammed systems are activated when the individual is placed under a situation of threat (Heard, Lake, & McClusky, 2009). One can see how the care-seeking and care-giving models fit that of the secure template, and the interest-sharing system is the PLAY circuit. The sexual system is the LUST circuit, and the self-defence system is the insecure template leading from PANIC into LOSS. Thus, their view is consistent with the model proposed here.

The secure attachment neural template, comprising SEEKING, CARE, PLAY, and LUST (see Figure 11, p. 62), provides the underpinning for secure adult loving relationships, which continue to enhance the survival and reproductive fitness of the species (Hazan & Zeifman, 1999). Such secure couples can move freely between being dependent in their relationship to being depended upon (Cudmore & Judd, 2001), according to the situation and need at the time. They can move from being two independent people with a strong sense of self, to being a cohesive couple unit with a strong sense of togetherness. It may be that the SEEKING circuit operates differently for men and women, as it was originally designed with very specific sets of tasks (Cosford, 2009). A man's SEEKING system is designed to search the world through the visual pathways, looking on a macrocosmic horizon. Thus, their eyes operate differently to a woman's, who seeks the world through potential threat to her microcosmic relationships, using more than just visual pathways, but also the prosody of sound and tone from her somatic senses. This may account for why these gender differences manifest so radically when the SEEKING circuit drive predominates and the individual spirals into addiction. More will be discussed about this in Chapter Eleven.

The ability to SEEK CARE from the partner when the PANIC circuit is activated is just as important as the ability to provide CARE and support when the partner needs it (Davila, 2003). When feeling safe and well-cared for, sex between the couple falls naturally into place. Holmes (2007, p. 21) suggested that secure couples can "make love freely, spontaneously, safely, excitingly, harmonically, tenderly and empathically".

However, if the initial attachment template follows the PANIC, FEAR, and RAGE circuits, and later LUST becomes incorporated into this, the person develops an inner working model of relationships based on an early threat to survival where needs are not likely to be met. Thus, loving relationships inevitably are affected. The power of the inner working model is that it elicits behaviours from others that act as self-fulfilling prophecies (Shorey & Snyder, 2006). This produces inappropriate and sometimes manipulative behaviour in the partnership, with the unconscious desire to have the early (missing) attachment needs met. The inevitable paradox with this behavioural manipulation, however, is that it often provokes the outcome most feared: rejection and abandonment. For example, when the SEEKING CARE is bypassed, the person with a preoccupied style will demand so much CARE that that her partner feels totally overwhelmed and backs off, fearing engulfment. Similarly, the person with an avoidant style will not SEEK CARE, as he will not feel it is necessary, and then his partner may leave because she feels she is never "let in". In addition, the PLAY circuit in these scenarios is totally bypassed, as the individual never feels sufficiently safe to relax into it.

Bartholomew (1990) simplified attachment styles for adults into two dimensions: low and high avoidance, and low and high anxiety, leading to four attachment styles:

- secure (autonomous): low avoidance, low anxiety (positive self, positive other);
- preoccupied: low avoidance, high anxiety (negative self, positive other);
- dismissing–avoidant: high avoidant, low anxiety (positive self, negative other);
- fearful–avoidant: high avoidant, high anxiety (negative self, negative other).

This quadrilateral approach is seductive, as it allows therapists a user-friendly method of working in a couple dynamic. However, it does have flaws: both the ambivalent style and the disorganized style are missing, and these clearly manifest from other research studies. We also know that sometimes a person with a preoccupied style is so fearful that they may avoid. Similarly, we know that although avoidants tend to use cognitive strategies to avoid accessing their emotions, their physiology would actually measure high anxiety levels. It may be preferable, therefore, that instead of the therapist trying to categorize individuals into compartments, they consider attachments styles as an adaptive flexible strategy. They are developed in the person's childhood for good reasons as a result of the dynamics of her family of origin. But, as the person moves into adulthood, sometimes still using these strategies is no longer functional in a new relationship with different dynamics.

Adults, building on their childhood attachment templates, construct expectancies related to these attachment systems. Thus, the person with a preoccupied style hyperactivates their attachment system with anxious rumination about the security of the relationship, whereas the person with an avoidant style deactivates theirs by placing a barrier around themselves and not letting people into their vulnerable emotional core, switching their security fears off. What underpins all insecure attachment styles, however, is sensitivity to rejection and a fear of abandonment, which has been laid down as a default pathway at an early stage of neural development. This pathway provides the template for how the adult will behave within close friendships, with acquaintances and work colleagues, as well as within intimate relationships. In general, insecurely attached individuals are unable to moderate or regulate the intensity of their emotions, including excitement, shame, rage, disgust, panic–terror, and hopeless despair (Cassidy, 1994). The stress responses that an infant produces are appropriate responses for an immature brain. However, if an adult with a mature brain still produces the same infantile, unregulated emotional responses, it is possible that under certain stressful conditions promoting insecurity, the insecure person may regress into an infantile state (Nijenhuis, Vanderlinden, & Spinhoven, 1998). As such, these adults are not responding via their thinking cortical areas, but via their subcortical limbic system, in particular, the "quick and dirty route" (LeDoux, 1996) to the amygdala, which specializes in processing unseen fear (Morris, Ohman, & Dolan, 1999).

Insecure adults may also display empathy disorders, demonstrating a limited capacity to understand the feelings of others with an inability to accurately read facial expressions (Schore, 2003b). In addition, they tend to be hypersensitive to criticism, which may be interpreted as another form of rejection, and they often have an overdeveloped sense of shame and feelings of worthlessness. There are physical consequences, too; people with insecure attachments are twice as likely to develop severe illnesses like coronary heart disease or cancer, and have five times greater risk of premature death compared to those with close and supportive families (Reynolds & Kaplan, 1990; Russek & Schwartz, 1997). The different manifestations of insecure attachment are complex behavioural repertoires, so it is worth spending time elaborating on each style in turn, although it is important to note that a person can have a dominant attachment style, with a coexistent, less dominant style (Mikulincer & Shaver, 2003; Shorey & Snyder, 2006).

Preoccupied attachment

Adults with a preoccupied attachment style are constantly worrying about their relationships, which often manifest very obviously as insecure; they are needy and greedy for reassurance and overt demonstrations of affection and attention:

"You do love me, don't you? You won't leave me, will you? Have you thought about me today? Why did you not call me or send me a text? Have you been thinking about me at all? Are you seeing someone else?"

This enmeshed and preoccupied individual does not have the ability to soothe herself from stress, and lacks the capacity to seek appropriate support from others. She needs constant attention and reassurance and can become endlessly clingy and demanding in relationships. She will precipitate conflict in her relationship, and will tend to blame her partner for any difficulties arising. She may remember her parents as unfair in their dealings between herself and her siblings, and is often overwhelmed by painful memories of perceived or actual rejection or abandonment in her history. She may, therefore, actively seek to gain her partner or friend's (attachment figure) approval in order to validate her tenuous sense of self worth. She may have a negative view of herself in contrast to a positive view of others (you're OK, I am not OK (Berne, 1964)) and may struggle at spending any substantial period of time alone without getting positive feedback from the company of friends or lovers.

Thus, a woman with a preoccupied style may be very demanding, constantly wanting attention and reassurance, and may become very jealous. Her feelings of unworthiness and needy desires are associated with high levels of negative affect, including anger and fear, in intimate relationships. She will get angry quickly and precipitate demands leading to arguments. She will struggle with her sexuality as her sexual functioning and sexual satisfaction will be significantly impaired (Birnbaum, 2007) and her anxiety will impede her ability to achieve spontaneous orgasm (Bartels & Zeki, 2004). Interestingly, Verny and Kelly (1981) found a correlation between feelings *in utero* and adult sexual behaviour. Those who recalled being terrified pre-birth were less able to express themselves sexually and were more prone to sexual dysfunctions than those who described the womb as a good and peaceful place.

Men who are preoccupied in their attachments often report later sexual dysfunctions, particularly premature ejaculation and hyposexual desire. Indeed, Kinzl and Mangweth (1996) report that aversive family attachment relationships are more influential to later sexual dysfunctions than childhood sexual abuse. Poor sexual functioning reinforces his sense of personal inadequacy, which, in turn, reinforces his fear of the loss of the relationship. As a consequence, he may become very controlling, holding on tightly to his partner to try to feel secure. He will want to be dominant in the relationship, demanding to be in charge of money, household decisions, and where they live. He may dictate with whom his partner is allowed to have friendships and what sort of leisure activities she may pursue. If challenged, he will always point out that this behaviour is because he loves her and because she needs protecting. He may perceive any rebellion against this protection as a transgression that may threaten the relationship, and may consequently lead to his disproportionate reactions of anger, which may spill into violence. Some of these men may also move into viewing violent pornography as a way of expressing or projecting their feelings.

Avoidantly attached

Adults who are avoidantly attached desire social contact and intimacy, but also experience pervasive interpersonal distrust and fear of rejection. They often suppress difficult memories and cannot access them, so they tend to downplay past traumas as character-building. Their hypersensitivity to rejection leads to an active avoidance of close and intimate relationships. At times of conflict in the relationship, they will actively withdraw physically and emotionally. They may use expressions such as "I need my space" as a way of keeping control of the emotional distance between themselves and a partner. They will choose relationships that offer mechanical, emotionless sex without the threat of intimacy. The paradox of this attachment behaviour is that they lose relationships because the partner feels that he or she can never get close, and can never receive a full commitment. This provoked abandonment leads to further tendencies to behave in ways likely to induce rejection, again leading to withdrawal accompanied by anxiety and anger and a stronger need for attachment.

Avoidant adults often remember their mothers as cold or rejecting precisely at the time they were most needy (Izard, 1991). Seventy-five per cent of people with an avoidant style had a parent who was dismissive (DeMaria, Weeks, & Hof, 1999). As a consequence, they prefer to maintain a distance from others, and may find closeness or intimacy threatening and engulfing. They are distrustful of the motives of others, especially those who profess to care for them, as their self-esteem is so low that they cannot offer a rational explanation as to why anyone would love or care for them. Brennan and Shaver (1995) found that avoidant adults were more likely to engage in one-night stands and to advocate sex without love, being more accepting of casual sexual relationships. They are also likely to report low psychological intimacy and less enjoyment of physical contact. Women with this attachment style are less likely to engage in any form of sexual relationship, whereas for men, the Internet would provide a safe place for sex without fear of rejection (see Chapter Eleven), again suggesting an interaction between attachment style and gender. Interestingly, Fossati and colleagues found that men are more likely to have this form of attachment style than women (Fossati et al., 2009).

Ambivalent attachments

Individuals with an ambivalent attachment style swing between the neediness of the preoccupied and the aloofness of the avoidant, so their partners are never really sure where they stand in the relationship. As with all insecure attachment styles, those who are ambivalent fear rejection and abandonment and are preoccupied with worrying about their relationships. They often remember their parents as unpredictable and unfair, tend to have experiences of trauma or abuse, and may, therefore, disassociate from the painful memories. As a consequence, they may turn to addictive behaviours as an attempt to soothe themselves, as these distract from the mental pain and humiliation of the abuse.

Sexually, females with this style may report involvement in exhibitionism, voyeurism, and domination–bondage, whereas the males are more sexually reticent. They both enjoy intimacy, but less clearly enjoy sexual encounters. Holmes (2001) suggested that compulsive sex might be a manifestation of ambivalent attachment, clinging on to gratification without the threat of abandonment.

Attachment style of older adults

If this book is taking a developmental perspective, then we should also consider the attachment styles of the elderly. The older person of today was a child growing up between the two world wars. Times were harsher in those days and parenting styles were different. In Western culture there was a philosophy of "spare the rod and spoil the child", and in the UK there was a post Victorian ideology of "stiff upper lip", not allowing one's internal emotions to be expressed. Home birthing was common, but as childbirth became more medicalized, babies were born in hospital and kept in a nursery away from their mothers, and only returned at feeding time for the first ten days to two weeks of their lives. Mothers were encouraged not to spoil their babies with too much attention, and it was suggested that a crying baby should be placed in a pram at the end of the garden or in a spare room and left to get on with it. Feeding times were ruled by the clock rather than by the babies' demands. During the years of the Second World War, children roamed the streets, as mothers were working and fathers were away at war, and death and destruction became a familiar sight. Many young children were removed from their parents in an evacuation process designed to keep the children away from the bombs. For most of these children, it was a major attachment trauma; some never saw their parents again. Unsurprisingly, in studies comparing the attachment style of the older generation than with younger people, a trend of a higher rate of avoidant attachment style has been consistently found (Diehl, Elnick, Bourbeau, & Labouvie-Vief, 1997).

As people grow older, their memory for events in the past becomes more consolidated, thus memory for past events becomes clearer, while the ability to store more recent information becomes more difficult. With age, they experience greater loss as members of their family and friends die (Webster, 1997). Secure adults take bereavement in their stride, whereas insecure adults will start activating (or deactivating, in the case of avoidants) their attachment systems.

When elderly people develop dementia, their capacity to store new information and to retrieve recent events from memory degrades (Browne & Shlosberg, 2005). As they become more disorientated with their present reality, their early childhood memories become more activated. This triggers their early childhood attachment patterns, sometimes leading to their thinking that their deceased parents are still living. Browne and Shlosberg (ibid.) found that this fixation was more for the mother than for the father attach-ment figure. Those who had secure childhood attachments are going to feel more secure at this time, thus making them less likely to respond to strong feelings of FEAR or RAGE. These elderly indi-viduals will be easier to look after, less likely to be searching for support, and will have closer relationships with their current care-givers. However, if their early attachment styles were insecure, then that insecurity will be revisited. They are more likely to act out their emotional dysregulation, are likely to be more difficult to look after and become more demanding or more dismissive, and may be considered by family members to be a burden or a liability (Magai & Cohen, 1998). Magai and colleagues found a greater incidence of avoidant (dismissive) attachment among their sample of elderly people with dementia compared to a younger sample (Magai, 2001). They found that the attachment styles of these elderly patients had a lower proportion of ambivalent attachment, yet these ambivalent people had more depression and anxiety than the secure and avoidant patients. This is consistent with a hyper-acti-vating attachment system. Avoidant patients experienced more activity disturbance and were more paranoid than securely attached persons, suggesting that they continue to deactivate their attach-ment system as distrust comes to the fore.

There is an interaction effect between the attachment style of the elderly person and the attachment style of the care-giver, showing how attachment styles still have an effect on familial and social rela-tionships. Care-givers of securely attached individuals experienced less feelings of burden than did care-givers of both the insecure groups (Magai, 2001). Perren and colleagues found that the higher the level of avoidance in the care-giver, the greater the level of agita-tion and aggression shown by the elderly person. They interpret this interaction as the avoidance producing ineffective or ambiva-lent caring, resulting in stubbornness and resistance to being helped (Perren, Schmid, Herrmann, & Wettstein, 2007).

Therapeutic work with insecure attachment

In having a clear understanding of attachment pathology, the psychotherapist has a strong therapeutic tool with which to work (Brisch, 1999). Main (1995) developed a semi-structured interview technique to help (particularly researchers) determine the attach-ment style of the adult, called the Adult Attachment Interview (George, Kaplan, & Main, 1985). The interview includes

- adjectives to describe each care-giver;
- descriptions of anecdotal incidents to demonstrate these adjectives;
- descriptions of significant losses or separations in childhood;
- descriptions of feelings of threat from parents when a child;
- assessments of how childhood experiences have effected him or her as an adult;
- assessments of why they think their parents behaved the way they did.

Main held that having a difficult childhood did not necessarily make the adult insecure; what was more important was the person's internal representation of his history. What distinguishes the secure from the insecure adult is how he describes his represen-tations of his childhood attachment relationships in a coherent and collaborative fashion. If the representation is secure, he will exam-ine the early relationships and life events with insight and humour, and will consider his own past thinking processes reflectively, re-evaluating the story as he is telling it. Insecure preoccupied adults, alternatively, are often overwhelmed and flooded by painful memo-ries of childhood events as if they occurred recently. They will tell long, rambling stories and will be preoccupied with the detail. Peter Fonagy suggested that these people are particularly difficult to treat in therapy, as they jump from one issue to the next without any internal consolidation or integration of cognitive or emotional processes (Fonagy, 2001). Insecure avoidant adults will try to avoid discussions about attachments, and may appear dispassionate when they describe painful childhood events, being rigid with the detail, or may even idealize their relationships with their mothers as a way of avoiding the pain of past rejections. Individuals with unresolved trauma or disorganized attachment style can tell some of their story, but large and essential gaps appear, especially if discussing attachment figures. Their memories are chaotic and frag-mented, as is their sense of self.

Chapter Eight reviews how insecurely attached adults formu-late intense, sometimes addictive, relationships, which may be long-lasting, but not necessarily happy. The next chapter, however, looks at a personality style that appears the antithesis of attachment: narcissism.

Gordon's review

As Gordon moves from adolescence into early adulthood, he has developed an avoidant attachment style. He finds that the girls he knows from school are too pressurizing and wanting to get too involved in his affairs, when all he is interested in doing with them is experimenting with different types of sex. He has lost respect for his mother, and in doing so has lost respect for most women in general. Therefore, he chooses not to have a regular girlfriend, even though he has had opportunities. His childhood interest in centrefold pornography has now matured into regular evening autoerotic behaviour with the aid of the Internet, which gives him instant gratification without the threat or hassle of intimacy. In addition, every Friday night after he has been paid, he finds himself a prostitute and tries a different sexual position that he has seen from his cyberviewing. He has little interest in these sex workers as individuals, and does not care if his explorations or objectifications hurt them. If they complain, he retorts that pain is one of their occupational hazards. As Gordon's LUST circuit has been integrated into his insecure attachment template, he is has developed a side circuitry that revolves around PANIC, LOSS, and RAGE, and has developed the expectancy that no woman is capable of meeting his needs.

.

CHAPTER SIX

Narcissistic personalities

Gordon is in a small, dingy bar on the other side of town from where he lives. He prefers to drink at a place where he is not known and where others will not stop to ask him questions about the problems with their cars. He is standing leaning on one elbow against the bar, with his foot up on the foot-rail, his leg bouncing up and down in jerking repetition, and he is drawing heavily on his cigarette through nicotine-splattered fingers as he watches the small television positioned on a bracket above the optics. The programme he is watching is *Only Fools and Horses*, which he enjoys even though he has seen the episodes numerous times before. On hearing another insignificant and corny joke, he emits a loud guffaw. Conscious that his laugh may have been heard by others in the bar, his gaze turns away from the television to another man, also standing alone at the bar, who is looking at Gordon after being distracted from his own thoughts by the laugh. Gordon's eyes narrow harshly at the man, and, throwing his half-smoked cigarette on the floor, he demands, "What the fuck do you think you are looking at!"

The man abruptly looks away, but still feeling the intensity of Gordon's stare, pours the remainder of his drink down his open throat, pulls his jacket collar up around his burning face, and hurries out of the pub without giving Gordon another glance. Gordon, however, is now burning with rage at the affront from the stranger. He quickly finishes his own drink and seemingly saunters outside into the dark evening air. He can see the stranger in the distance, scurrying away into the darkness, and, with a swift, deliberate stride, Gordon follows. The man's pace seems to quicken, even though he does not look around, which makes Gordon chuckle at the stranger's obvious discomfort. The man turns into a pathway through a nearby park, and Gordon seizes his moment. Picking up a rock he sees as he passes a flower border, he lobs the rock at the man. The rock strikes the man a glancing blow to the side of his skull and he collapses to the ground. Gordon smiles widely, mutters "Wanker!" under his breath, thrusts his hands into his pockets, and ambles off. He whistles the signature tune to the television programme as he idles away.

The story of Narcissus

In the classic myth, Narcissus is the child of the rape of a beautiful nymph, Leiriope, by the river-god Cephisus. Leiriope had consulted the seer Teiresias, who predicted that if the boy ever really knew himself, he would die. Everyone loved Narcissus, including a beautiful nymph called Echo, who could only repeat what she had heard, thus could never tell Narcissus how she felt. She became so unhappy in her unrequited love that she pined away until only her voice could be heard. Narcissus, however, eventually found himself in his reflection in the pool, and when he realized that the only person he did love was himself in the reflection that gazed back at him, he plunged a dagger into his breast, and as the blood soaked into the soil he was transformed into the beautiful flower, the narcissus.

Although not commonly considered an attachment style, narcissism develops within a child during the same physiological process of attachments and may be linked to an avoidant/dismissive attachment style (Slade, 1999). Indeed, Bowlby highlighted the processes of narcissism in his original work as a person who "may attempt to live his life without the love and support of others, and may later be diagnosed as narcissistic" (Bowlby, 1988, pp. 124–125). Narcissism is also linked to the development of shame, the function of which is to reduce the arousal caused by elated, grandiose, euphoric, excited, or manic states (Tomkins, 1963). In the story of Narcissus and Echo, one can clearly identify the avoidant style of Narcissus, who was not interested in any form of intimacy except with himself, and the preoccupied style of Echo, whose only focus was on her unrequited love for Narcissus. Echo is the hyper-vigilant thin-skinned narcissist (Rosenfeld, 1971, 1987), and Narcissus is the oblivious thick-skinned narcissist. As is discussed in Chapter Eight, this relationship formulates a classic co-dependent model. How does this classic story relate to our contemporary understanding of child development?

Parenting styles and the development of narcissism

As infants reach the end of their first year, the emphasis of parenting shifts from primarily providing nurturance and protection to providing support, boundaries, and limits, and teaching effective control strategies (Sroufe, Egeland, Carlson, & Collins, 2005). The practising period of an infant at ages 12–24 months is particularly significant, although later years are also important. It is also a significant time when the attachment to the mother becomes less important, and the attachment to the father and significant carers, such as grandparents, becomes more important. Freud considered that all infants are born with primary narcissism, as they feel omnipotent and powerful in their symbiotic connection with their mother (Freud, 1914c). But that connection needs to be broken if the child is going to develop a strong sense of self and other in a social milieu. This break occurs at the time the child develops a sense of self separate from the mother, thus parenting styles at this critical time will determine how the child develops strategies of social coping. Research has shown that parents who have firm and clear boundaries, combined with warmth and support, produce children who are the most socially confident, and this has been shown cross-culturally (Carlson & Harwood, 2003). Boundaries are essential at this time, as it is through the imposition of limits that the child learns frustration tolerance and mastery over disappointment

(Levy & Orlans, 2003). But these limits need to be imposed in a sensitive way to prevent the attachment relationship becoming damaged or damage to the child's self esteem.

Consider a developing infant who has now learnt to pull himself up on to his feet and has started to explore the world by toddling away from his mother. His sympathetic arousal system is engaged as he is learning that he is separate from her and is developing a sense of autonomy. He is excited by his forays into the world, and will turn to look at her face for confirmation of his mastery of it. At last he rushes back to her embrace (the safe base) for reconciliation and reinforcement of security. Secure mothers will be attuned to the excitement of his exploration, but will also give him some support to bring his arousal back down to a baseline, thus teaching him how to regulate the intensity of his exciting emotions. Sometimes, however, mother may not be so readily available. Perhaps she is busy with domestic tasks, and therefore when he rushes back, he does not receive her eye contact or the warm reconciliation that he had expected. His heightened sympathetic nervous system will crash down into a parasympathetic flop; his muscles will lose tone, his gaze will be averted to the floor, his stomach will feel empty, his face will burn red in the blush of shame. This mirrors Erikson's proposals of the second stage of a child's social development that he called "autonomy versus shame and doubt" (Erikson, 1963). A secure mother will soon notice this change in posture in her child, and a warm hug and soft voice tone will provide rapprochement (Mahler, Pine, & Bergman, 1975) as his autonomic balance is promptly restored. However, for a mother who is preoccupied with her own emotional turmoil, or who is physically absent, this parasympathetic flop becomes a learnt response to the breakdown of his own omnipotence. It will condition him to how fearful and scary the world really is, and imprint on to the amygdala a ready response to threat. Consequently, the child learns that a passive, depressive style is linked to stressful or fearful situations.

In some situations, however, the maternal response to a returning infant in the height of his elated exploratory arousal is neither absent nor calming. Through constant stimulation and activity, the parents maintain the high levels of arousal in his system (Goldberger, 1982), so the child does not learn to modify his omnipotence or sense of separateness from his mother. Indeed, his omnipotent and primary narcissism moves him into a power struggle with his mother, who, instead of moderating and balancing his demands, indulges his every whim. This indulgence, emanating from what Broucek called "adoring, doting, narcissistically disturbed parents" (Broucek, 1991, p. 60), continues throughout the child's formative years to overstimulate and indulge him without boundaries or rules. This produces children who are self-centred and controlling, who lack respect for, or trust in, authority (Levy & Orlans, 2003). The parents become enslaved to the unregulated extremities of the child's expressed emotion, manifest in infantile rage responses as he continues to exert his power over everyone. Shame dysregulation leads to bypassed shame, as the child starts behaving in a shameless way, and will rage against any shame-inducer to protect himself from humiliation. The child has not learnt how to moderate his own emotional intensity, has not learned to balance his needs with the needs of others, has no concept of social hierarchy or respect for authority, nor has he learnt to consider how other people may feel by developing empathic responses. He is at the centre of his own universe and never loses the infantile grandiosity and omnipotence. He expects everyone to respond to his instant desire for gratification, and will fly into a rage when he perceives his needs have not been met. This is the development of the narcissistic style, and it is thought that this may underpin some of the frustration-triggered responses in children and adolescents and their consequent narcissistic rages. Indeed, it has been argued that overstimulation of the child as described can have an aversive effect on a child that is just as serious, if not more so, than understimulation or neglect.

The child who has a secure and appropriate relationship with his father can ameliorate some of this pathology of narcissism. It is dad's role to introduce authority concepts and boundary setting. He helps a male child to attenuate his anger and aggression and encourages sport, exercise, and rough and tumble play as a method of emotional regulation. By encouraging positive behaviours and constructively disciplining, he eliminates negative behaviours in the child in the warmth of a secure environment. Antithetically, a distant or critical father is likely to exacerbate the pathological development of the potentially narcissistic child, and if both mother and father are physically or emotionally abusive, the child is more likely to develop a subsequent personality disorder. For example, Adolf Hitler was said to have had an extremely indulgent mother and an excessively punitive, brutal father, which may account for his narcissistic personality (Miller, 1990).

Classic narcissism

There are two forms of narcissism: the classic narcissist and the compensatory narcissist, which relates to the previously discussed thick-skinned and thin-skinned narcissism, respectively. Both styles manifest a pervasive sense of grandiosity, self-absorption with displays of arrogance, omnipotence, a lack of spontaneous empathy, and an unreasonable expectation of entitlement. In addition, the classic (egotistical) narcissist develops fantasies of specialness, success, and achievements in her constant need for attention and admiration (Broucek, 1982). As such, she tends to be manipulative and envious, and responds to real or implied criticism with uninhibited anger. The interpersonal strategy is, therefore, to demand and to compete. The classic egotistical narcissistic personality is one of an insecure–resistant attachment style, which Kohut (1972) argued developed because of a lack of frustration tolerance; when a child never experiences frustration because parental pandering means that every need is met, then the person is incapable of a true development of the self in resourcefulness. She will always look for perfection, never find it, and will never have the skills developed to deal with the discrepancy between the two. This may also make her relentlessly self destructive, without fear of the process or the consequences.

Compensatory narcissism

Compensatory narcissism is also sometimes known as dissociative narcissism. Such individuals are shy, self-effacing, and self-conscious. They have low self-esteem and a vulnerability to overt shame, making them hypervigilant to perceived criticism or rejection. They avoid being the centre of attention alongside a subtle form of superiority and entitlement. The development of this style differs from the classic narcissist described above, although it can still be traced back to the affective overstimulation from parenting. Johnson (1987) suggested that people with compensatory narcissistic personality styles typically had a parent who humiliated the child with "harsh, continuous or massive exposure", perhaps being themselves the child of a narcissistic parent. Feldman (1982) contended that such parenting would create a narcissistic weakness leading to blocked empathy and hypersensitivity to criticism, which is defended against with narcissistic rage, producing cognitive distortions and conflict escalation, often over insignificant issues (DeMaria, Weeks, & Hof, 1999). And Klein (1957) discussed how the invasion of someone else's personality into the child can lead to an evacuation of the unwanted parts of the self, and, thus, the adoption of a new one. Thus, a compensatory narcissist covers himself with a cloak and a mask, to make himself into something that deep down he knows he is not.

Again, consider an infant in the height of his exciting exploratory foray into the world. Instead of being supported and encouraged in his developing independence, he is constantly attacked, either verbally or physically, for his misdeeds. He is commanded not to touch this, not to go there, or not to do that. The eyes that watch him are angry and distrustful, and accuse him repetitively of being bad or being naughty. This is a child who is learning that he is constantly under a negative gaze because he always behaves negatively. This child may subsequently develop into a passive (compensatory) narcissist who avoids being the centre of attention and whose grandiosity is hidden behind a façade of shyness and compliance. The explicitly expressed self-deprecation coexists with an implicit sense of entitlement and superiority (Broucek, 1991), as the only way of defending against repetitive negative approbation. He will over-regulate the high levels of sympathetic arousal of FEAR states, leading to an avoidant attachment style.

To summarize the difference between these two narcissistic styles, the classic narcissist tends to have a more endogenous malevolent style (thick-skinned), with no consideration for other people's feelings, whereas the compensatory narcissist actively takes on the style to compensate for the perceived inadequacies in his own ego-strength (thin-skinned) and low self-esteem. Thus, the grandiose style becomes a cloak that the person wears to cover up his lack of self-worth. Otway and Vignoles (2006) distinguished the core of these two styles through the recollections of people with narcissistic disorders: the classic or overt narcissists recollected their parents as overvaluing and excessively admiring, whereas the compensatory or covert narcissists recollected their parents as cold and exploitative. For a narcissist, the safe base means constant attention, either from fame or infamy.

Masterson (1981) believed that the grandiosity manifest in these styles serves the function of minimizing the experiences of depression; it is a defence mechanism against the potential annihilation from the critical or indulgent parent and the onset of the parasympathetic flop. The narcissistic fantasy is based on a survival mechanism to protect from a dysfunctional family system. Fearful of further rejection or abandonment, the person uses avoidance of intimacy and close interaction, and builds a grandiose fantasy of the self who is always loved and admired and self-sufficient. Thus, with narcissism, the grandiose self becomes the secure base. More recently, however, Lara and colleagues have shown that grandiosity comes from the dysregulation of the basic emotional states of low FEAR and high RAGE linked with the dopamine pathways (Lara, Pinto, Akiskal, & Akiskal, 2006). Chapter Nine elaborates on this concept.

Empathy

One deficit the narcissist demonstrates is his ability to empathize, because empathy requires the ability to look at another individual and, using the emotional database of facial expressions stored in the right brain, to make an assessment of how that person might be feeling. In addition, the person makes a person-analysis of how an event makes the observer feel under similar circumstances. Empathy creates social connection and prosocial behaviour; the lack of empathy promotes social alienation and antisocial behaviour.

Empathy is also related developmentally to time and maturity. Thus, the older and more experienced one becomes in life, the more empathetic, theoretically, one can become. Parenthetically, this accounts for why many clients do not wish to have young therapists, because their experience of life and, thus, their empathic stance would be limited. Rich (2006) points out that empathy has cognitive (in perceptual interpretation), emotional (feeling the pain of another), and motivational elements. A classic narcissist particularly lacks the motivational aspects of empathy because the other is not the priority; the self is the priority.

Symington (1993) points out how damaging narcissistic individuals are to both people around them and to society in general. From a transgenerational transmission perspective, if they ever have children, they are incapable of helping the child to develop a strong sense self, and the child can become disempowered (Brown, 2001). Any success the child experiences will be seen as an extension of the parent's specialness, and any failure will be denigrated and despised in the child.

Working in therapy with narcissism

The window of opportunity when working therapeutically with a classic narcissist will be at a time when he is actually able to see himself as who he is; that is, when he looks at the reflection of himself in the pool and realizes that the person reflected back is himself. As he has not developed the necessary coping strategies (resilience) to deal with stressors as an adult, he will not know how to deal with such a discrepancy between his idealized self and the realization of his real self. This will be the narcissistic collapse, and makes the person at greatest risk of suicidal behaviour.

The *modus operandi* of a person with a narcissistic style is their denial of dependence and retreat into omnipotence. Their hypersensitivity to perceived criticism or rejection elicits the humiliation and shame of childhood that is defended against with rage. It is this inability to cope with any form of perceived rebuff or abandonment, alongside an inability to regulate the extreme emotion of anger from affronted entitlement, which is channelled into narcissistic rage responses. Thus, when working with such clients in a right-brain-to-right-brain process (see Chapter Fourteen), that rage will be ubiquitous in the therapy room. Many classic narcissists will not consider that they need therapy unless they meet a specific external threatening situation, or, alternatively, they may be using therapy to manipulate a situation to "prove" that they are trying to change. Compensatory narcissists will be more open to change, but will be hypervigilant to implications from the therapist that they are lacking in some way. It is not unusual for a narcissist to unexpectedly leave the therapy, or even to commit suicide, when the therapist thought the process of therapy was going reasonably well. These are the critical times in the therapy, because it is the time that Narcissus looks into the pool to see himself.

To appeal to the grandiose side of their presentation, the client with a narcissistic style will either revere the therapist, as being the best therapist in the whole world, or, following challenge and disappointment, will subsequently denigrate the therapist as totally incompetent and unfit to practise. Complaints against the therapist's competency, or sneering remarks to colleagues or other clients, erodes the confidence of the therapist and his or her peers and, in a self-fulfilling way, taps into the therapist's competency. This desire to hurt, control, or destroy the therapist represents the abusive attachment figure who will eventually abandon and reject him, and, thus, restores the narcissistic fantasy. The client has no concept that the grandiosity behind these attacks is a defensive mental state used to define the self, and that just like all other mental states it can be confabulated and distorted. It is really important, therefore, not to use a purely humanistic method of working with such individuals, otherwise the therapist becomes Echo in therapy, purely reflecting back what is heard instead of moving the situation on. Remember, if Narcissus had learnt in his history how to self-actualize, he would have found a way. In contemporary narcissism, if the client did not learn empathy in the first place, no amount of therapy is going to help him find the way without a few road maps. It is vital, therefore, for the therapy to strike a balance between support and challenge of a client who may be very difficult or even highly punitive in the therapy room, and to encourage him to mentalize (Bateman & Fonagy, 2006) the process that is occurring. In the dynamic between client and therapist, there may be a tendency for the client to lead in his narcissistic fantasy, which does not give the therapist time to think or respond, and that would keep the therapist as Echo in a co-dependent relationship (Chapter Eight). Alternatively, if the client's narcissism is punctured too brutally by the therapist, there is a danger of the therapy becoming persecutory. So, it needs to be supportive and creative without colluding with the narcissistic myth. The next chapter will discuss how the narcissistic style may develop into a personality disorder.

Gordon's review

Gordon is starting to act out his avoidant attachment and his compensatory narcissistic style. He chooses to spend time drinking alone instead of meeting up with friends and developing intimate friendships. His heavy drinking and smoking are the commencement of addictive processes that he uses to change the way he feels, as he fails to get the endogenous opiates from a secure attachment template. The cigarettes calm much of his anxiety, and the alcohol disinhibits his tendency towards freeze–fear responses in awkward situations. He always feels angry, and sometimes he struggles to suppress it sufficiently to be civil to people he is close to, as his anger bubbles out in derision and contempt. He is hypervigilant to any form of criticism, so has developed a perfectionist tendency in his work. He works long hours, so that each car engine he maintains leaves the garage with everything checked and double-checked. He is not prepared to leave anything to chance lest he is criticized, because he is hypersensitive to the shame of making an error. But this also makes him angry with himself, and he has split his contempt and derision for his own weakness and inadequacy, alongside his grandiose concept of being the best mechanic in the area with everyone searching for his services. He is also angry with his boss, who is making a good profit on the back of Gordon's addiction for work.

In the scenario at the beginning of this chapter, Gordon is giving himself one of the few indulgences of pleasure that he rarely enjoys. He is away from everyone he knows, so his narcissistic cloak can be set to one side as he relaxes to watch a comfortable and familiar television programme in a familiar pub. But his enjoyment suddenly becomes public as the stranger hears his laugh and turns to look at Gordon. The shame response is one of feeling naked in a crowded room. Gordon cannot bear the gaze (which he interprets as negative) looking into his unprotected self. The emergence of his narcissistic rage is neither proportionate to the "offence" nor does it have a coherent, verbal explanation. It is a surge of pure, un-regulated rage that spills out on to a stranger, who is in the wrong place at the wrong time. Gordon has no empathy for the stranger's position or the extent of his injury, nor any interest in mitigation for the stranger's visual offence. Only Gordon's punishment of the observer will lower his pumping adrenaline and appease his narcissistic rage.

CHAPTER SEVEN

Psychopathology, personality disorders, and schizophrenia

"'Ere, Gov. Come and have a look at this." The garage manager, absentmindedly, looks up through the office window, still preoccupied with the invoices he is reading. "'Ere!" Gordon insists.

With a sigh, the manager heaves himself out of his chair to look at yet another engine that Gordon has finished servicing. He gets frustrated with Gordon's constant need for approval of his work, and has told him so a couple of times. But Gordon reacted so angrily that he threatened to leave there and then and go to work for his competitor around the corner. Gordon may be obnoxious at times, but he is a damned good worker, and does a brilliant job on the engines. The customers often ask for him, too, because, even though he is brusque and sometimes rude to them, he gets to the heart of the problem quickly, and no one has ever brought a car back that Gordon had serviced saying the problem had not been fixed. And that is more than can be said for his fellow mechanics.

The garage owner peered at the engine of a classic car, which purred contentedly as Gordon meticulously cleaned his spanners.

"Sounds good, Gord." He nodded his approval and noticed how the engine sparkled where it had been thoroughly cleaned.

"'Course it's good, Gov. You ought to get rid of these other tossers calling themselves mechanics." He added, loud enough for the others to hear, "One day I'll own this garage and all that's in it, and more besides. Then they will be looking for work!"

The boss tries to appease with, "Everyone has different skills Gordon. No need to be like that."

Laughing at their scowls, Gordon sneers at his colleagues, "Some people are still looking to find what skills they have got!"

Personality disorder

Personality disorder is a controversial diagnosis covering a wide range of presenting difficulties and behaviours. Although not uncommon, there is great variation in severity. The varying types of personality disorder do tend to share the following features: individuals with a personality disorder hold a narrow range of entrenched attitudes and behave in ways which cause difficulties for themselves and others who have contact or care for them. They have multiple vulnerabilities and needs, and experience extreme emotions that they are unable to soothe. The symptoms or signs most often appear in late childhood or adolescence and continue into adulthood. As in childhood, the presenting behavioural problems and dysfunctions are often described as conduct disorders. Having said that, not all conduct disorders in children necessarily lead to adult personality disorders.

Current classification systems divide personality disorders in the following modality:

CLUSTER A: (the "odd" or eccentric types), paranoid, schizoid, and schizotypal personality disorders

CLUSTER B: (the dramatic, emotional, or erratic types), histrionic, narcissistic, antisocial, and borderline personality disorders

CLUSTER C: (the anxious and fearful types), obsessive–compulsive, avoidant, and dependent.

It may be that cluster B personality disorders, which may underpin the majority of offending behaviour, demonstrate a disorganized or unresolved attachment style, leading to the hypoactive emotional responses found in antisocial and psychopathic personalities. Indeed, there is evidence linking maternal abuse and childhood neglect with adult antisocial personality disorder (Hildyard & Wolfe, 2002). In contrast, the type C personalities tend to demonstrate those who run around the FEAR and RAGE circuits of preoccupied (anxious, dependent, and obsessive–compulsive) and avoidant attachment styles.

There is a variable gender ratio for specific types of personality disorder; antisocial being more common in men and borderline commoner in women. Indeed, Saltaris (2002) suggested that antisocial personality disorders and their consequent behavioural disorders and psychopathy are five times more prevalent in men than women, accounting for why the vast majority of offending is conducted by men. Afro-Caribbean populations seldom seem to attract this diagnosis, and are more likely to be classified with schizophrenic-type diagnoses, but it is unclear if this is a true difference in culture or due to diagnostic practice. It is not within the scope of this book to overview the differing presenting styles of each personality disorder, especially as many individuals fit the criteria for at least two different types. However there are many good texts to which the reader can refer to get a summary of the various classifications and assessment criteria of personality disorder (Beck & Freeman, 1990; Tyrer, 2000).

Some people with a personality disorder are able to cope with daily living and function without too much difficulty, although they often manifest extreme difficulties with relationships and social acquaintances. However, many others suffer great emotional distress, are debilitated, cannot function in various areas of their life, and place a heavy burden on those around them. Some of the consequences of these personality problems are as follows:

- self harm and impulsive suicide attempts;
- accidents from impulsive and dangerous behaviour and increased mortality;
- violent and/or criminal behaviour;
- predisposed to suffer from other mental health issues like depression, anxiety disorders, obsessive–compulsive disorder (OCD), post traumatic stress disorder (PTSD), and phobias;

- more likely to suffer from alcohol and drug addiction problems;
- more likely to experience adverse life events, including housing difficulties, long-term unemployment, and relationship
breakdown.

Individuals with a personality disorder demonstrate difficulties
in social interaction and an inability to cope with stress (Kernberg,
1975; Rich, 2006). They also manifest an inability to sustain a sense
of self and a sense of relatedness with significant others during
stressful moments. This leads to identity diffusion as the primary
symptom of the person's presentation. They demonstrate frequent
expressions of emotion and depressivity, and an insufficient capacity to regulate shame (Schore, 2003a). Even minor threats to a tenuous attachment bond, like to a psychotherapist, can be experienced
as devastating and disequilibriating to such individuals (Holmes,
2001), yet they repeatedly behave in ways that provoke rejection
and abandonment as the self-fulfilling paradox.

The majority of distressed individuals with a personality disorder are cared for in primary care settings, as many are unable to
access the care they need from secondary mental health services.
This is due to some mental health professionals in the UK being
reluctant to work with people with personality disorder, because
the professionals believe they neither have the skills nor resources
to offer adequate services. These clients provoke high levels of anxiety in professionals and carers alike, and make heavy demands on
services by frequent and escalating contact.

Attachment dysfunctions

There is little consensus about the causes of personality disorder,
although increasingly researchers are suggesting that personality
disorders are disorders of attachment (Shaver & Clark, 1994; West
& Sheldon-Keller, 1994). It is generally recognized that early childhood experiences such as abuse, inadequate parenting, neglect, and
trauma all have an impact, although neurological and genetic
factors such as brain damage and low serotonin levels are also
thought to play a part. Solms (1996) suggested that an individual

child who failed to experience appropriate right hemisphere development at the critical time may experience difficulty in building appropriate representation, or schema, of the external world, leading to fragmented object relations. This may predispose this individual as an adult into developing personality disorders.

As discussed in Chapters Three and Four, by the time a child reaches two years old, the maternal and paternal attachment systems are in place. If the mother cannot meet the toddler's needs, the child will turn to the father to search for a secure base. If the father is absent, mocking, abusive, or emotionally unable to meet that need, personality disorders in the child are more likely to develop, as he will be unable to learn how to moderate or regulate his fearful affective states. There is no evidence that an individual with one specific attachment dysfunction will present with a specific personality disorder, although trends can be identified. Shorey and Snyder (2006) elaborated that each personality disorder is a more severe manifestation of an attachment style, with the following examples:

Avoidant attachment style → obsessional, paranoid, schizoid, or schizotypal personality

Preoccupied attachment → dependent or histrionic personality

Disorganized attachment → borderline personality (Fonagy et al., 1996).

Interestingly, the avoidant attachment style is not usually associated with an avoidant personality disorder, as people affected by the former actively withdraw from social contact, whereas those affected by the latter want more contact but are fearful, so avoid it (Westen, Nakash,Thomas, & Bradley, 2006). The adult with a disorganized attachment style, who may have childhood experiences of trauma or abuse, disassociates from painful memories (Lyons-Ruth & Jacobvitz, 1999), and Brisch (1999) argued that this becomes a risk factor for the development of later psychopathological symptoms. Children who have been physically abused may become aware of the anger and disgust in mother's "terrifying eyes" (Peto, 1969) that burn into the child, promoting a sympathetic state of shame. In her rage, mother will not re-engage with the child to moderate the painful negative feelings, and the snapshot memory of the eyes will be stored in the right hemisphere with the response of terror, anger, and fear attached to it. Repeated rejection or ridicule from mother or father to the child may lead the child to internalize himself as not worthy of comfort, warmth, or attention, and would increase his sense of shame. These children may then turn to substance abuse or to self-harming, both of which elicit dopamine and endogenous opiates for pain relief, as an attempt to soothe themselves, which distracts from the mental pain and humiliation of the abuse.

Levine (1997) argued that people who experienced childhood trauma have residual snapshots in their memory of their unsuccessful attempts to defend themselves. When a child experiences abuse, the sympathetic nervous system is highly activated in preparation to flee, but if she is restrained from doing so, or is frozen in the face of terror, the threat response becomes truncated and remembered in the body. Thus, the desire to remember the details of the abuse may be the desire of the body to complete its aborted or truncated physiological response.

People who present with borderline personality disorder tend to show a disorder of the regulation of affect, particularly of fear and rage. They seem to have a misconnection between the amygdala (the threat system) and the orbitofrontal cortex (the attenuating system). Indeed, many people with borderline presentation have amygdalae that are reduced by up to 16% in volume, probably as a result of *intra utero* stress or damage from the first year of life (Gerhardt, 2007). They demonstrate frequent expressions of emotion and depressivity from their over-reactive amygdalae (Donegan et al., 2003) and an insufficient capacity to regulate shame. As children, such individuals can demonstrate difficulties in social interaction and an inability to cope with stress. The pathway between their right brain emotional circuitry and their left brain prefrontal problem-solving capacity seems to be interrupted. As Cozolino (2006) put it, they become unable to think about their own thinking and their emotional turmoil leads to decompensation. They also manifest an inability to sustain a sense of self and a sense of relatedness with significant others during stressful moments, and have difficulty in making trusting and rewarding relationships. Some studies have identified that their brains have a small hippocampus (Johnson, Hurley, Benkelfat, Herpetz, & Taber, 2003), which is thought to have developed as a result of the parents being neglectful, inconsistent, or abusive (see Chapter Three). Indeed, Lake (1981) argued that the first trimester of pregnancy is the time and place of origin of many personality disorders, as well as some somatic illnesses such as asthma, migraine, and allergies to food. However, Herman (1992) placed the development of borderline personality squarely on the shoulders of severe and prolonged childhood trauma, although rarely as dangerously extreme as for those who later develop multiple personality disorder. From her studies, Herman argues that the earlier the onset of abuse to the child and the greater the severity of the abuse, the greater the likelihood of the child developing symptoms of borderline personality disorder in adulthood (*ibid.*). Certainly, this view would fit with the physiological changes in the child's brain as described above and also in Chapter Three.

Schore (1994) suggested that the development of the borderline disturbance is due to a mother who cannot tolerate independence in her child, which may revive old feelings of inadequacy or abandonment in her own childhood. The mother, unable to cope with a distressed or intense child, emotionally abandons the child, leaving him feeling empty and hollow. The response will be an avoidant style covering unmodulated aggression, together with a lack of the development of empathy (Trevarthen, 2001). The child will then turn his attachments needs to the father; if the father is not available, the borderline pattern commences as a serious disturbance in attachment and compensatory narcissism may ensue.

Splitting defences are developed between twelve and eighteen months old, and protect the child from these unregulated arousal states. Parental disgust and anger combined often promote a defensive attack position in the child, and may lead to personalities who are pathologically hostile and aggressive (Rich, 2006). Glueck and Glueck (1966) identified a cluster of behaviours in two-year-old children, which included vindictive destructiveness, physiological hyperactivity, hostile or indifferent attachments to parents, and a lack of submission to parental authority, that are indicative of later delinquent behaviour. These children may have alcoholic or criminal parents who may be abusive towards their children. The children, therefore, develop a template of the world as hostile and unsafe, and develop an aggressive behavioural repertoire in order to protect themselves from it.

Substance abuse and psychosis

Insecure attachments lead individuals to search for external methods of security, and using substances or self-harming are both common maladaptive strategies to deal with the intensity of extreme emotions in an attempt to change how one feels. Substance abuse is a form of self-harming where the individual becomes deluded into thinking that the temporary high or the temporary peace from negative thoughts brought on by the substance outweighs the detrimental consequences. Van der Kolk suggested that women with a history of abuse or rape often use alcohol and substance abuse as a means of emotion-focused coping and have comorbid PTSD. He continued, "The relationship between substance abuse and PTSD is reciprocal: drug abuse leads to assault, and assault leads to substance abuse" (van der Kolk, 2003, p. 170). Alternatively, substance abuse is seen by Schore (1994) as the addict's inability to self-regulate or tolerate his emotion with consequent demonstrations of impulsive behaviour. Recreational drugs provide temporary relief from the pain, and arouse narcissistic states of grandiosity and omnipotence.

Substance abuse has always been associated with both general and violent offending. Goldstein, Glick, Irwin, Pask-McCartney, and Rabama (1989) distinguished three ways in which substance abuse and violence might be causally related:

- psychopharmacological violence—the effects of the drug *per se*;
- economically compulsive violence—the need to support the habit leading to crimes such as mugging;
- systemic violence—the system of drug distributing and dealing.

Alcohol has equally been implicated in many violent crimes. Shupe (1954) found, in his large sample of men arrested for a crime, that 88% who had been charged with cutting were intoxicated, as were 67% charged with murder and 45% charged with rape. However, it is not clear if the alcohol changed an otherwise passive person into a violent offender, or whether the alcohol was taken to disinhibit and provide "Dutch courage" for the pursuance of the crime.

As discussed in Chapter Three, recreational drugs such as cocaine, cannabis, and amphetamines stimulate the D_2 (or second) dopamine pathways of the brain. The subjective feeling state that these external substances produce resemble the energizing of antici- pation of a reward (Panskepp, 1998), which is part of the SEEKING circuit. As tolerance develops towards a regularly-used drug occurs, larger doses are required, resulting in long-term over-activation of the D_2 system. This can precipitate a drug-induced psychotic inci- dent, such as cocaine intoxication or amphetamine psychosis, producing frequent, vivid, and bizarre hallucinatory dreams, which mirrors paranoid schizophrenia. This provides insight into what might be occurring with the false beliefs of people diagnosed with schizophrenia, and how their affect-seeking system is in overdrive (Turnbull, 2003). The positive symptoms of hallucinations, paranoia, delusions, and bizarre thought patterns can be helped by neuro- leptic medication (e.g., Haloperidol), which targets the D_2 system, but not the negative symptoms of cognitive deficits, depression, loss of motivation, or social isolation. Contemporary theories about the contribution of dopamine in the precipitation of schizophrenia are that D_2 receptors in the basal ganglia (brain stem) are overactive, but the D_1 receptors in the prefrontal cortex, which contribute to the negative symptoms, are underactive (Friedman, Temporini, & Davis, 1999). Modern antipsychotic medications may help with the positive symptoms, but leave the negative symptoms untouched, and, unfortunately, also deaden the personality (Panskepp, 1985). More is discussed about psychosis later in the chapter.

Self-harm

It is suggested that each year 400–1,400 per 100,000 of the popula- tion will intentionally hurt themselves (Favazza & Rosenthal, 1993). One in 600 people harm themselves sufficiently to need hospital treatment (Tantum & Whitaker, 1992). Many under twenty-fives are admitted to hospital after an overdose or self-injury (Hawton, Fagg, Simkin, & Bond, 1997) and, although self-harm is highly predictive of future suicide (Appleby, Kapur, Shaw, & Robinson, 2003), many do not intend to kill themselves, but see their behaviour as a form of self-preservation (Herman, 1992).

Self-harm can commence at an early stage of a child's life, and is very common in abused children, usually presenting with behaviour such as headbanging, biting, burning, and cutting (Green, 1980). Studies of people with borderline personality disorder suggest that 70–80% will self-harm and 60% of those will report feeling no physical pain while doing so (Bohus et al., 2000). A highly significant correlation between early childhood sexual abuse and later self-harming behaviour occurs, especially cutting and self-starvation, and there are consistent reports of people who self-harm having histories of physical or sexual abuse, or repeated surgery (van der Kolk, 1989). Hawton and colleagues found that adolescent girls engage in more self-harming than boys, but, as age increases, so does the proportion of men who self-harm (Hawton, Haw, Houston, & Townsend, 2002). Attachment dysfunction can produce self-injurious behaviour, such as self-harm, substance abuse, compulsive eating disorders, or compulsive masturbation, which are characteristic of borderline personality disorder (van der Kolk, Perry, & Herman, 1991) and characteristic of a preoccupied attachment style.

There are also physiological processes to the addictive side of self-harming behaviour. When people harm themselves, endogenous peptides, like opiates, are released into the body to anaesthetize it, which reinforces the pathological behaviour, as the relief from real pain may feel better than the constant ache of emotional pain. Often, these people will go into a dissociative state prior to harming themselves, together with the restless irritability found in addictive states. The compulsion to self-harm becomes overwhelming; thus, the safe place, or secure base, may be the physical body, because the mind feels like torture. Many will describe the feelings of relief or calm when they see the blood after cutting themselves, or the feeling of being washed-out out after a drug overdose. For the anorexic woman with an avoidant style, the paradox of wanting to eat yet not allowing herself to do so gives her feelings of control, which, of itself, provides security and comfort. Or the man with a binge-eating disorder who has an ambivalent attachment style, who compulsively eats when his FEAR circuit is activated, but then purges and vomits when the RAGE circuit fires.

Self-harm comprises much more than the usual considerations of cutting, burning, head-banging, or hair-pulling. People with personality disorders may display a mixture of self-harming and suicidal tendencies. By the injudicious use of drugs, alcohol, food, or erratic driving, they may play Russian roulette with their lives, leaving it to chance as to whether they will be discovered and saved or remain undiscovered and die. Others may self-harm by risking attack from others by walking alone late at night, working in the sex industry, getting drunk and picking fights, or living in abusive relationships.

Confusing terminology, such as focal suicide, self-injury, self-abuse, and self-mutilation, can hamper understanding self-harm as a concept *per se*. Bunclarke (1999) suggested that we should see self-harm as somewhere on a continuum between socially acceptable behaviours, such as tattooing and body piercing, to suicide at the other extreme. She argued that it is the intention behind the act that is important rather than the method, and pointed out that repetitive self-harmers often find verbal communication difficult, hence the expression through their bodies (Crowe & Bunclark, 2000).

Crittenden argued that maladaptive behaviour from childhood trauma causes harm, generating danger and discomfort when safety and comfort could have been possible. Those who harm themselves are diagnosed with psychopathology, most commonly a personality disorder, and assigned to the secondary mental health services. Those who harm others are judged to be criminal and are assigned to the criminal justice system (more is discussed about these individuals in Chapter Thirteen). Yet, the underlying processes between them are exactly the same (Crittenden, 2008). Many people with personality disorder become repeat attenders at GP surgeries and A & E departments, and there may be an ambivalent response from medical staff, who identify the damage as self-inflicted. It can lead to abusive physical interventions, such as harsh and critical treatment, or suturing without anaesthetic. This self-fulfilled response reinforces the person's belief about herself as bad and worthless, and that there is no one who will care for her. She may be discharged without follow-up or psychiatric support; others may be viewed as dangerous, and may be sectioned into secure environments, which again reinforces the person's previous experiences of rejection or abandonment, so, circularly, they will seek comfort through their usual method, i.e., self-harm. Van der Kolk (1988) has pointed out that a person's propensity to self-harm can be reduced when they are prescribed naltrexone, an opioid receptor antagonist that blocks the reinforcing effects of the endogenous opioids, forcing the person to find another means of getting their pleasure centres stimulated.

Comorbidity with other problems

Personality disorder is rarely identified as the primary problem needing treatment. People with a personality disorder usually seek therapeutic treatment for reasons other than personality problems (Layden, Newman, Freeman & Morse, 1993). They may present with depression, anxiety, panic disorders, eating disorders, deliberate self-harm, substance misuse, bipolar disorders, or vague complaints of emotional malaise that are difficult to diagnose. As mentioned above, there is a high comorbidity of mood disorders and substance misuse with personality disorder and it may be that personality disorder is the primary disorder from which the others manifest. Consider a domino effect, where the primary condition is the dysregulated emotional system in an insecure attachment style that leads to the acting out, as is common in most personality disorders. This may, in turn, lead to substance abuse in a desperate attempt to relieve their extreme feelings of discomfort or distress. As a consequence, they develop anxiety and depression as a result of their poor impulse control and unsatisfactory relationships. Alternatively, it may be that these disorders naturally co-exist.

Personality disorders and belief systems

Core beliefs can start to develop in the first year of life, when children are starting to develop schemata of the world. These are often bipolar, like hot and cold. Core beliefs are developed by the child's experience of the world, and may sometimes be negative even if they are brought up in a positive environment. For example, "I am not as good as my older sister" can lead to the core belief of "I'm no good", or "I'm never good enough". This may precipitate feelings of shame, guilt, depression, and anxiety. However, as the child develops, she will start to learn nuances in these beliefs; the shades of grey that comprise our world.

People with a personality disorder often have unipolar core beliefs about themselves that are rigid and inflexible and cannot be changed quickly. These beliefs, which should be paired; e.g., I am lovable–I am unlovable, are often unbalanced. Often, the positive side is weak, missing, or impaired, leaving the person disadvantaged in the ability to generate a more functional belief system. Sometimes, if a therapist can understand the beliefs that underpin the impulsive behaviour, then the person's behaviour makes more sense. By not focusing on the negative behaviour *per se*, because of the strong feelings of shame, but instead talking about their beliefs about their behaviour, then greater insight is found into the maladaptive coping strategies: we all do things for good reasons (Padesky, 2003). Therapy encourages an understanding of these good reasons collaboratively (Greenberger & Padesky, 1995).

Many clinicians in the UK are sceptical about the effectiveness of treatment interventions for personality disorders and are, hence, reluctant to accept individuals with a primary diagnosis of personality disorder for treatment. However, a growing range of treatment interventions is available, including psychological treatments and drug therapy. It helps to work on the secondary problems of depression and anxiety first, as these individuals often appear more dysfunctional when they are distressed. It is also better for the therapeutic alliance, as it gives the client the chance to get to know the therapist and learn to trust him or her.

Bateman and Tyrer (2004) reviewed the available outcome evidence on treatments and concluded that, in general, a combination of psychological treatment reinforced by drug therapy at critical times is the consensus view. They also identified key guiding principles for effective therapy:

- being well structured in the therapy;
- devoting efforts to achieving adherence to treatment interventions;
- having a clear focus;
- being theoretically coherent to both therapist and client;
- being relatively long term;
- being well integrated with other services;
- involving a clear treatment alliance between therapist and patient.

In therapy, clients with a personality disorder are skilled at projection, so their transference reactions to the therapist are likely to be immediate. However, negative transference reactions are common, and any semblance of a good therapeutic alliance would be easily fractured by the therapist being unavailable for an appointment (rejection), or going on holiday (abandonment).

The preoccupied insecurely attached may test boundaries and raise anxieties in the therapist by becoming increasingly more self-injurious to themselves, demanding the therapist break out of boundaries to provide continual ongoing support and help, becoming the twenty-four-hour unconditional mother. Despite the challenges of working with people with a personality disorder, it is useful to remember that there is nothing pathological about a personality disorder if it is viewed as a problem of attachment, and the behaviour as the client's desperate attempt to find a secure base (Holmes, 2001).

Schizophrenia

Goodman and colleagues have emphasized that physical and sexual abuse in children is highly correlated with adult psychosis, schizophrenia, borderline personality disorder, and dissociative identity disorder, in a range of 51–97% of cases (Goodman, Rosenberg, Mueser, & Drake, 1997). Although childhood sexual abuse tends to be considered a female issue, there are many boys who experienced it, too, and they are just as deeply psychologically affected (Ahmad, 2006). Boardman and Davies (2009) agree, and have criticized some studies that have proposed that a large percentage of adults are unaffected by childhood sexual abuse, which take a narrow range of asymptomatic victims, and do not consider the very common developmental delay that occurs following trauma and abuse. Interestingly, studies have found a statistically significant link between birth complications and later schizophrenia (Verny & Kelly, 1981).

More recent research has emphasized the risk of psychotic experiences as a result of trauma experienced before the age of sixteen (Bak et al., 2005). Kahr (2007b) developed this link to psychosis by observing from many years of working with people with schizophrenia that they all have insecure attachments. He elaborated a further attachment style, which he called *infanticidal attachment*, resulting from premature morbidization in children, which later developed into adult schizophrenia,. In these individuals, he noticed that they all had received either covert or overt death threats from their parents ("I could kill you"), parents destroying the child's precious teddy bears or real animal pets, or threats to the parental self ("you'll be the death of me"). These threats often took three forms:

- actual death threats or death wishes from the parent; depriving the child of the basic sustenance of life, such as food, water, light, or medical attention. Killing the child's pets in front of the child, either their teddy bears or real animal pets;
- replacement child syndrome, where the child is born to replace a dead sibling, and may even be given the same name as the dead sibling. Linked to this might be a situation where the child was born with another sibling who died *in utero*;
- aborted abortion, where the mother informs the child of her unsuccessful attempt to terminate the pregnancy.

Kahr suggests that this can produce a death of the soul of the person, leading to adult psychosis, and he emphasized the importance of listening to the story or symbolism of the delusion or hallucination to hear what cannot otherwise be told (Kahr, 2007a). He also pointed out that psychotherapists may have countertransference responses of either being attacked by such clients or fantasies of "hurling these understandably demanding and frightening individuals out of the window" (Kahr, 2007b, p. 125). Sachs elaborated on Kahr's proposals by suggesting that the infanticidal attachment has two forms: a symbolic form of death threat, which leads to the highly symbolic language of schizophrenia, and the concrete acts of torture that, if a child is forced to endure, witness, or commit them, can lead to the concrete language found in people with dissociative identity disorder (DID) (Sachs, 2007). She argued that this was consistent with Ross (2004), who found that individuals with DID had the greatest severity of abuse in their histories.

The role of oxytocin and vasopressin in CARE and, thus, attachment was discussed in earlier chapters, and for people with psychopathology where the person is clearly unattached or disconnected, one could hypothesize that there might be a subsequent correlation of a reduction in oxytocin. This is indeed the view of Insel (2000), who proposed that there might be a reduction of oxytocin in the brains of people with conditions such as schizophrenia or autism. Panskepp also pointed out that schizophrenics may develop their delusional insights and persistent thoughts because of poor regulation of the neural firing in the SEEKING circuit (Panskepp, 1998). He noticed that antipsychotic drugs that reduce schizophrenic systems block the dopamine receptors and reduce the self-stimulation that occurs from the SEEKING system. In addition, he observed that there was a fundamental relationship between schizophrenic process, the SEEKING system, and REM sleep, through which much (but not all) of our dreaming occurs. Solms and Turnbull (2002) agree that the positive symptoms of schizophrenia seem to be generated from an overactivation of the SEEKING circuit. They also pointed out that the SEEKING circuit is the primary driving force behind dreams (Hartmann, Russ, Oldfield, Falke, & Skoff, 1980), and hypothesized that one of the functions of dreaming may be to protect us from the delusory activity experienced within schizophrenia. Panskepp hypothesized the intriguing prospect that the symptoms of schizophrenia might be alleviated by the person focusing on the SEEKING circuit and providing more outlets with emotional exercises (Panskepp, 1998, p. 163).

Violence and psychopathy

The fundamental difference between people with other forms of personality disorder and those with sociopathic or psychopathic personality styles is their complete lack of empathy. Insecure attachments and their consequent developmental neural impairments make some adults unable to process appropriate autonomic responses to social stimuli, and, thus, may impede empathic responding (Damasio, Tranel, & Damasio, 1990). It also produces a demand for instant gratification irrespective of negative consequences, even if those negative consequences have occurred in the past; what Bechara, Tranel and Damasio (2000) called "myopia for the future".

Bowlby (1984) said that those with insecure attachments either shrink from the world or do battle with it, and people with an attacking or aggressive style may be using the maladaptive strategy of attack being the best form of defence. Bandura (1973) saw aggression as socially learnt by modelling on the behaviour of others; vicarious reinforcement would emphasize the rewards of violence, increasing the likelihood of imitation. Researchers have added cognitive elements on to the social learning theory, making it more cognitive–behavioural. For example, Slaby and Guerra (1988) found that violent people generate fewer solutions to interpersonal conflicts. Thus, a person may feel his violent response was justifiable in a hostile world, and he may lack the skills to behave differently, having modelled from the behaviour of his parents. Zillman (1979) agreed with this cognitive approach by suggesting that people do misattribute their internal arousal under specific conditions, and, thus, the normal sympathetic system adrenaline surges of fight and flight can be misinterpreted as anger. So, could these cognitive processes have anything to do with IQ? Heilbrun (1982) found that less intelligent psychopaths had a history of impulsive violence, whereas intelligent psychopaths are more likely to be sadistic.

Neuroscience now shows that in secure people, the anterior cingulate of the brain's prefrontal cortex would be activated at the sight of another's pain or distress, this being the centre for empathy. However, in the bully, the nucleus accumbens of the midbrain is activated, which is the reward centre, suggesting that bullies feel excitement from seeing others hurt. Interestingly, Raine and colleagues found that the frontal lobe volume in the brain of psychopaths was reduced (Raine, Lencz, Birhie, LaCasse, & Colletti, 2000). Recall, the frontal lobe is the part of the brain where the "volume switch" to reduce the extremity of emotions is stored. Raine and colleagues also found anatomical differences in brain structure between "unsuccessful psychopaths", that is, those who faced convictions for their offending, and "successful psychopaths", who had managed to evade the law. They found that the former had less grey matter in the prefrontal cortex, while the latter performed better than average on a number of neuropsychological assessments (Raine et al., 2004).

So, there are cognitive and physiological differences in people who are aggressive. What about attachment histories? A study by Yates, Beutler, and Crago (1983) compared murderers and violent offenders with property offenders. They found that violent offenders were more likely to have histories of severely impaired relationships or to be labelled as emotionally disturbed or learning disabled at school. Clearly, this shows attachment difficulties, although it is unclear whether the disturbed relationships and school labels were a consequence of the child's violent tendencies, or whether the violence was a form of frustration due to their inability to learn or lack of social skills.

De Zulueta (1996) agreed that violence occurs as the result of insecure attachments. She elaborated that the trauma of loss, deprivation, or abuse creates potential for violent behaviour. As psychological trauma is defined as the sudden uncontrollable disruptions of affiliate bonds (Lindemann, 1944), there is an overlap between attachment disorders and psychological trauma. This can lead to narcissistic rage derived from psychological defence mechanisms such as denial, dissociation, splitting and projection. Renn (2007) agreed that most of the "serious incidents" committed by offenders occur in the context of the loss, rejection, and abandonment trauma they have experienced in their lives and the activation of their FEAR and LOSS systems. He criticized contemporary complacent over-reliance on actuarial risk assessment tools (see Chapters Eleven and Thirteen) at the expense of the clinical understanding of the individual in the context of his attachment template. One of the consequences of such trauma is PTSD, leading to re-enactment of the trauma using the victim or persecutor (see Figure 15, p. 162: the Karpman drama triangle; Karpman (1968)), which was a common phenomenon with Vietnam veterans. Van der Kolk also viewed much violence as re-enactment, not only from a psychological sense of repetition compulsion, but also from a physiological sense, as the endogenous opioids released during acts of violence are addictive and produce a feeling of well-being and calm (van der Kolk, 1989). This was demonstrated in a study by Bach-y-Rita (1974), who studied men in prisons who were habitually violent. He found that when they were removed into a situation where there was no one else to get violent with, they started to self-mutilate. Thus, the acts of violence may, in fact, produce, for the perpetrator, an inner calm.

Finally, social cultural factors influence situations of violence. Just as society's view of homosexuality has changed from something to be abhorred and punished into something that must be accepted and not discriminated against, so there have been similar changes over domestic violence, marital rape, and childhood abuse. Institutional violence in wars gives people a mixed message, as society chooses to praise and celebrate some forms of violence if it is for their Queen and country, and to discredit and punish others. Godsi (1999) contended that the increase in violent crime in Western society is directly related to the introduction of free enterprise, creating a greater gap between "the haves" and the "never-will-haves", that is, in terms of relative poverty. He also blamed society that wants to turn violence on and off when the country needs to go to war, but abhors and condemns violence at other times. Godsi also blamed the lack of support and preponderance of abuse in families. As the majority of violence is conducted in the home, it is producing a damaged adult and, thus, an insecurely attached population. Citing many famous cases of extreme violence, and without condoning the crimes that were committed, Godsi highlighted that virtually all of the offenders were themselves the victims of abusive upbringings, either from their families of origin, or from the care of the State. He argued that these abusive situations damaged the persons' sense of self, and, in doing so, created the psychopathic style.

Gilligan (1996) agreed with Godsi's view of the damage of the individuals' psyche by childhood abuse and neglect, but he went into deeper psychoanalytical depth by proposing that the reason why these individuals create acts of violence is that when they become damaged, they develop an inner sense of shame and guilt (compensatory narcissism). So, Gilligan, like de Zulueta (1996), viewed violence as a defensive act and, therefore, preventable. We return to the issue of violence in Chapter Eleven. In the next chapter, we examine the most common form of violence: violence in the home.

Gordon's review

Gordon is now starting to demonstrate a narcissistic personality disorder. Still able to function well on a working level, Gordon has no social skills with his colleagues, has no sense of empathy in the importance of their jobs, exploits his boss to achieve his own ends, and is unwilling to identify with the feelings and needs of the others. He has made himself unpopular at work because he is arrogant and self-important, and has fantasies about unlimited success and potential achievements. He believes that he is special and that only other special people understand him, like his boss. He often feels envious of his boss, however, and wants to be in his place. Even so, he shows a constant need for attention and admiration from him. He has become rigid and stubborn in his outlook, and pedantic about how he conducts the tasks in servicing the car engines. This is the only way he can protect himself from any fear of criticism, and it also protects him from potential failure.

Gordon rarely bothers to see his mother these days. She remarried, but he has contempt for the man she has chosen and regards him as a rival for her attention. Equally, he has contempt for his mother for choosing her new husband instead of her son. So, Gordon now lives alone in a small apartment and, when not working spends vast amounts of time surfing the Internet. He drinks heavily and smokes even more. He is still uninterested in relationships, so he satisfies his sexual desire with compulsive masturbation. His friendships are few, as most people cannot cope with his arrogance or his cynicism. However, Gordon is becoming aware of his loneliness, and is starting to make plans to find himself a woman who will be good enough to bear his children.

CHAPTER EIGHT

Relationship dynamics and co-dependent relationships

ordon was in his usual place, standing at the bar in the pub,
when the sound of laughter from the corner of the bar
caught his attention. He dragged his eyes away from the
television above the bar, and looked with disdain in the direction of
the happy conversationalists. He recognized two people from when
he was at school in a group of five sitting around a table. Facing him
sat a girl he particularly remembered, with fair hair to her shoulders and a thin, pale face. He remembered she had been in the year
below him at the same school. Her laughter did not seem as ebul-
lient as the others, and she seemed nervous and shy in the
company. As there were two men and three women in the group,
Gordon checked now and again to see if she was attached to either
of the men, but it seemed she was accompanying two sets of
couples. Gordon was pleased by that, and resolved to speak to her
if she walked past him to go to the ladies' room.

Once, when he looked at her, she caught his eye at the same
time. He stared at her coolly, and she blushed at their mutual eye
contact and she abruptly looked down at her hands in her lap. Her
friends spotted the blush, teased her, and looked across to see who
had caught her eye. However, when they saw who it was, the smile

fell from their faces, as they leaned closer and whispered to one another. But Gordon had made up his mind. Rachel. Her name had come to him. Rachel was going to be his girl.

Attachment and couples

The attachment template developed during childhood and adolescence formulates the working model of expectancies in adult relationships. In the dynamic between two partners, expectations can precipitate healthy, loving, secure relationships, unhappy yet stable relationships, or precipitate the ending of relationship in a self-fulfilling paradox. In general, secure adults tend to feel more satisfied in their relationships (Feeney & Noller, 1996), show greater trust, commitment, and interdependence, and are more willing to use their relationship as a secure base from which to explore the world (Fraley & Waller, 1998) than insecure adults. A secure couple will operate on the secure template: they will SEEK to be in each other's company, SEEK loving CARE from one another, PLAY together, and have sex (LUST) together. When threats occur to either partner, the PANIC circuit will prompt them to SEEK CARE and loving support from one another.

Crowell and Treboux (2001) conducted research with couples to look for which attachment pairing might place a couple at risk of relationship breakdown. They found that when both partners were insecure, couples were significantly more likely to break up than other couples. Mutual love and support is vital in maintaining the security of the relationship. If partners stop SEEKING CARE from one another or fail to give each other appropriate support at times of distress, then the PANIC system pushes them into distress and physical pain. The secure template will be broken (Figure 14), and the other partner will fly into PANIC and FEAR of LOSS, manifesting as FEAR or RAGE (or possibly both). Beck (1988) pointed out that underneath the trivia of couples in conflict lies the feeling of hurt or fear. Hurt can be manifest in the wound-licking of LOSS or in defensive RAGE, again showing an insecure template. Cobb and Bradbury (2003) suggested that preoccupied partners demand too much CARE but never feel satisfied with the support they receive, avoidant partners will feel they do not need support at all, whereas

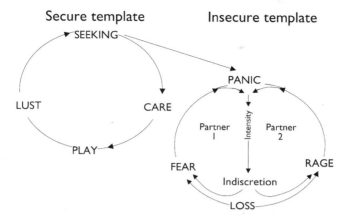

Figure 14.   In co-dependent relationships, each partner behaves in one half of the insecure attachment template, maintaining the position of the partner in the other half.

ambivalent partners would SEEK CARE and then reject it or turn to someone else for support, like a parent.

Insecure couples may also cease to PLAY or have sex (LUST) together. This is common in relationships where the children become the predominant focus of the family unit. Children can have a bonding effect for a secure couple, but for a couple who are insecure, the arrival of a child can destabilize the relationship. For a husband, it may mimic when he was a toddler / young child looking back for support from his mother only to find her attention is focused on a new baby sibling on her knee or at her breast. This may account for why so many divorces occur within two years of the birth of a child (Pacey, 2004). For the wife now mother, it may precipitate memories of her own childhood, and if she had unresolved difficulties or a traumatic infancy or childhood, can precipitate her tumbling into post-natal depression. As a consequence, she becomes emotionally unavailable either for her partner or her child, and provides the gateway for transgenerational transmission.

Common couple dynamics

What do we know about couples in distress? Anxious women and avoidant men tend to have relatively stable relationships, but maintain a negative view of it (Kirkpatrick & Davis, 1994). In these types of relationships, partners tend to attribute negative intent, especially selfishness and malice, to each other when they would not do so to someone else (Fincham, Bradbury, & Scott, 1990). They offer each other less positive behaviour and more negative ones. They respond disapprovingly to perceived negativity or criticism, and they underestimate the nice or positive things they do for each other. It is not just conflict that causes the distress; all couples argue. It is whether they interpret the conflict as a threat to the security of the relationship and how they try to repair the rift that matters. When couples engage in pernicious dynamics of demand and with-draw, criticize and complain, or defend then distance, it is these behaviours that threaten the happiness of the relationship. This is the behaviour that partners have learnt from their parents in their early years, re-enacting their childhood attachment styles. The capacity to reconnect after conflict and emotionally re-engage with one another will predict the success of the relationship (Gottman, 1994).

Couples often present to a therapist with a list of minor complaints, like him not picking up his socks, her not taking out the rubbish, or either keeping the other waiting. What is often underlying their conflict is the different perceptions of how things "should", "ought" or "must" be, which have been learnt at a cogni-tive and emotional level from their families of origin. Much of the literature on couples has focused on such cognitive distortions that individuals become trapped into, which maintains the distress in their relationships. For example:

• negative labelling: "you did this, so therefore you are a bad/angry/evil person";
• tunnel vision: only seeing what fits with his own point of view, and ignoring it if it does not;
• mind reading: "I know what you are thinking of me";
• over-generalization: "this always happens. All men are the same".

The eye of the storm in a row is not the inconvenience of being kept waiting, or having to pick up dirty socks from the bedroom floor, but the belief that these events "prove" that the partner is irresponsible, insensitive, or disrespectful, or does not respect the other. It is these misinterpretations that people make that cause many of the problems in the relationship.

There is also negative framing—the flip-flop factor (Abrams & Spring, 1989). Often the attribute that attracts one partner to another in the early stage of the relationship becomes the part that is most criticized later, as all attributes have a downside. For example, Deborah was attracted to Simon because he was strong, solid, and reliable (like her father); later, she complained he was boring and rigid. David was attracted to Julia because she was bubbly, gregarious, and always laughing (the opposite of his mother). Later, he complained that she was flirtatious and untrustworthy. Dealing with these cognitive distortions are essential in working through dysfunctional couple dynamics, irrespective of the sexuality of the couple.

However, although cognitive distortions must be considered, they are not sufficient to deal with the whole presenting problem of couples in distress. Increasingly, couple therapists have been looking not just at cognitive distortions, but at the preprogrammed emotional and attachment styles developed in childhood that they are bringing into their relationships (Atkinson, 2005; Clulow, 2001; Johnson, 2002). Most difficulties could be alleviated if the partners would turn their attention away from their preoccupation with "injustice" or "impropriety" and focus on the preceding hurt. If partners could recognize that it is not what their partner does so much as what they are sensitive to as a result of their histories, and that it is the personal pain that loads the anger, then they are better prepared for dealing with the conflicts of the future.

Co-dependency

The term co-dependency was originally developed in discussion regarding a complex set of behaviours exhibited by the partners and children of alcoholics. These partners were viewed as neurotic, poor copers, and obsessed with controlling the behaviour of the addict (Dear, 2002), and it became a pejorative term used for (usually) women who were accused of sabotaging their husband's potential sobriety in order to meet their own pathological neediness

(Kalishian, 1959). Subby and Friel later described co-dependency as:

> an emotional, psychological and behavioral condition that develops as a result of an individual's prolonged exposure to, and practice of, a set of oppressive rules—rules which prevent the open expression of feelings as well as the direct discussion of personal or interpersonal problems. [Subby & Friel, 1984, p. 26]

Early discussions on co-dependency suggested that the wife of an alcoholic had a disturbed personality (Edwards, Harvey, & Whitehead, 1973), and, less pejoratively, that the stress caused by the drinking affected the wife's or partner's psychological functioning (Watts, Bush, & Wilson, 1994).

More precisely, a co-dependent relationship comprises two insecurely attached individuals, irrespective of sexual orientation, who may be in a loving or familial relationship. Interestingly, insecurely attached partners are drawn together into relationships like magnets. For example, a meta analysis of research, conducted by van IJzendoorn and Bakermans-Kranenburg (1999), found that more unresolved individuals form into partnerships with each other than would usually occur by chance. Insecurely attached individuals will meet with a strong and intense attraction to one another; "the eyes across a crowded room", as the excessive eye-contact mimics the child–parent protoconversation. In doing so, they perceive in the other the missing parts of themselves. There follows a very intense sexual relationship with heightened arousal and heightened FEAR of LOSS, often creating intense jealousy. A minor indiscretion in the relationship can precipitate one partner to rush around the insecure template, creating intense reactions of FEAR or RAGE. What is interesting, however, is that in a co-dependent relationship, each partner seems to revolve around the template in opposite directions, making two halves of a whole (see Figure 14, p. 151). So, if one person hits the RAGE circuit and gets coldly angry, the other is pushed into intense FEAR that the relationship will fail. Thus each partner circles around their respective parts of the circuit between PANIC → LOSS → RAGE, or PANIC → LOSS → FEAR. When the PANIC circuit is activated and the real threat to the relationship becomes apparent, they bounce back together in an intense reunion.

The dynamics of the co-dependent relationship will vary according to the attachment style makeup of the dyad. Relationships involving an avoidant male and anxious–ambivalent female can be stable, although not necessarily happy. Very often these couples will act out what Mellody and colleagues called the co-dependent dance (Mellody, Miller, & Miller, 1989). Similar to Lerner's pursuers and distancers (Lerner, 1985), the preoccupied partner (sometimes called the love addict) pursues and demands constant reassurance and protestations of love, and feels hurt or rejected if the partner has been at work all day and not sent her an email or text, does not want to meet up for lunch, or wants to spend an afternoon with other friends. So, she will pursue her partner even harder, fearful of potential rejection and abandonment. The partner who is the avoidant (sometimes called the sex addict) backs off, fearing being completely overwhelmed and engulfed. There is a lot of self-fulfilling behaviour in these co-dependent relationships, as they confirm each other's expectations. His avoidance confirms her neediness, which in turn confirms his belief that getting too close can lead to being overwhelmed. The more she clings on, the more likely he will want to break free, the even greater she will cling on.

Eventually, the preoccupied partner angrily and abruptly withdraws, which taps directly into the avoidant's fear of rejection and abandonment. So, the roles reverse: the avoidant pursues, and the preoccupied distances. Eventually, the preoccupied will rationalize that the partner must love her after all, as he is pursuing, so, after a passionate reunion, the dance reprises its original sequence: preoccupied pressures while the avoidant distances.

As the sexual passion starts to wane in the relationship over time, as it does in all relationships, the intensity of the passion in this co-dependent dance is replaced by either partner in precipitating squabbles and bickering, and sometimes ferocious rows, where one partner or the other will threaten to leave. Thus, either intense sex or intense fighting provides the adrenaline rush that people soon become addicted to within their partnership. Subsequently, they move into a dynamic of not being able to live with each other, yet not being able to live without each other either.

The avoidant partner in such relationships likes to call the shots and set the pace of the relationship, often not turning up to dates or being involved with other things. Yet, if he (often it is he, but not always) thought his partner was out without him, a pathological jealousy may take over with demands to know where she is and whom she is with. He will make rules about what she can or cannot wear when she is out without him. Although he is drawn to the overt displays of affection from her, his avoidance is based on his fear of her neediness and fear of being overwhelmed and engulfed by it. In turn, his aloofness exacerbates her neediness, making her anxious and fearful that he might leave her. She will become clingy, possessive, demand overt displays of affection and demand verbal reassurance of his love for her, which, in turn, confirms his belief that getting too close can lead to being overwhelmed.

An interesting study by McKibbin and colleagues looked at the way (insecure) men have a tendency to insult their partners, which can predict an escalation into domestic violence. They found that men who habitually insult their wives or girlfriends do so, para-doxically, to prevent them from leaving for someone else (McKibbin et al., 2007). By putting the partner down and insulting her looks, behaviour, or figure, he is perversely hoping to maintain her attach-ment to him. The link between an insecure attachment style and the perverse self-fulfilling prophecies are clear from this study.

Co-dependent relationships are not confined to heterosexual couples, as attachment dynamics are equally important in couples of the same sex. Johnson (2002) argued that in homosexual couples, the need for attachment is heightened, whereas the ability to achieve trust and intimacy is more difficult. Josephson (2003) agreed, proposing that it may be even harder for gay men and lesbian women to achieve secure attachment following all the shame, fear, threat, and homophobia they may have experienced.

Attachment trauma

Relationships involving partners who are insecure may remain stable, despite the unhappy dynamics. Davila (2003) pointed out that attachment insecurity binds people together in chronically unhappy partnerships, and that insecurity increases the likelihood of staying together, yet decreases the likelihood that these partner-ships will be happy. She elaborated that in these unhappy relation-ships, the female partners showed the highest level of depressive symptoms compared to happy couples, and that the husbands of chronically depressed women were particularly insecure, predicting their maintenance of their wives' depression. She also found an interaction between those who were preoccupied and those who were avoidant; the former were overtly concerned about abandonment, whereas the avoidant did not appear so. This, of course, fits the pattern of behaviour, as for the person with a preoccupied style, their conscious fear is rejection and abandonment, whereas their unconscious fear is intimacy and sex; for the person with an avoidant style, the conscious fear is intimacy and engulfment, whereas their unconscious fear is rejection and abandonment.

An attachment injury (Johnson, Makinen, & Millikin, 2001) can destabilize a relationship. For example, when one of the partners feels an urgent need to connect (SEEKS CARE) and her partner does not respond (e.g., a woman is about to give birth and the partner goes out with his friends). An affair can also create an attachment injury that can destabilize the relationship. Johnson (2002) calls these incidents trauma with a small "t", and they may elicit responses similarly found in post trauma stress. This can produce somatic responses in the injured partner, like disturbing memories, vivid images, hypervigilance, excessive rumination, and a lack of appetite and sleep (Makinen, 2006). Such injuries confirm each other's expectancies about the relationship in terms of rejection or abandonment, and maintain the distress in the relationship as the injured partner consistently views the partner as unreliable (Davila, 2003). Johnson (2003) argued that such injuries can emerge in therapy like a traumatic flashback, even if they occurred many years previously, and can create an impasse in couple therapy, particularly for a preoccupied partner, who will want to go over and over the event, reliving the minutiae of the trauma.

Anger

Partners in loving relationships often use the conflict resolution strategy that they learnt within their family of origin, like shouting or door slamming, even though these methods might be counterproductive. They often persist in using them, either because they have not considered other approaches, or because they are convinced of their effectiveness. Kobak and Hazan (1991) viewed these angry, blaming, reciprocal conflicts as distorted expressions from attachment threat as they see their partner as unavailable or not providing CARE (Kobak & Hazan, 1991). One can see how they are actually distress vocalizations when the PANIC circuit has been triggered.

Some people do not realize that it is possible to be assertive without depending on anger to fuel their assertion. Anger comes from the preprogrammed emotional RAGE circuit, and, as such, is not negative *per se*, but it needs to be expressed in appropriate ways by understanding what triggers it rather than just acting it out. When we do erupt in anger, however, not only does our body stiffen in a sympathetic RAGE, but so does our mind, as we develop a cognitive rigidity as the link between the right hemisphere emotion and the left hemisphere prefrontal logic is bypassed. Partners in a relationship are least likely to express their true thoughts and feelings at times of high intense emotion or strong conflict. What they often express is the automatic thoughts generated by the primitive thinking programme, between the right brain amygdala and the left brain prefrontal cortex. These flash-thoughts fire through the "quick and dirty route" (LeDoux, 1996) down the HPA axis, triggering huge sympathetic arousal, while the left hemisphere tries to make some form of rational sense of what is being said or done. Instead, distortions, catastrophizations, and overgeneralizations twist it, and words come flying out which are not at all what the person would think or say in a calm state. The power of such a single unpleasant event can erase many positive ones, and is an important principle contributing to the problems of misinterpretation, miscommunication, and conflict between the couple.

Domestic violence

In the 1980s, Bowlby wrote about the high prevalence of violence in the family and the far-reaching consequences it would have on the family (1984). Still, today, the most common place for violence to occur is within the home (Godsi, 1999), and much of it still goes unreported. The 2005/2006 British Crime Survey showed that reported domestic violence was three times higher for female victims than for male victims: 0.6% of women had been a victim of domestic violence, compared with 0.2% of men (Walker, Kershaw, & Nicholas, 2007). In a survey of child custody referrals where allegations of partner violence had been made, Bow and Boxer (2003) found that more than half were male perpetrators of the violence, with a further 17% bidirectional but male instigated, whereas 11% were female perpetrators, with a further 7% bidirectional but female instigated. The rest were bidirectional and mutual. Graham-Kevan (2007) emphasized that although the incidence of men being victimized in intimate relationships may be less, they can still be the victims of a battering partner in the same way as women, and she argued that they are not best served by taking only a feminist perspective of domestic violence. However, male partners consistently under-report violent attacks by women and are less likely to consider it a crime. Indeed, it may be that women may not engage in as many overtly violent attacks as men to both male and female partners, but they are capable of manipulative, controlling, and emotionally abusive behaviours as well as physical assaults (Dutton & Nicholls, 2005). In addition, a woman's potential for violence would be increased if she had a narcissistic style or borderline personality disorder. It has also been shown that women who hit their partners are more likely to hit their children (Margolin & Gordis, 2003).

What makes some people more prone to violence in relationships, and what makes others more vulnerable to abusive relationships than others? For the perpetrators, Holtzworth-Munroe and Stuart (1994) proposed a typology of men who were violent in their own homes, and proposed three distinct categories: family only (FO), generally violent/antisocial (GVA), and dysphoric borderline (DB). They proposed that 50% of men who exhibited domestic violence fell into the FO category, and these men differ from the other two categories in that they are less likely to escalate their violence, and it may, indeed, cease over time (Holtzworth-Munroe & Meehan, 2004). Dixon and Browne (2007) proposed that this may be due to their poor communication skills, mild impulsivity, and their (co)dependency on their partner. The remaining sample of perpetrators fell equally into the other two categories. The GVA group were characterized by an avoidant attachment style, with high levels of impulsivity, antisocial personality, substance abuse, and criminality, whereas the DB group demonstrated a preoccupied attachment style, with high levels of depression and anger, who react angrily when they feel rejected, abandoned, or slighted (narcissistic rage).

For the victims, Alexander (2003) highlights that a disorganized and unresolved attachment style are intricately linked with subsequent vulnerability to violence, and, as already discussed in Chapter Three, disorganized styles are synonymous for people who have experienced abuse or trauma in their childhoods. One in three women and one in ten men have experienced some form of sexual contact in their childhood (Loeb et al., 2002). Such individuals who were abused as children are more likely to enter relationships where they become victimized, as this fulfils their expectancies and perceptions of themselves (Carmen, Reiker & Mills, 1984). Revictimization is a consistent finding. Girls who were sexually abused as children are more likely to be raped as adults, more likely to become prostitutes, more likely to pose for pornography, and are twice as likely as other women to report violence in their relationships (van der Kolk, 1989).

According to Few and Rosen (2005), violence occurs within 30% of dating relationships, 50% of which remain intact, thus leading to chronic abuse. They suggested two dimensions of vulnerability: relational vulnerability and situational vulnerability, which may be offset by protective factors such as high self-esteem. Relational vulnerability refers to whether a woman was exposed to family violence in her childhood, and whether she developed a care-taker identity that stemmed from growing up too fast, or having to move swiftly into a caring parental role while still a child. In these circumstances, the woman may feel a responsibility to rescue and protect her violent partner. Situational vulnerability refers to a woman's current life circumstances, such as being lonely after moving away from her family, or feeling the need to be in a serious relationship, or losing her virginity at too early an age.

The analysis of Few and Rosen can be reframed to suggest that the situational vulnerability is an insecure attachment, and that the care-taker mentality is a manifestation of preoccupied attachment. Such a woman may be drawn to the antithesis of her own attachment style; a man (or a woman) who is avoidant and aloof, but who also may have a narcissistic overlap which would predispose him to narcissistic rage and possibly even violence. Clulow (2001) describes this as an existential dilemma "between longing for intimacy yet dreading the possibility of loss of the self through merger, and longing for independence yet dreading the loss of self through isolation" (p. 133). Such is the development of a co-dependent relationship.

People with a preoccupied style repeatedly show a tendency to aggressiveness towards others (Moretti & Holland, 2003). Similarly, domestic violence is consistently associated with preoccupied attachment, either for the aggressor or the victim (Bartholomew, Henderson, & Dutton, 2001), and can be found in both heterosexual and homosexual couples (Landolt & Dutton, 1998). This is especially the case if both partners of the couple have an insecure attachment, as this produces the greatest negativity toward each other. Indeed, having just one of the dyad with a secure attachment can have an attenuating effect on the heat of the conflict, although if the insecure partner is a male with a partner (whether female or male) who has a secure style, then this represents the most negative and volatile combination, as these insecure men express more anger towards their partner than other men. Cowan and Cowan (2001) suggested that these men seek women whom they perceive as qualitatively different from their mothers, yet subsequently displace their anger towards their mother on to their partner. In return, the secure woman who has chosen a vulnerable, insecure man may have done so to make him feel more loved and secure. But in her attempt to rescue him, invokes the Karpman drama triangle and becomes persecuted as a result of rescuing the victim (Karpman, 1968) (Figure 15).

The trigger for the abuse is the FEAR state, often from jealousy, triggering the LOSS, FEAR, and RAGE circuits from the threat of rejection or abandonment (Dutton, 1995). Thus, the aggressor becomes overly dependent on his partner and takes ownership of her: "you are mine"; "you belong to me". His FEAR of LOSS makes him very controlling within the relationship, laying down rules about whom she can speak to, where she can go, what she is allowed to wear. This sense of control is related to a sense of entitlement, particularly from narcissistic expectations, and is evidence of coercive, aggressive, and disordered personality traits (Graham-Kevan, 2007). Meanwhile, the needy, preoccupied partner interprets this control as evidence as to how much he loves her, and fails to

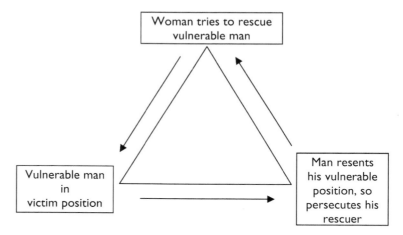

Figure 15.   The Karpman triangle, after Karpman (1968).

object or assert herself at the early manipulative attempts. She may even feel that his violence is justifiable, and may respond positively to any expressions of remorse following the abuse (Walker, 1979). It has been shown that such aggression in relationships serves to strengthen the attachment bond rather than weaken it, albeit at the expense of the victim's psychological and physical wellbeing (Dutton, 1999).

As a couple, they will fall into a pattern of his dominance and her subservience. Any attempt at her autonomy will elicit sudden and often disproportionate rage to the perceived "offence", and he therefore uses violence to maintain the status quo. The intensity and adrenaline surges that such outbursts produce has an addictive quality *per se*, for both of them. The intensity of fights replaces over time the intensity of what was a very passionate and sexual relationship in the early stages. Often, the abused partner will refer back to that early time as justification for staying, in the hope that things will go back to where they were. But, like other addictions, tolerance develops towards the violent behaviour and the strength of the violence subsequently escalates. This may continue to occur even if the relationship ends. Tjaden and Theonnes (1998) found in their American study of stalking by ex-partners that 81% had been physically assaulted and 31% had been sexually assaulted. This stalking behaviour is addressed further in Chapter Twelve.

If a child is born into this dynamic, the child becomes another threat to the security of the relationship, particularly to the preoccupied partner, who tends to feel his needs are never sufficiently met anyway. He may view the child as replacing him as the primary attachment figure, and may, therefore, perceive the child as a rival. For the child living with battling parents, his attachment security is obviously going to be deeply affected by what is going on (see Chapter Three), and he will feel the stress and trauma of living in a battle zone with divided loyalties. Dixon and Browne describe three patterns of intra-familial violence. First, a paternal pattern, where the husband is violent to the wife in sight of the child, who may also mirror the father and be abusive to the mother. Second, a hierarchical pattern, where the husband is violent to his wife, who, in turn, is violent to their child. The husband may also be abusive to the child. Third, a reciprocal pattern, where both parents abuse each other and abuse the child (Dixon & Browne, 2003). They argue how imperative it is in assessing risk to children living with intra-familial violence that consideration is given not only to the spouse-abusing male of the household, but equally the victimized female and the risk she may pose to her children post separation from the violent partner (Dixon & Browne, 2007).

Thus, the aggressor in a co-dependent relationship lashes out from an insecure base. Dear (2002) vehemently disapproved of using the concept of co-dependency when discussing domestic violence, as he saw it as denigrating women with their own pathology and, thus, blaming them for their abuse. However, it is important not to throw the baby out with the bath water. Co-dependency pathologizes the woman only if one considers her as the victim of the abuse. But, as discussed above, co-dependency is a dynamic within a relationship, where neither partner can happily live with each other, nor can they live without each other. Interestingly, if one reads the stories of the victims of domestic violence without knowing the gender of the protagonists, one could not determine whether the victim was male or female. The only difference seems to be that a fearful (preoccupied) man is more likely to be violent than a fearful woman. A fearful man is more likely to attack externally, whereas a fearful woman is more likely to attack internally, thus demonstrating another interaction between gender and attachment style (Bartholomew, Henderson, & Dutton, 2001).

Gordon's review

Gordon and Rachel do, indeed, embark on a very intense and very sexual relationship. For both of them, it is their first real relationship, but not their first experience of sex. Gordon had developed his sexual expertise by visiting prostitutes; Rachel had been sexually abused by her grandfather between the ages of nine and thirteen. Although Rachel was much more reticent sexually than Gordon was used to with the sex workers, he liked having sex with her on a regular basis, and she was keen to comply with all his wishes. Although they had been going out together for less than three months, he decided to move her into his flat, as this way he could monitor where she was and what she was doing.

Rachel was excited by his proposal, and to her it showed how much he loved her and how much he wanted to make a long-term commitment to her. Rachel's friends tried to caution her to take it slower, but when she shared that with Gordon, he became angry and accused her friends of trying to come between them. He suggested that she should stop seeing her friends, as they had a disruptive influence on their relationship. Rachel reluctantly agreed, as she rationalized that it is a normal progression to leave one's friends to make a home and family of your own. She liked the feeling of being taken to work in the morning, knowing that he would be waiting for her outside when she finished. She liked the interest he took in her clothes, and the advice he gave her about what is and what is not appropriate for her to wear when he is not around. She liked the freedom he gave her in the kitchen and for her watching her programmes on television while he was working in his study on the computer. And she liked going to bed at night, knowing he would follow some time later and be very sexual with her when he got there. She forgave him the one time when his love got the better of him, and he lashed out at her outside the pub because the barman had given her a friendly wink. Gordon's intensity makes Rachel feel attractive and alive, in a way that she has never felt before.

CHAPTER NINE

Cyclothymia and the bipolar spectrum

R achel sighed and lay back in bed as Gordon left for work. She had been feeling low for a couple of weeks now; since that last fight that they had. Now, she felt so down, she could barely get out of bed. She had always slept a lot, and gets very irritable if she cannot get ten hours a night. Gordon does not seem to mind her having time off work, but he gets annoyed if she is still in bed when he gets home from work and she has not got his tea ready. She has had these lows before, which she experienced regularly throughout her childhood and teens. She has never had the mania that her mum used to have, except once when they put her on antidepressants. Then she became really agitated and did not sleep for days, so they took her off them again. Doctors have watched Rachel with a knowing look. Her mother had been a manic–depressive and was sectioned three times before she was killed in a car accident three weeks after her last release from hospital. Rachel's father had left them when Rachel was little because her mother kept having affairs, and he never bothered to keep in touch. When mum was in hospital, Rachel went to stay with her Nan and Granddad, which she hated. They have both died now, so all she has in the world is Gordon.

Bipolar disorder

Bipolar disorder, or manic–depression, affects about 1% of adults during their lifetime. Not all bipolar states are alike, although traditionally, three major forms have been identified: cyclothymia, bipolar II, and bipolar I.

- Cyclothymia is when mood swings from moderately depressed states to mildly manic and back again, and is most likely to be unrecognized and undiagnosed. Such people are considered by family members to be moody, unpredictable, or petulant.
- Bipolar II clients have much deeper depressive episodes where they feel hopelessness, lose interest in work and life, have reduced libido, and experience suicidal ideation or sometimes make suicidal attempts, although the manic phase stays moderate.
- Bipolar I clients have the full swing from the most deeply depressed, and very often suicidal, to the highest of mania when people rarely sleep, can become aggressive and impulsive, grandiose, delusory, drive too fast, indulge in indiscriminate sex, spend money wildly, or make irrational decisions.

Research has shown that episodes of bipolar swings are unpredictable, and may produce mood swings that are days, weeks, or months apart, with no particular sequence of episodes, although it has been noted that the average time between episodes decreases as the number of episodes increases (Post, Rubinow, & Ballenger, 1986).

More contemporary thinking about bipolar disorder, however, has criticized the current categorical models of mood, personality, and behavioural disorders as distinct entities without clear evidence that this is the case (Lara, Pinto, Akiskal, & Akiskal, 2006). Akiskal and colleagues have published widely elucidating the complexity of the bipolar presentation, which they called the bipolar spectrum. This is because bipolar presentation may not necessarily be on a neat continuum between the unipolar depressive state to the bipolar swings of highs or lows. It is now identified that there might be a mixed state of bipolar disorder, where people can experience manic symptoms and depressive symptoms at the same time. This mania can be positive in elation or negative in self-criticism and self-destruction. Or there can be hypomania, where the individual experiences a manic episode without experiencing delusions. The concept of a mood spectrum (Akiskal, 1983) provides a better model for the variety of bipolar presentations, which often may go undiagnosed in primary care. This concept has been further elaborated into an understanding of "soft" bipolar disorders (Akiskal, 2003), which are versions of depression without any hypomania, as found in bipolar II, where the person commonly responds to mood stabilizers but not to antidepressants. These might be people experiencing depressive episodes with comorbid extreme anxiety, severe insomnia, or extreme irritation with angry outbursts. They often have extremely negative responses to antidepressant medication (Ghaemi, Ko, & Goodwin, 2001). Bentall (2003) agreed that mania and depression may not be at the opposite ends of an emotional continuum, but that mania may be a psychic defence from the person's desperate attempt to escape from the depressive mood, and what actually fluctuates is the person's self-esteem and positive or negative evaluation of self. Thus the therapist working on the client's perception of self and self-worth may be valuable in helping the person moderate the swings.

Lara and colleagues have synthesized clinical and theoretical literature to demonstrate that temperament can form the basis of mood, behaviour, and personality manifestations, and in doing so indicated that fear and anger are the most basic regulating emotions: fear as an inhibitor of behaviour and anger as an initiator (Lara, Pinto, Akiskal, & Akiskal, 2006). Early life events will influence the biological regulators of anger and fear traits, which interact with the genetic influence on a person's temperament. They argue that dysregulated or accentuated anger or fear traits lead, in various permutations, to the major mood and personality pathologies (Figure 16). For example, anger involves the aggressive behaviour one usually associates with the emotion, but also the impulsivity, extravagance, and goal-directed behaviour one finds in mania and the dominance one finds in psychopathy. Fear is related to anxiety, as one might expect, but also related to pessimism, timidity, and chronic fatigue. They also point out that there can be two types of cyclothymics: a person who demonstrates high fear

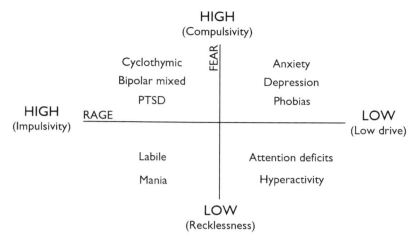

Figure 16.   The emotional dimensions of FEAR and RAGE underpin many psychopathologies, after Lara, Pinto, Akiskal, & Akiskal (2006).

and high anger, or a person with low fear (reckless) and high anger, whom they called labile.

As cyclothymic temperaments predispose to bipolar disorder, they conclude that high anger is a distinguishing feature of bipolar spectrum disorders, which is consistent with other research showing that depression with anger and hostility is characteristic of bipolar depression (Benazzi & Akiskal, 2005). Similarly, soft bipolar or bipolar II, which manifests more depressive states and the absence of mania, are related to high fear and high anger states with a cyclothymic temperament (Lara, PintoAkiskal, & Akiskal, 2006).

Lara, Pinto, Akiskal, and Akiskal's research clearly links with the FEAR and RAGE of an insecure template bouncing between PANIC and LOSS, with the inability to regulate the extremes of emotions due to lack of security. Figure 17 shows how the synthesis of temperament, mood, and psychopathology can be linked into a predisposing insecure attachment template. Individuals who are preoccupied and have high FEAR will be predisposed to general anxiety disorders, compulsive eating, obsessive–compulsive disorders and cluster C personality disorders. Individuals who are avoidant and have high RAGE will be predisposed to bipolar spectrum states, anorexia, conduct disorders (oppositional defiant disorder is commonly found in children with ADHD), cluster B

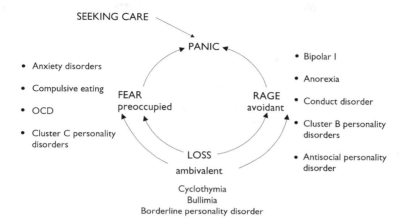

Figure 17.   Insecure attachments predispose emotional dysregulation, which in turn, predisposes psychopathology.

personality disorders, and antisocial personality disorder. Individuals who swing between high FEAR and high RAGE have an ambivalent attachment style and will be predisposed to cyclothymia, bulimia, and borderline personality disorder.

Children of people with bipolar disorders

Individuals who have a family member with a mood disorder are at greater risk of developing similar behavioural styles (Kochman et al., 2005). The children of mothers with bipolar disorder often demonstrate a difficulty in regulating their emotions, which can be identified in the child at twelve months old (Gaensbauer, Harmon, Cytryn, & McKnew, 1984). They tend to show disturbance in the ability to regulate their emotions that manifests at twelve months, which increases in prominence by eighteen months to two years of age. By two years, they may already be showing problems with aggression (Zahn-Waxler, McKnew, Cummings, Davenport, Radke-Yarrow, 1984). Schore (1994) suggested that this predisposes the child to later vulnerability to stress-triggered bipolar illness, although this is not true for all children of manic–depressives. But it may account for the reason that not all children will also become manic–depressives like their parents; they need the interaction between the genetic predisposition and the toxic environment.

Bipolar attachments and narcissism

There tend to be elements of narcissism in an individual who is bipolar that link with the grandiosity during times of mania. Schore (2003b) suggested that people with bipolar disorder are notoriously irritable after mild frustration, are readily provoked by seemingly harmless remarks, and react with rage to minor provocations. The links with narcissism discussed in Chapter Six again are clear, and may relate to the disruption in the development of the self at the critical time. Individuals with a fragile or fragmented sense of self may adopt grandiose or narcissistic methods of coping with their lack of self-worth (compensatory narcissism). Pao (1968) conceptualized the depressive phase of bipolar disorder as the passive re-experiencing of a "narcissistic wound", and pointed out the importance of non-verbal behaviour in the understanding of mania. People who are bipolar also tend to manifest an ambivalent attachment style. They show impairments in interpersonal relationships; when manic they demonstrate a neediness for contact, and when depressed, slip back into an avoidant pattern and withdraw. This ambivalent attachment style can be very difficult in trying to maintain stable relationships, and may account for the push–pull process found in co-dependent relationships (see Chapter Eight). As discussed, Lara, Pinto, Akiskal, and Akiskal (2006) proposed a model that suggests that what underpins the diversity of the presenting mood states are dysregulated FEAR and RAGE systems. They argue that fear and anger are an individual's most basic emotions which initiate or inhibit a person's behaviour. In particular, for many bipolar conditions, the person would have an anger system that is too high, and a fear system that is too low. This model provides a useful focus for therapeutic work, which can concentrate on the dysregulated or accentuated FEAR or RAGE states.

Recent research by Miklowitz and his colleagues undertaking the Systematic Treatment Enhancement Programmes for Bipolar Disorder (STEP-BD) compared the two treatment models: intensive psychotherapy and cognitive behavioural therapy (CBT) *vs.* "collaborative care" in a randomized controlled trial. They found that participants receiving intensive psychotherapy were 1.58 times more likely be clinically well in a given month and had higher rates of recovery than individuals only receiving collaborative care

(Miklowitz et al., 2007). There are two implications from this study. First, the use of medication may not necessarily be the best way of managing bipolar spectrum disorders. Antidepressants do not tend to relieve the pits of the depressive stages in bipolar disorder, which are notoriously difficult to treat, and may sometimes even trigger manic states (Phelps, 2006). Although the more severe forms of the disorder may involve the client being medicated with a mood stabilizer, such as lithium, Depakote or carmazepine, many clients feel unhappy with being held in artificial stability, which gives none of the normal highs and lows of human experience. Indeed, as many people with bipolar disorder are able to access creative aspects of themselves, which others cannot attain (Andreason & Glick, 1988), some clients are very unwilling to have their creativity taken away by the medication.

Second, the intensive psychotherapy, which included some family systems therapy, highlights the importance of the family in treating people living with bipolar disorder. People who have supportive relationships with family members had better long-term results with the involvement of their family members. Similarly, work conducted by Miklowitz and colleagues also highlighted that high expressed emotion from critical family members can have a detrimental effect on the morbidity of the person's presenting problems for up to a year later (Miklowitz, Wisneiwski, Miyahara, Otto, & Sachs, 2005).

Therapy with these clients will involve support through the depressive and self-harming phases, establishing support networks and keep-safe agreements. It is unlikely that a client will attend for therapy when manic, as the client's grandiosity will pervade and there may be a perception that it is unnecessary, as things are "great". Afterwards, however, there will be a need for support through the aftermath debris of the hurricane of inappropriate and indiscriminate behaviour and risky decision-making. In between episodes, some really useful therapeutic work can be done by focusing on preparation strategies for dealing with the highs and lows: seeking help, developing support networks, and recognizing prodromal experiences or triggers and relapse prevention strategies. Sorensen (2005) has developed a really useful workbook for clients to develop their own relapse prevention strategies, which can complement the therapy.

Rachel's review

Rachel demonstrates some of the signs of bipolar spectrum disorder. She has had repeated episodes of major depression since her mother was first hospitalized when Rachel was five years old. The familial link and her negative response to antidepressant medications are strong indicators of her condition. However, her GP presses her to try different forms of antidepressants until they find the "right" one. He never considers offering her a mood stabilizer as she has never had a manic episode, so cannot be like her mother. After her one negative experience with an antidepressant, Rachel is extremely resistant to any form of medication, as she was so scared by how she felt on the occasion that she did try it. She is also terrified that she will end up being sectioned like her mother. Rachel knows by experience that the mood will not last longer than a month, which is the longest it ever lasted, after her Nan died. She and Gordon have talked about it, and he said he will look after her, and that she does not need to go and see the doctor because he, Gordon, will look after her now.

CHAPTER TEN

Sexual addiction

Gordon and Rachel have been living together for a year now, and the intensity of their sexual relationship is reducing. He finds her neediness overwhelming at times, so he lashes out at her in rage. For a time this precipitates a distance between them that feels more comfortable to him. Then he reclusively stays in his study for hours, compulsively masturbating to the memories of previous sexual encounters. At times, he goes out to visit prostitutes, as he used to before he and Rachel met. Unlike the dominant and sometimes aggressive role he takes with Rachel, with the sex workers he adopts a passive role, where they seduce him and take what they want. Sometimes, he pays for two at once, and watches them having sex with each other before they turn on him. He plans each encounter in great detail, taking them outfits to wear, and extra sex toys. He enjoys the intensity, and the secrecy makes it even more intense. It is a dimension of sex that he knows Rachel could not participate in. And, in a way, he would not want her to be like that. This is his fun, and Rachel would spoil it for him.

Introduction to sexual addiction

When sexual behaviour becomes obsessive and compulsive, and continues in the face of negative consequences, then that behaviour is defined as sexual addiction (Carnes, 2002). The concept of sexual addiction is controversial, and some argue that calling it an addiction is an excuse for not controlling inappropriate and indulgent behaviour. A major problem with some of the literature surrounding sexual addiction, and whether it is considered compulsive, impulsive, or obsessive–compulsive, is that a sex addict is not necessarily someone who wants a lot of sex. Goodman proposed the following diagnostic criteria for sexual addiction:

- recurrent failure to resist impulses to engage in a specified sexual behaviour;
- increased sense of tension immediately prior to initiating the sexual behaviour;
- pleasure or relief at the time of engaging in sexual behaviour;
- symptoms persisting for more than one month;
- at least five of the following:

  o frequent preoccupation in preparation for sex;
  o frequent engagement in the sexual activity or extending over a long period;
  o repeated efforts to reduce, control, or stop the sexual behaviour;
  o a great deal of time spent on it or recovering from it;
  o being sexual when the person should be doing other things (like working);
  o giving up other activities to make time for sex;
  o continuing despite negative consequences;
  o tolerance—need to increase the intensity to get the same thrill;
  o restlessness or irritability if not engaging in sex (Goodman, 1992).

Of course, there have been criticisms of these proposals, as these criteria may fit any couple in the first flush of an intense sexual relationship (Mosner, 1992). Patrick Carnes, who is considered the leading authority on sexual addiction, described addictive behaviour as progressing through three hierarchical levels. He argued that as people become more desensitized to their own sexual behaviour, they need greater levels of stimulation to get the same thrill. Thus, tolerance and escalation, the same as any other addiction to an external substance such as drugs or alcohol, appears to become a common factor. The three levels are graded from behaviours that are generally socially accepted, so have public tolerance even though they are regarded as unseemly, to those that are overtly illegal. The lowest level are behaviours such as compulsive masturbation, multiple simultaneous relationships, browsing visual stimulation: centrefolds, paper, video, and Internet pornography, strip shows, sex shops, using prostitutes/sex workers, having anonymous sex, or numerous one-night stands. The next level usually involves behaviours with legal sanctions, like exhibitionism, voyeurism, offensive phone calls, and illicit frottage (rubbing against people in crowded places). The highest level, level 3, is where all boundaries of society are swept away as the person moves into needing to maintain the highest levels of sexual excitation and fulfilment by indulging in bizarre or illegal activities (Carnes, 2001).

However, it is important to stress that not all sex addicts go through this progression from Level 1 to Level 3. Many have their own inhibitory levels over which they cannot cross, and the conflict between their needing to escalate further or to cross their own value system may precipitate a psychological breakdown. Alternatively, they indulge in behaviour that means they inevitably "get caught" at what they are doing, either by their partner, their boss, or the police. This is a subconscious miscalculation (Freudian slip?) in their behaviour that leads them to be found out; for example, leaving an explicit CD or DVD in someone else's laptop, leaving telephone numbers of sex workers on a family mobile phone, or easily traceable pornographic websites in the computer history at work. Very often, the person will later confide that when he was "caught" indulging in his inappropriate behaviour, he felt relief more than shame, as the other person would make him stop in a way he could not stop himself.

My understanding of sexual addiction steps away from the more classic views of addictive processes. You will recall from Chapter Three that infants rub their mouths and their genitals when they are trying to soothe themselves and reduce their arousal.

Secure infants will stop this behaviour as they learn alternative ways of soothing themselves with the support and encouragement of their parents. Others, through their insecure attachments and later vandalization of their sexual template, have not developed the emotional and sexual maturity to adopt alternative ways of soothing themselves through their negative feeling states. Some of these individuals started viewing pornography at a very early age and indulging in genital manipulation as means of calming themselves; sometimes prepubescently. Thus, by the time they reach adulthood, genital stimulation, that is, masturbation, and other sexualized behaviours become compulsive and addictive. Thus, a sex addict actually is someone who has an inappropriate relationship with sex. He may not be having a lot of sex, but he will be compulsively thinking about it and planning it a lot of the time. He will use sex to change the negative way he feels, searching for comfort. But, instead of getting comfort and gratification from the act of sex, pleasure is transient, so he will feel bad, disgusted, and often despise himself. Just like other addictions, he becomes desensitized by the compulsive and repetitive behaviour, develops a tolerance to his repertoire, and so will have to escalate his "fix" to get the same turn-on factor. It is this escalation that gets people into difficulties. So, a sex addict may not be always having a lot of sex, but he will:

- compulsively ruminate about it;
- ritually make plans for his next sexual adventure;
- indulge in repetitive behaviour until desensitisation occurs;
- increase the diversity of his experiences because of increased tolerance;
- escalate his activity to make it more exciting;
- experience a huge anti-climax because he feels bad instead of satiated;
- search for comfort because he feels bad, leading back to sex again;
- deny the consequences and lie about the extent of their behaviour.

This concept of denial is important in all areas of addiction, as addicts tend to minimise the importance of the amount of time, money, and aversive consequences of their preoccupation. Female partners of male addicts, who have a different approach to, and relationship with, sex often feel let down and betrayed by a partner or a spouse (Schneider, 2003) who would rather spend time looking at pornography, finding prostitutes, or calling sex phone lines, than having "real" sex with them. However, the men themselves argue that it is natural and demand to know what all the fuss is about. They will suggest that if it is the use of the phone or pornography via DVDs or the Internet, then it is fantasy and not real. If it is the use of prostitutes or sex workers, it will be rationalized as "just sex", whereas they "make love" with their partner, again trying to minimize the impact.

Incidentally, there is an interaction between sexuality and gender in the presentation of sexual addiction. I have rarely come across a gay man whom I have considered a sex addict, as gay men in general tend to be much more frequent, more open, and more adventurous in their sexual activity, and may, therefore, be less inhibited about it. Similarly, it seems to be a rare presentation in lesbian women, too. A heterosexual man is more likely to present to a therapist and be more distressed about his behaviour, especially when he is in a relationship with a woman who has made it clear that she will not tolerate further "acting out". Similarly, a heterosexual female sex addict in a relationship with a dissenting male partner is likely to feel more distress from derogation and criticism she may receive from her partner. Heterosexual men and women who are not in relationships are less likely to present with this problem unless their escalation has got them into acute difficulties either with their employer or with the police.

The addictive cycle and an insecure template

Carnes, Delmonico, and Griffin (2001) proposed that the behaviour of a sex addict forms a cyclical pattern (Figure 18). The individual becomes preoccupied in thinking about sex. This obsessive rumination leads to plans of ritualized behaviour, for example scanning the telephone numbers in phone booths to search for a prostitute, or walking through a red-light area where the "right" person might be. This may lead to sexual behaviour. Yet, instead of feeling warm and comfortable with sexual satiation, the person feels bad about

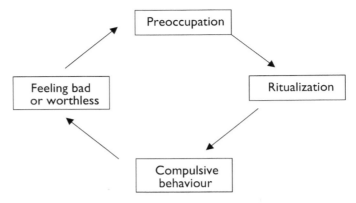

Figure 18.   The addiction cycle, after Carnes, Delmonico, and Griffin (2001).

themselves, and feels shame and guilt. These negative feelings make the person want comfort, so leads back to rumination about sex, and starts the person going back around the cycle again.

However, there are physiological as well as psychological processes with sexual addiction. Repetitive sexual behaviour is intense and invokes the sympathetic nervous system, producing an adrenaline surge. Ejaculation and orgasm evokes the release of endorphins, enkephalins, vasopressin, and oxytocin, all connecting with the dopamine pathways to provide physiological addiction as well as psychological dependency.

In addition, as discussed in Chapter Four, there are no endogenous opiates produced by insecure attachment template (Figure 19). In the secure template, the brain produces dopamine and endogenous opioids with the SEEKING and PLAY circuits, opioids, dopamine, and oxytocin with the CARE circuit, and dopamine, opioids, and vasopressin with the LUST circuit. These make the person feel pleasure, warmth, comfort, confident, and hopeful. However, in the insecure template, the brain produces adrenaline, cortisol, acetylcholine and glutamate with the RAGE circuit, cortisol, and glutamate with the FEAR circuit, and inhibits the production of opioids and oxytocin while producing cortisol with the PANIC circuit, causing physical pain. Thus, the pleasure centres are not being activated when insecurely attached, and, indeed, when the PANIC button is pressed, it makes people feel physically ill from opioid withdrawal. Additionally, glutamate has now been

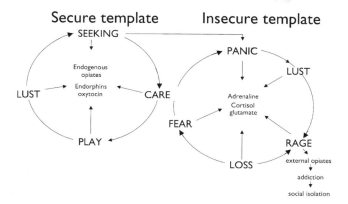

Figure 19. A secure attachment bond produces endogenous opiates in the brain and peptides that stimulate the pleasure centres. The insecure attachment template produces only stress hormones, so people search for pleasurable feelings externally.

shown to be neurotoxic and to promote cell death, and has been linked with strokes, traumatic brain injuries, and dementia (Nutt, 1999).

Thus, individuals living within a perpetual state of insecurity reach for external opiates to stimulate their dopamine pathways to invoke the pleasure centres and reduce the pain of LOSS. In the orbitofrontal areas of the cortex, dopamine excites neural activity, whereas noradrenaline inhibits it, facilitating the opposing mechanisms of excitation and inhibition (Aou, Oomura, Nishino, Inokuchi, & Mizuno, 1983). So, insecure individuals may use all sorts of behavioural processes to stimulate their dopamine pathways: drugs, alcohol, sex, work, shopping, gambling, food, or religion. But they all produce an addictive quality because they provide feelings that cannot be accessed from internal sources. This why addicts will often describe their fixes on external opiates as "womb-like experiences", or feeling great warmth and comfort, so much so that it is worth the risk of bad trips. It can also account for why so many sex addicts have comorbid alcohol or drug addictions (Schneider & Irons, 2001). However, the paradox of this external addictive search for reaching our pleasure centres is that these lead to social isolation, whereas the endogenous opiates from the secure template enhance social bonding.

Maladaptive coping mechanisms

As discussed in the previous chapters, an individual who has an insecure attachment, or has pre-existing emotional trauma that has not been resolved, has inefficient emotional regulatory systems and is predisposed to maladaptive methods of coping with situations of stress (Kernberg, 1975; Rich, 2006). They will also have a predisposition to adult post trauma disorders (Schore, 2003a). As the "quick and dirty" (LeDoux, 1996) neural pathway through the amygdala down the HPA axis is hypersensitive, the cognitive processes cannot moderate the extreme feeling of emotion. Under conditions of extreme or chronic stress, the right brain goes into overload and shuts down. It is at this stage that the individual will step out of their insecure template to search for the external opiates in order to numb the pain and activate the pleasure centres. It is in this way that individuals start developing dysfunctional and addictive behaviour patterns that are not only maladaptive, but also self-destructive.

Rich argued that it is not surprising that so many individuals with insecure attachments develop maladaptive sexual strategies as a way of coping with their inability to regulate the extremes of their emotions considering how contemporary western society uses sex as a commodity. "Sex is desirable, and endows special properties onto those who engage in and control it, including power, adulthood, masculinity, special knowledge, pleasure and prestige" (Rich, 2006, p. 227). And in Western society, women are trying to attain the same power and prestige as men, and thus have become more sexually demanding. Rich agreed with Prendergast, who argued "society is preoccupied with sex" (1993, p. 6). Society in general, and the media as the voice of society, idealize great sexual ideals and multiple orgasmic experiences as not only every "right-thinking" person's desire, but also their fundamental right. Youth and beauty are idealized as a sexual model (Smallbone, 2006). Sex is also used as a powerful marketing tool, as provocative semi-clad women are draped over powerful fast cars, as if one automatically arrives with the other. In using sex as a commodity that everyone should aspire to, it has been brought outside of the concept of the fulfilment of loving attachment relationships. Why are we surprised, then, when fundamental religious societies demonize such behaviour, and swing the pendulum in entirely the opposite direction, demanding that sex objects (women) are completely covered to prevent objectification? And why are we surprised when insecure, lonely, stressed, or depressed individuals use sex as a way of trying to change how they feel about themselves? Working therapeutically with sexual addiction is covered in the next chapter, where I also examine how one particular sexual addiction, using the Internet, has destroyed many people's lives.

Gordon and Rachel's review

As Rachel has become more depressed, she has become less interested in sex, so Gordon has taken to compulsive masturbation as a form of self-comfort, and the use of sex workers to enhance his fantasies for his autoerotic activities. At one level, Gordon is angry with Rachel for no longer wishing to be sexual. It feeds his insecurities about the relationship and he flies into unnecessary intense jealous rages if the postman smiles at her, or her boss rings her to have long discussions about how her health is progressing. He even goes with Rachel on her visits to her GP in case the doctor wants to make examinations of Rachel that Gordon would not consider appropriate.

On another level, however, Gordon is relieved from the monotony of having sex with Rachel, which had become boring and routine. He wanted more excitement than she was able give him; she just did not seem capable of the raunchy, hot sex that he enjoyed when watching pornography.

So Gordon felt that Rachel being *in absentia* from sex gave him permission to find it through other means. He would spend many hours thinking through and preparing for each encounter with a prostitute. He was no longer so thorough at work, and would often cut corners with engine repairs so that he could leave work early for a specially planned encounter with a sex worker. He spent a lot of money on choosing more high-class women, and also buying more outfits for them to wear. And, of course, the cost was doubled if he hired two at once.

Rachel, on the other hand, was relieved that Gordon no longer pressed her for sex. She had found more recently that he wanted to keep penetrating her for hours on end. She would get very sore and sometimes she would bleed with his constant vigorous thrusting. The more painful the sex became, the more turned off she became. She wanted to get medical attention for the sores that she had developed, but Gordon would not allow her to be vaginally examined by her GP. These days, though, Gordon does not ask her to be sexual. When he comes into bed in the early hours of the morning, she pretends to be asleep and he leaves her alone instead of starting to have sex with her anyway. Sometimes he will start masturbating in bed and would ejaculate over her, but she would still pretend to be asleep. She was too tired to be bothered with the time and energy it required these days, and was more demoralized by his violent rages which left her bruised and cut for weeks on end. Thus, Rachel colluded with Gordon's sexual addiction. She knew him well enough to know he was getting it somewhere else, because Gordon could not be without sex, but she chose not to ask.

CHAPTER ELEVEN

Internet addiction and offending

Gordon and Rachel have been together three years, and she is now pregnant. The pregnancy was not planned, but Rachel conceived during a time when she was feeling down and stayed in bed a lot. She did not go to work, but Gordon would get take-away meals, which they would eat in bed, then he would smoke pot and have sex with her because he had run out of money to have more interesting sex with prostitutes. During one of these sessions, she must have forgotten to take her contraceptive pill.

"Stupid cow!" he thought. He did not want a child. He knows nothing about children and does not like them when he meets them. He has no knowledge of them, either. He had no brothers or sisters; his mother had become pregnant again when he was two, but it had died before it was born.

Gordon did try to suggest to Rachel that she get rid of her baby, but she freaked out in hysteria and cried for days, so he said she could keep it so long as it didn't get in his way. Rachel was so pleased; she rushed around cooking his favourite meals, hugging and kissing him (which he didn't like), and giving him lots of sex (which he did like). But now she has a big swollen belly, and he does not like that at all. He does not fancy her like that, and the times when Rachel has offered to have sex with him, he has made excuses about not wanting to hurt her, and has gone off into the spare room, which he calls his study. There he can have as much sex as he likes without any hassle, because there is his computer and his instant access to the Internet, which he has discovered never bores him and never makes demands on him.

Internet pornography

Although constituting less than 1% of Internet usage, since the Internet was introduced internationally in 1985, the incidence of websites offering images of sexualized children has increased exponentially (Jenkins, 2001). But why are so many individuals, who are not paedophiles, yet have hitherto been ordinary heterosexual or gay men in long-term and loving relationships, presenting to therapists after being discovered compulsively viewing abusive images of children on the Internet? This chapter proposes to take forward the processes of sexual addiction discussed in the last chapter, going beyond the established theories regarding addiction, to offer some hypotheses synthesizing the neurological development of the brain and the processes of compulsive Internet viewing. In presenting neuroscience literature, I offer some suggestions that may predispose men to become addicted to Internet pornography, along with suggestions of precipitating factors to the Internet addiction process. I then move on to discuss the contentious issue of abusive images of children on the Internet, and whether all viewers of this material are actually paedophiles.

Contemporary website browsers can view any form of sexual repertoire, paraphilia, unusual or deviant sexual practice on the Internet in graphic detail, either as pictures, stories, live sex shows, or animated movies, online from the world-wide web, in the comparative privacy of their own home. Cooper described the process of exponential interest as turbocharged from a Triple-A engine: it is affordable in that most people now own a personal computer (PC); it is accessible, in that this information can be accessed from one's own home (or even on a 3G mobile phone); and in theory it is anonymous; no one knows what websites an individual may visit. However, every time a person logs on to the Internet, cookies are embedded on the computer from marketing companies, which view the search engine usage of that individual and use information in order to target appropriate advertising or spam (Cooper, 1997; Cooper, Putnam, Planchon, & Boies, 1999; Young, Cooper, Griffin-Shelley, O'Mara, & Buchanan, 2000).

In a classic survey conducted by Cooper and colleagues of a self-selecting sample of 10,000 men and women, they found that 15–20% of Internet users engaged in some form of sexual activity via their computer. Thirty-two per cent acknowledged that their activity jeopardized at least one important area of their life; 20% of men and 12% of women admitted using their work computer for some form of sexual activity (Cooper, 2002) with 70% of Internet pornography traffic occurring between the hours of 9.00 a.m. and 5.00 p.m. Eight per cent showed signs of sexual compulsivity (Cooper, Boies, Maheu, & Greenfield, 1999). Since this survey was conducted, the use of the Internet has massively increased, and a survey these researchers conducted in Sweden showed an increasing trend of women (55% male and 45% female respondents) whose major sexual activities were either seeking partners or accessing erotica (Cooper, Månsson, Daneback, Tikkanen, & Ross, 2003).

One activity that is very popular on the Internet is the viewing of pornography. Men have always been very visual with their sexual arousal; pornography has been drawn on cave walls. However, the Internet provides access to sexually explicit material in way that has never been available before. But the overuse of Internet pornography can lead to relationship regression; the more time a person spends on the Internet, the less time for real intimacy and real relationships. It can also lead to other inappropriate behaviours, such as stealing or embezzling money to pay for the costs of website memberships. It may be a catalyst, and precipitate real off-line sexual behaviour as desensitization and tolerance occurs, and the computer and Internet *per se* may become a fetish and create arousal at the tap of a keyboard or the click of a mouse. But why do some people develop such intense relationship with their PC whereas others can take it or leave it alone?

The development of the infant brain

Let us review where the preceding chapters in this book have been leading us. You will recall from Chapters Two and Three that brain maturation starts in the last trimester of pregnancy, although most of the development of an infant's brain occurs post natally. Within minutes of birth, the infant is preprogrammed to use his SEEKING circuit to search for his mother's face, communicating with her via the visual neural pathways using the retinae (Hess, 1975). Thus, one could argue that the SEEKING circuit is the primary driver to the other emotional circuits, both in providing vigilance against danger and the need to focus and attach to mother, both of which are essential to the survival of the infant. The SEEKING circuit uses the amygdala as its means of searching, always scanning out into the world like a human periscope, never inward-looking. SEEKING orientates the baby to search for faces, to process the non-verbal emotions, and to learn and search for new experiences (George et al., 1999). To motivate and provide curiosity, SEEKING elicits endogenous opioids via the dopamine pathways for excitement and reward, and oxytocin during attachment, the pathways of which cross at the ventral striatum of the brain. These feelings of search and excitement and the desire to explore have, no doubt, been responsible for moving our species forward from living in caves to accessing our modern technological systems.

Predisposing factors: Phase 1—insecure attachments

In Chapter Three, we discussed the development of an infant's attachment style, which develops at a critical period between the twelfth and twenty-fourth month of life, called the practising period (Schore, 1994). The child, who hitherto had been egocentric and narcissistic with a sense of omnipotence, develops a sense of separateness from his mother, learning autonomy, empathy, shame, and a sense of self. If mother provides secure, loving, and predictable parenting, again mediated by visual, tonal, and somatic communication, the child develops a secure attachment style. This is a neural template that formulates the working model of how the child, on becoming an adult, will respond in his adult attachments within loving relationships, friendships, and collegiate relationships.

Those infants who did not have access to their biological mothers, or for those whose mothers were depressed, emotionally disturbed, victims of domestic violence, or whose working life made their parenting unpredictable, were more likely to develop an insecure attachment style. For these children, the first spontaneous emotion learned outside of the mother is a fear of rejection or abandonment, which I have called a LOSS circuit. They will constantly search, unsuccessfully, for a safe and secure base. Their sense of fear is so great that they struggle to tolerate the extreme emotions triggered by the amygdala. These extremes of FEAR, RAGE, and PANIC will be readily expressed (Cassidy, 1994), producing the counter-response of frustrated and irritated parenting. Such children will be labelled as difficult or demanding, even though essentially they are infants trying to get their needs met.

Predisposing factors: Phase 2—the sexual template

Recall that the right hemisphere stays dominant in development from birth through to three years old (Chiron et al., 1997). When the child obtains about seventy words or so (Schore, 2003c), the development of the left hemisphere comes online for the learning of language and school skills. Then, at age 5–9, depending on the developmental capacity of the child, the right hemisphere has another growth spurt. This is the time a child develops his lovemap (Money, 1986). It is at this stage that the right brain starts developing the neural pathways in preparation for puberty and sexual play and adolescent sexual experimentation; the LUST circuit or sexual template comes online. For a securely attached child, the LUST circuit becomes incorporated into the secure attachment template (Figure 20), making sex a part of SEEKING CARE and PLAY in terms of the development of later adult loving relationships.

For an insecurely attached child, however, the LUST circuit is incorporated into an insecure circuit, so sex becomes part of PANIC of LOSS, and an appeaser of FEAR and RAGE. Any awareness of sexual diversity may start emerging into conscious awareness this early. As Money proposed, vandalization by sexual molestation or abuse at this stage can also have critical consequences. However, it appears that the vandalization of the sexual template is not just from sexual abuse. When the right hemisphere is online, and the amygdala pathway triggering extreme and unregulated emotion is open, any severe aversive situation corrupts the construction of an appropriate sexual template. In addition, it is known that childhood

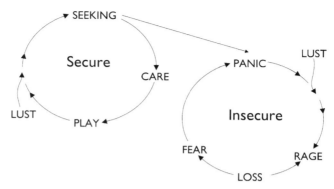

Figure 20. At prepubescent right-brain development (around six or seven for girls, eight or nine for boys) the LUST circuit, or sexual template, is activated and attaches to either the secure or insecure attachment template.

trauma affects the formation of the HPA axis, predisposing the child to addiction disorders (DeBellis, 2002). A securely attached child would respond to aversive experiences differently; he would have a clearer understanding of the nature of his emotions and know how to get them soothed, and it would not affect his later sexual repertoire. An insecurely attached child, however, will act up and act out, at the mercy of unregulated emotions, and incorporate the aversive experience into his own sexual template. So, any event that elicits extreme emotions of fear, rage, panic, anxiety, etc., within a child who has not pre-learnt the coping strategy for regulating or controlling them, is vulnerable to the corruption of their sexual template. They do not know how to soothe themselves or where to turn to for soothing, as their early parenting has not equipped them with this knowledge. They feel that their parents would respond in a negative or unpredictable way to the requests for comfort. Thus, they turn to their only known method of self-soothing: oral and/or genital soothing, which turns into sexual soothing while they suppress, repress, and turn their negativity on to themselves. It is very common for sex addicts to report that pornography had become an important feature of their life from eight or nine years old. For example, Delmonico (2004) highlighted that 90% of 8–16-year-olds have viewed pornography online while doing their homework. For some, this is a habit that never stops, even into their adulthood.

Predisposing factors: Phase 3—adolescence

Adolescence is the time when the child makes preparation for adulthood through behavioural practice and experimentation. It is also the time when the brain starts to reorganize itself (Spear, 2000), as discussed in Chapter Four. Securely attached adolescents become proactive in planning their futures, responding appropriately to the excitement and challenges of their future autonomy as an adult. They respond to aversive events in an appropriate way, turning to established support systems for help and protection.

For the insecurely attached adolescent, excessive neural pruning when brains have not sufficiently developed adaptive coping strategies can lead to later amygdala-driven fear states without having the cortical inhibition. This can feel emotionally over-whelming and disorganizing (Schore, 2003b) and can lead to dys-regulated aggression. These adolescents become passive responders to their internal fear states, and their behaviour promotes what they most fear: parental rejection and abandonment. Even low-level stressful events can elicit huge fear responses (Corodimas, LeDoux, Gold, & Schulkin, 1994) based on the individual's early history, stored in the right brain as snapshot memories. To cope with emo-tional dysregulation, the drive of the SEEKING system compels contemporary adolescents, who are already extremely IT literate, to search the Internet. Computer games become a ready escape, and sites like Battle.net for WarCraft or Sandbox.com become their first addiction. Hours on end spent compulsively playing games via the Net means that their spontaneous sexual arousal will occur while they are online, so pornography to feed the arousal of the moment is only a click away. And so is the addiction.

Sex becomes a means of comfort and a search for attachment (Smallbone, 2005) and can lead to inappropriate sexual behaviour. As mentioned, so many youngsters under the age of seventeen have visited a porn website, with the average age of initial Internet exposure being eleven years old. Abel and Osborn (1992) found that a large proportion of the paraphiliacs they investigated reported that their behaviour had commenced during adolescence.

Any further emotional trauma at this adolescent stage may facil-itate psychopathology. For example, witnessing parental violence has a detrimental effect on an adolescent (Mahoney, Donnelly,

Boxer, & Lewis, 2003) and increases the risk that he might perpetu-ate partner abuse in adulthood. Similarly, sexual abuse in adoles-cence may precipitate later inappropriate sexual behaviour and paraphilias in adulthood. Smallbone (2006) highlighted that sexual offending peaks during adolescence, and there is a second, more prominent, peak in the mid to late thirties, suggesting that these may be two distinct populations and that offending in adolescence may not necessarily lead to adult offending. Miner and Munns (2005) also suggested that what separates juvenile delinquents from juvenile sexual offenders is their perception of their social isolation and their inability to experience satisfaction in social relationships.

Awad, Saunders, and Levene (1984) found that the parents of adolescent sexual offenders were often abusive, rejecting, and emo-tionally detached from their offspring. Moultrie (2006) made a comparison of adolescent Internet offenders compared to other adolescent sex offenders. She pointed out that the literature is rife with both populations having experienced family violence, abuse, and family dysfunction, and that they present with a constellation of psychological and behavioural problems. She found that in the majority of her (small) Internet group, however, there was less abuse or family trauma, higher IQ, and that the majority believed that they did not "fit in" with their peers and regarded their rela-tionships as superficial.

As discussed in Chapter Four, Schore (1994) suggested that inse-curely attached individuals develop addictions in an attempt to regulate the extreme emotions triggered by the amygdala, because they do not have the internal capacity to self-soothe. Indeed, the PANIC circuit induces endogenous opiate and oxytocin with-drawal, causing physical pain and making it more likely that the individual will SEEK external and often addictive processes to replace the missing opiates. This process over-regulates the SEEK-ING system, and makes the person more driven in the desire to SEEK, overloading it into a primary focus of NEED rather than desire. As the brain matures into its adult capacity, the neural path-way interconnections become more complex and layered, mirroring the bottom-up developmental process. As can be seen in Figure 21, the primacy of the SEEKING circuit, driven by a need to replace missing opiates, and fed by curiosity, interest, stimulation, and excitement, focus the search into a narrow tunnel of NEED into

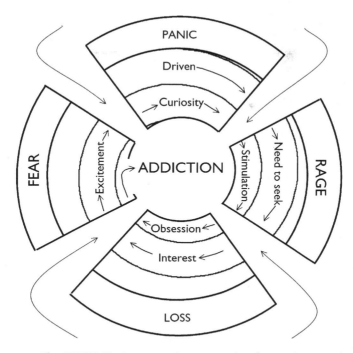

Figure 21.   The SEEKING circuit produces peptides that make an individual feel aroused and curious. For Internet addicts, the SEEKING and the LUST circuits merge until the SEEKING system predominates into a NEED to look at sex. Thus, individuals spiral from natural interest and curiosity into obsession and addiction.

obsession and addiction. (My son, Darren Hudson, whose expertise in multidimensional computer modelling enabled him to visualize the process of neural connections, proposed this concept.)

Internet sexual addiction

It has been argued that the Internet cannot be an addiction, because there is no evidence of a physiological dependence (Davis, 2001). However, this is far from the truth, as physiological dependence is endogenous, as this chapter will endeavour to describe.

Internet sexual addiction is a manifestation of sexual addiction discussed in the last chapter, which Galbreath, Berlin, and Sawyer

(2002) describe as a paraphilic disorder of voyeurism. Whereas most men can ordinarily view pornography on the Internet within limits and boundaries, there are some who are "at-risk users" (Cooper, Putnam, Planchon, & Boies, 1999), who have insufficient control over the level of Internet pornography they use which continues in the face of negative consequences.

In the previous chapter, I discussed the addictive cycle of Carnes. Applying this to Internet sexual addiction, the individual becomes preoccupied in thinking about sex. This obsessive rumination leads to plans of ritualized behaviour, for example, spending hours scanning the Internet for the "right" arousing image. This may lead to sexual behaviour, either with oneself or another in cyberspace. However, instead of feeling warm and comfortable with sexual satiation, the person feels bad about themselves, and feels shame and guilt. These negative feelings make the person want comfort, so leads back to rumination about sex, and starts the person going back around the cycle again, and back to their computer.

Thus, Internet sexual addiction, as mentioned, is a dysfunctional relationship with sex. These men and women choose to spend time online viewing pornography, or talking in chat rooms, rather than doing other things, like working, or having a sexual relationship with their partner. At first it starts as a fascination, which Careaga (2002) called the "newbie syndrome" (Careaga, 2002). Like a child with a new toy, the individual spends vast amounts of time and energy exploring the new world. But the enthusiasm wanes and obsession takes over. There becomes consistent preoccupation with, preparation for, and ritualization about, a sexual repertoire, but sometimes little sexual behaviour *per se*. This is because masturbation and orgasm tends to end the process of Internet viewing, whereas the addictive quality of the Internet is the stimulation it provides as it animates the dopamine pathways in the brain. Particularly for men viewing pornography, they are curious and stimulated by the knowledge that there is always another picture that one has not seen before. This preoccupation of sexual behaviour mirrors addiction to alcohol, drugs, or nicotine. It involves using sexual behaviour as a form of comfort from painful internal processes in order to change how one feels (Galbreath, Berlin, & Sawyer, 2002). The paradox, however, is that Internet addiction produces a small

but statistically significant increase in mi&
(Careaga, 2002).

Individuals tend to be in a trance-like st&
computer or television screen, which accounts for
iour perpetuates in the face of, and in denial of, r
quences. Like the use of addictive substances, tok
pornographic images develops, so it requires an inc   &ne
stimulus in order to achieve the same arousing effect; tł &s, escalation is a facet of this problem. In addition, the person is often split-
off from other aspects of their life, developing a fantasy life and a
real life, with the former eventually engulfing the latter. As a consequence, in his relationships he may start manifesting increased
aggression, distorted beliefs and perceptions about appropriate
sexual activity with his partner, or increased isolation as he buries
himself away with his computer (Maltz & Maltz, 2006). This is an
implicit, or sub-conscious, process, so that the individual will not
be overtly cognizant of the two sides of himself or of the damage
he is doing to his own life, or to others.

The theoretical addictive cycle of Carnes (2001), described
above, provides a very sound description of the maintaining process of online sexual addiction. But what creates Cooper's concept
of the "at-risk user" (Cooper, Putnam, Planchon, & Boies, 1999)?
Why do some men become addicted to the Internet and not others?

Back to the brain

The Internet, and, to a lesser extent, the television, opens up the
visual pathways through the thalamus, with direct access to the
amygdala when viewing pornography. Individuals tend to be in a
trance-like state, with eyes locked on to the screen of a computer or
television, fed by the driven need of the SEEKING system. In
Chapter Three, we discussed the two routes to the amygdala: the
"quick and dirty" route triggered by the sensory thalamus, and the
"slow and accurate" route via the thinking cortex (see Figure 7,
p. 34). These two routes work antagonistically with one another. So,
for the thalamus route to operate, the thinking system closes down,
and vice versa (LeDoux, 2002). The Internet viewer, operating on
his primary driver, the SEEKING circuit, therefore feels aroused,
stimulated, and curious, while his thinking cortex is bypassed. The

se proximity to the computer screen (which mimics the visual proximity of a mother and infant), with the multiple, graphic three-dimensional images, triggers the SEEKING circuit and orientates the amygdala, mimicking the early developmental process of infant learning. These primitive neural pathways reprocess the images, each with an emotional tag. The bypass of the thinking cortices, using the quick and dirty route (LeDoux, 1996), offers an explanation as to why Internet addicts scan the pornographic images for hours, losing a sense of the consequences of their behaviour, spiralling down into obsession and addiction, as demonstrated in Figure 21 (p. 191). They are operating on a preverbal, automatic process hardwired into the neurological system. They are disassociated in a massive autoregulatory mode for long periods of time, closed and impermeable to interactive regulations (Schore, 2003b). No wonder these individuals can offer no explanation for why they do what they do; the right brain has few words, and the system was developed long before the cognitive processes came online.

As the cognitive system is switched off, it accounts for why this Internet behaviour perpetuates in the face of, and in denial of, negative consequences. As already mentioned, tolerance to the pornographic images subsequently develops, requiring an increase in the stimulus and inducing escalation. The Internet facilitates the addictive process. Pornography provides information in graphic detail. It visually demonstrates all forms of unusual sexual behaviours and offers support groups and social networks for those with the same interests. The flash of images on the Internet mimics the preverbal memory process of flashbulb images stored in the right hemisphere through the orientation of the amygdala from the SEEKING circuit, creating arousal, stimulation, and curiosity. Panskepp described the feeling from this circuit as "a psychic energization . . . akin to that invigorated feeling of anticipation we experience when we actively seek thrills and other rewards" (Panskepp, 1998, p. 145).

This interacts with the visual pathways of male sexual arousal systems. Hiller (2004) proposed that the strong sexual urges at puberty, which interact with the heightened male sensitivity to visual stimuli, may be due to the increased vasopressin manufacture in the preoptic area of the hypothalamus, stimulated by elevated levels of testosterone. Through this process, Solms and Turnbull (2002) proposed that the LUST system is supposed to switch the SEEKING system off when the inner need has been met. With Internet addiction, however, the LUST circuit and SEEKING circuits intertwine, feeding each other. Listen to a client discussing his viewing of online videos of male to female transsexuals before surgery:

Therapist:	So, did these pictures sexually arouse you? Did they turn you on?
Client:	Well, I had a hard on. But I didn't want to masturbate, in case I ejaculated. Cumming would mean stopping. I wanted to stay stimulated.
Therapist:	What was it in the pictures that stimulated you? Did you want to be like them?
Client:	Hell, no. I was just fascinated with the bizarreness of them. It seemed the best of both worlds to have big breasts and a penis.

It has been established that when viewing erotic movies, the cingulate cortex and the insular cortex of the brain of the viewer are highly activated (Damasio, 2003). The arousal that the viewer feels is being heightened via the dopamine pathways in the orbitofrontal cortices. Interestingly, a gender difference has been found with brain activity when viewing erotic films: with men, the hypothalamus is significantly engaged, but not so for women (Karama et al., 2002). Considering how important visual feedback is for the role of male sexual arousal, it could be hypothesized that men use the episodic memory potential in the hypothalamus to recall the visual information for later sexual fantasizing. As women are less interested in visual feedback in sexual arousal, and have more cognitive arousability linked with relationships, the use of the hypothalamus would be less necessary.

Female internet addiction

So far, the discussion regarding the use of the Internet has been predominantly regarding men viewing pornography. However, we know from Cooper's studies that a large proportion of women get addicted to using the Internet too (Cooper, 2002). In the early

Cooper studies, a gender interaction was found as men confided that they accessed erotica and porn, whereas women accessed chat rooms to build sexual relationships (Cooper, 1997, 1998). Schneider (2000b) reported that 80% of female Internet addicts would seek real off-line encounters with their online sexual partners. This mirrors the different arousal systems of men and women: where men tend to be very visual with their sexual arousal, women tend to be cognitive and interested in relationships, although Schneider did find some women who were very visually orientated consumers of pornography and identified with the more traditional male stereotypes. However, women's Internet addiction tends to focus on chat rooms and relationships (e.g., Facebook, MySpace, Twitter, Second Life, Friends Reunited, Match.com), falling in love with, and sometimes being sexual with, men they have never met. As Careaga (2002) pointed out, the Internet is a social community where people gather to meet, talk, argue, spend time, construct avitar pseudo-personas, develop relationships that are pseudo-intimate (Ferree, 2003), and to have sex and make virtual love. People can do anything in cyberspace that they can do in reality, without their physical bodies. Men and women can also become very addicted to cybershopping and websites such as eBay, which offers retail therapy and a form of gambling from the front room. Another maladaptive way of self-soothing.

Avoidant attachment style

Often men addicted to Internet pornography will manifest an avoidant attachment style developed from a fear of getting too close and thus being hurt, or from being overwhelmed or engulfed from over-intrusive parenting. The Internet means that a man can develop a sexual repertoire without the threat of intimacy, and without fear of rejection. The Internet will never abandon; it will always provide more. Cooper, quoted in Careaga (2002), expressed his view that the Internet is an avoidance activity, and if the Internet did not exist, other avoidance activities would be found. This is due to the behavioural style of the individual who avoids rather than faces, hides instead of confronts, inwardly covertly seethes, instead of actively exploding from their RAGE circuits.

Precipitating factors: stress burnout and post traumatic
stress disorder (PTSD)

An individual who has an insecure attachment, or has pre-existing emotional trauma, has inefficient emotional regulatory systems and is predisposed to maladaptive methods of coping with situations of stress (Kernberg, 1975; Rich, 2006). They will also have a predisposition to adult post trauma disorders (Schore, 2003a), and some consider insecure attachments as the cornerstone of PTSD (Allen, Coyne, & Huntoon, 1998). Parenthetically, researchers have discovered that when a person experiences the flashbacks symptomatic of PTSD, there is intense activation of the right visual cortex of the brain, and deactivation of the left verbal area (Siegel, 2003), again, images without words. Listen to a client talk about looking at images of abused children on the Internet:

Therapist: You described these painful flashbacks of hurt, damaged, and disabled children you saw in orphanages in Kosovo, yet you constantly observed hurt and damaged children on the Internet.

Client: I know, I know! (blusteringly bursting into tears, that he had been trying to suppress). I don't know why, but they were entirely separate in my mind. I hadn't connected the abuse side. They were just these poor little faces and I just kept looking and looking. I was fascinated, yet I was appalled at the same time. What was I thinking? What was I thinking! (sobs more).

As the neural pathways to the amygdala are hypersensitive, the extremes of emotion cannot be easily moderated. These emotional hyperactivating states can occur without the person having any overt knowledge of what has triggered them. Under conditions of extreme or chronic stress, the right brain goes into overload and shuts down. Using a computer analogy, it turns in on itself to operate a system analysis for repair. The result may be one of two responses: either the left brain takes over completely, and the individual throws himself into excessive working, or a defensive dissociative response is elicited. The former may account for why so many of the presenting clients are of professional status. When the left hemisphere is dominant and the right is inactive, the individual displays a flat, emotionless façade, with no access to empathy and no inhibitions. A closed right brain allows no enjoyment in art or crafts, music, poetry, or literature; all are squeezed out with the left brain logic of "there is no time for these". Years of left brain dominance will take its toll and lead to brain dis-ease and burnout.

The alternative process of disassociation is a result of the corrosive effect due to the hyperactivity of the HPA axis of sympathetic arousal, producing the freeze response in long-term shutdown, and feelings of excessive anxiety, hopelessness, defeat, and depression (Weinstock, 1997). The dissociative state is an appropriate response in infancy (mimicking death when there are no other developed coping strategies), but not for adults. An adult demonstrating the same infantile responses may be in danger of reverting into an infantile state (Nijenhuis, Vanderlinden, & Spinhoven, 1998). Schore (2003b) calls this a psychic-deadening defence, which puts people into a massive autoregulatory mode for long periods of time, during which they are shut out from the external environment. This is clearly seen in an emotionally blunted man sitting in front of a computer screen for hours on end, oblivious to his family surroundings. His only connection to the world is via the graphic images from the Internet, giving him a secure base while at the same time avoiding intimate or emotional contexts.

Serran and Marshall (2006) have highlighted how sexual offenders either hyperactivate or deactivate their emotional systems under times of stress. However, they pointed out that it is not the stress or depression *per se* that causes the risk of offending, but the change in mood, and presumably the person's inability to regulate it. Greenfield (1999) agreed and elaborated that when a person gets addicted to using the Internet, his browsing is not the only aspect of his life of which he feels out of control. Thus, current stress, depression, or trauma can reactivate the latent insecure templates (Mikulincer & Shaver, 2003; Shorey & Snyder, 2006).

Precipitating factors: mood and sexuality

Research undertaken at the Kinsey Institute looked at the relationship between mood and sexuality (Bancroft, Janssen, Strong, & Vukadinovic, 2003; Bancroft et al., 2003). In a clinical sample, fifteen out of twenty cases showed an increase in sexual arousal as a consequence of stress or depression on a Mood and Sexuality Questionnaire. Bancroft and Vukadinovic (2004) also conducted studies with sex addicts, and found that up to 25% of men experienced an increase in arousal at times of stress, depression, or anxious mood, with 54% of sex addicts studied reporting using masturbation as a way of relieving their stress. Galbreath and colleagues agreed that stress and anxiety increased the intensity of pornographic Internet viewing (Galbreath, Berlin, & Sawyer, 2002). The Internet provides a perfect outlet for those who are experiencing difficult times, yet have not learnt the appropriate strategies for self-soothing. Young (1998) described in her study of Internet addicts how many suffered with psychological, physical, and social problems, and she assumed that their feelings of depression, isolation, and low self-esteem are a consequence of obsessive Internet use. However, Careaga (2002) rightly criticized her conclusions, as she seemed to have failed to consider that these negative emotions may be a cause as well as a cyclical consequence of Internet addiction.

Impact of internet addiction on partners

As (male) Internet addicts spend hours online, searching for progressively more hard-core pornographic images, it erodes into time with their partners and the family (Manning, 2006). Sex in the relationship flounders, either because it becomes porn-like, male-focused, extreme, and lacking in intimacy, or because the man completely loses interest in real-life sex as he cannot get aroused to the same degree with a real partner (Bridges, Bergner, & Hesson-McInnis, 2003). Schneider conducted a survey on the impact of Internet addiction on relationships and the family. She found that partners (both male and female) felt shame, hurt, betrayal, devastation, loneliness, isolation, humiliation, jealousy, anger, rejection, and abandonment; all of these emotions can be placed into an insecure template. In particular, one-third of the women in Schneider's survey found her partner watching pornography on the Internet highly distressing. Thirty-two per cent said it had adversely affected their sex life, 39% said it had negatively affected their relationship, 34% had reduced self-esteem, 41% felt less attractive and desirable, and 42% said it made them feel insecure. More than one quarter responded in a similar way as if he had been having an actual affair (Schneider, 2000a,b).

Schneider found that partners held that the incessant secrecy and lying was particularly distressing, and it was not uncommon for either of the partners to lose interest in sex (Schneider, 2003; Landau, Garrett, & Webb, 2008). Female partners felt particularly betrayed and inadequate through their male partners watching pornography on the Internet. They felt under pressure not to appear controlling or unreasonable, as their partners argued that men's consumption of pornography is natural, and to judge it as anything but positive was to risk being labelled by their partner as a prudish (Shaw, 1999) or a nag (Schneider & Weiss, 2001).

As discussed earlier, this conflict between partners tends to occur due to the differences in how men and women respond to sex. Men tend to be very visual in their sexual arousal. When they view pornography, they enjoy the visual entertainment of watching the women (models) really enjoying the sexual activity and being very involved with their male and female partners. As Lindgren (2010) argues, pornography for men is homosocial; men watch porn to be men, not necessarily alone, but in a social and cultural context where the most important concepts are male pleasure through "wanking" and a reduction of women into a category of their specific sexual parts, and that wives and girlfriends may be present in some sense, but inherently marginal. Men tend to minimize the effect of their pornographic activity by saying, "Pornography is just sex, what I do with my wife is make love". Women tend to struggle with such compartmentalization. They are not so visual in their sexual arousal, hence the reason that most pornography targets male fantasies, although parenthetically, there is now a significant trend in female-owned pornography web sites (Attwood, 2010b). Most women are more concerned with communication and the quality of their relationships, which sex enhances. Thus, when a heterosexual woman views pornography, she is less likely to view the activities taking place, and more likely to focus on the women models, and to make a comparison between the model and herself. Thus, she is likely to feel that she cannot compete with the beautiful, long-legged, big-breasted, high-heeled, hypersexual woman her husband likes to watch. As a consequence, it is likely to lower her self-esteem and make her feel sexually inadequate. Some women try to compete with the pornography models by having vulval waxing (Brazilian style), breast implants, and other forms of cosmetic surgery to make themselves more alluring to their partners. Others find themselves tolerating sexual activity, like brutal oral sex, anal sex, or ejaculation on their faces, which has moved into mainstream Internet pornography within the past twenty years (O'Toole, 1998). These activities may be something that the women had not wanted or liked, and had not previously been usual in their loving sexual repertoire until their husbands started viewing Internet pornography, but then the husbands insist that such activities are normal and the wives are prudish not to want to accept it.

Young and colleagues discussed the process of what they called "cyberaffairs", which they held occurs because of the anonymity, convenience, and the ability to escape (Young, Griffin-Shelley, Cooper, O'Mara, & Buchanan, 2000), so a romantic or sexual relationship is developed via a chatroom or a news group They proposed a list of "at risk" features that may prepare spouses or therapists for warning signs of this covert activity. These were:

- a change in sleep patterns as people work late in the night or get up very early in the morning to engage in cybertalk;
- a demand for privacy as the computer or laptop is taken into a private space and suddenly becomes passworded;
- usual household chores or activities with the children are ignored;
- credit-card and telephone bills are hidden and lies are told to cover up extensive use;
- personality changes as the person becomes more withdrawn and sullen, and may resort to defensive attacks when questioned;
- loss of interest in sex with the partner, as masturbation may be occurring on a frequent level;
- usual intimate relationship activities, like shared baths, talking over dinner, or renting a video, are shunned (Young, O'Mara, & Buchanan, 2001).

Of course, this kind of relationship withdrawal can also occur in the context of a partner who is addicted to using prostitutes, addicted to pornography on the Internet, or who is having a real-life affair.

Summary of proposals

I have proposed a model of neural development that incorporates a psychological process of attaching to others and learning social support systems, and a physiological process of developing appropriate neural networks of emotional regulation using the preprogrammed emotional circuits. This process is diverted or corrupted over time during the critical periods of right-brain development. Figure 22 illustrates the model of predisposing influences. Individuals with insecure attachments are predisposed to vulnerability at later stages of brain growth when the sex template is being developed, which later becomes more reinforced during the adolescent pruning of unused neural pathways, leading to more entrenched repertoires that may become addictive.

Internet images offer a place where this right-brain development of snapshot memories is mirrored and potentially re-enacted

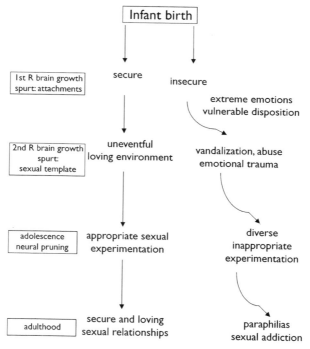

Figure 22. Predisposing factors contributing to the development of obsessive sexual practices.

at an implicit, preverbal level of processing. As men use their visual pathways in their sexual arousal, Internet pornography provides a graphic outlet. The addictive behaviour is maintained within the addictive cycle (Carnes, Delmonco, & Griffin, 2001) through the trance-like visual pathways in a paraphilic fugue (Money, 1986), with direct connection to the amygdala in the right hemisphere, using the SEEKING circuit. The sexual addict ritualistically searches for the "right" image on the Internet to seek comfort. Csikszentmihalyi argued that the time spent operating the SEEK-ING system was satisfying of itself, regardless of the external rewards achieved (Csikszentmihalyi, 1990). As he does so, the Internet viewer reconnects with images from his history. He feels alone, abandoned, and ashamed. This leads to a preoccupied rumination about the images, and a compelling desire to look again. Desensitization with familiar images provokes the desire to find more interesting and evocative stimuli, and, thus, escalation and even offending may occur.

Abusive images of children on the Internet

The Internet operates on market forces of supply and demand; if no one wanted to visit pornography sites, then few would be available. When Jenkins published his review of child Internet pornography, it was suggested that some pre-teen pornography websites got up to 7000 new postings each week, and that is likely to be an underestimate of the postings that occur nearly a decade later (Jenkins, 2001). So why is there so much interest in this material? Is society rife with covert paedophiles?

Some police operations have successfully targeted Internet offenders. Operation Starburst, directed by the UK police, started in 1995 and led to the identification of thirty-seven men internationally (Akdeniz, 1997). Operation Avalanche was a USA investigation into Internet abusive images of children that spanned three continents, identified some 250,000 website subscribers, and was providing a computer consultant, Thomas Reedy, with a turnover of 1.4 million dollars each month. He was jailed for 1,335 years in 2001, and his wife was jailed for fourteen years, although Reedy's sentence was later reduced to 181 years on appeal. The US Department of Justice identified 35,000 American users of these sites, and provided the UK police with a list of 7,250 UK suspects. Seventy to ninety-five per cent had no previous convictions and were not known to the law enforcement agencies (Carr, 2003). These people were not the stereotype of a computer "geek", but predominantly white middle- to upper-class professionals: paediatricians, teachers, judges, and lawyers, some of them quite elderly. Frei, Erenay, Dittman, and Graf (2005) conducted a study of the men investigated from this operation, and two-thirds gave their motivation as curiosity, fascination, or investigation. All of these are produced via the SEEKING circuit.

Operation Ore succeeded Operation Avalanche, and has precipitated many of the suspected individuals to seek therapeutic help, either because they are frantically searching for mitigation for court appearances, or because it has been a wake-up call and they really do want to change. But are all pornography viewers the same? Krone (2004) produced a typology of such men, which shows a progressive escalation in offending:

- *browser*: who comes across pictures accidentally and keeps them;
- *private fantasy*: purely played out in someone's head;
- *trawler*: the person trawling for any and all pictures, some of which are of children;
- *non-secure collector*: buys openly online from websites and chatrooms;
- *secure collector*: usually members of clubs with heavy security barriers;
- *online groomer*: initiating contact with a child;
- *physical abuser*: actively involved in the abuse of children;
- *producer*: provides images of the abuse for others;
- *distributor*: may not be interested in the material at all, but it is purely a commercial enterprise.

In another police operation, Operation Appal, a number of the suspects were children themselves, with one being only thirteen years old and having over 300 pictures of abuse of children and babies (Silverman & Wilson, 2002). O'Donnell and Milner (2007) argue that punishing this child and putting him on the Sex

Offender's Register for viewing the abuse of children of his own age does not seem an appropriate way of dealing with this issue.

The legal process for internet offenders in the UK

There are five classes of activities involving illegal Internet usage:

• downloading illegal child images;
• trading these images with others;
• producing illegal images of children;
• contacting children on the Internet for sexual reasons;
• off-line sexual activity with children.

Gallagher (2007) called for another category to be added to this list: those who incite or conspire with others to commit the sexual offence against the child, but may not actually contact the children directly. Although this offence is relatively rare, there is an awareness that it is on the increase as paedophiles gather together in cyberspace, brag about their exploits, and challenge and incite others to do the same. This offender–offender interaction online may lead to escalation in real time with real children.

When police seize the computer of a man suspected of viewing abusive images of children on the Internet, they use software, such as EnCase, which mirrors exactly the hard drive of the computer, preserving the original. This allows the IT forensic experts to trawl through the copy without the threat of allegations from defence barristers of tampering with the evidence. The computer intelligence officers (CIOs) have to count every image (which sometimes might be hundreds of thousands), and categorize each image according to its severity. This evidence is later presented to the Crown Prosecution Service (CPS) for a decision as to whether the person is to be charged with an offence. The CPS also prosecute men for making pseudo-images of children; that is, cutting and pasting pictures to create images, such as pasting a child's head on to an adult nude pose. These are not actual pictures of abuse, but are digitally synthesized to convey a similar scenario. However it is argued that such pictures may precipitate and perpetuate the actual physical abuse of children (Williams Committee Report, 1979).

It is also argued that downloading from the Internet and saving images of child sexual abuse on discs, memory-sticks, or hard drives creates new images for circulation. Thus, the courts have now opted to prosecute individuals with the more serious crime of "making" an indecent photograph (*R. v. Bowden* (2000) 1 Cr App R (S) 26), in an attempt to try to reduce the number of photographs in circulation, and also because "making" commands a higher sentence than "viewing" abusive images of children. This has been taken one step further to apply to a person simply viewing the images on the Internet without downloading, as he still gets prosecuted for "making" an image, because the image is automatically saved on to the computer cache to facilitate the speed of access should the person want to view it again (*R. v. Smith; Jayson* (2003) 1 Cr App R 1).

The UK Sentencing Advisory Panel (SAP), which gives advice to the UK Court of Appeal, created five categories of pictures of abusive images of children for law enforcement purposes (Sentencing Advisory Panel, 2002), which were an abbreviated version of the COPINE (Combating Paedophile Information Networks in Europe) scheme (Taylor, Quayle, & Holland, 2001). These categories were seen by SAP to be of increasing seriousness:

1. posing;
2. explicit sexual activity;
3. assault;
4. gross assault;
5. sadistic/bestiality.

Images in levels two to five in this taxonomy can be linked to specific offences involving children. Some images in category 1 may also be linked to criminal acts of indecency involving a child. The sentencing advice is that if the images found on a computer are essentially in categories 1 or 2, then the sentence is likely to be community service and/or fines, with registration on the Sex Offender's Register, and a requirement to attend a Sex Offender's Treatment Programme. As the categories become higher, however, the sentence is likely to be custodial. Bizarrely, although the age of the child being viewed is supposed to be relevant to the sentencing advice, in reality it often is not considered. So, a man who compulsively views pictures of babies or toddlers being abused would receive the same sentence as a man viewing pictures of sixteen-year-old girls or boys. Even more bizarrely, if a seventeen-year-old takes a photograph of his seventeen-year-old girlfriend on his mobile phone, and then sends it to her phone with her consent, he can be prosecuted for distributing abusive images of children, punishable by up to ten years in prison (Gillespie, 2005). In addition, their notion of increasing seriousness in these categories may be more controversial than the taxonomy suggests. Some off-line child sexual abusers may only use erotica or posing images in category 1 to facilitate their offending, rather than using images from the other categories (Krone, 2005). For example, a person with a paedophilic orientation may videotape television advertisements of children, which, although not unseemly or even pornographic, may be played repeatedly for masturbatory purposes. Howitt (1995) found that before the Internet made access to abusive images of children relatively easy, many paedophiles rarely used child pornography, many finding them positively distasteful.

There tend to be four predominant reasons that precipitate Internet offenders into therapy: they have been caught via the law enforcement process as described above (or feel they will be); they have been caught by their relationship partner and threatened with the loss of their marriage or partnership; they have been caught by their employer and have been threatened with the termination of their employment; or they have reached their own inhibitory level (discussed in the previous chapter) in their escalation of viewing material, which has precipitated a psychological breakdown, and, in a few cases, a psychotic incident.

Viewing abusive images of children is a child protection issue. These images of children consist of crime scene photographs of child sexual abuse and exploitation (Akdeniz, 1997). On becoming adults, these children may later recognize themselves online or be recognized by others. In addition to having to deal with their own personal abuse history, many of these victims later have to live with the knowledge that the recording of their personal trauma is augmented by the presence of a camera, and is still providing sexual gratification to a myriad of unknown voyeurs. Although it is argued that men who view these images have not participated in the sexual abuse of a child, they have certainly colluded with it. In addition, some people with a previous history of contact offences against children or easy access to children may be predisposed to acting out following stimulation from their viewing material. As far as Quayle and colleagues are concerned, there is no difference between someone who views child abuse images and someone who touches a child. They argue that one is a catalyst for the other, so they all should be treated as child molesters (Quayle, Erooga, Wright, Taylor, & Harbinson, 2006).

As sex addicts become desensitized to the images they view, tolerance develops, and there is a risk that this may lead to acting out. Men who are addicted to pornography on the Internet are the sex addicts, as discussed in the previous chapter, and it is via the Internet that their addiction is manifest. To reiterate, this is a dysfunctional relationship with sexual activity, rather than the usually implied definition of individuals who want a lot of sex. Often, men who are addicted to Internet pornography do not experience a lot of sex. They may spend a lot of time thinking about it, preparing for it, and ritualizing the process as they spend hours scanning for the "right" image. They are addicted to the arousal and stimulation that their viewing provides. Their visual life is so much more intense and exciting in comparison with their usual sex with their partner that they may start avoiding their partner and the opportunity to have real sex, in preference for many hours on the Internet seeing what else they can find, culminating in the viewing of even more deviant material (Barron & Kimmel, 2000). Thus, their fantasy life starts to engulf their real life. However, it is the nature of human beings that boredom and desensitization sets in, deviant sexual pornography becomes normalized (Krone, 2005) and the need to escalate from acceptable to unacceptable websites takes place.

Therapist: So, were you sexually aroused by these pictures of children? Did they turn you on?

Client: (expression of horror) God no! I wouldn't want to have sex with a child! But I couldn't stop myself looking. I was stimulated by them, but I was not aroused.

Therapist: What was it that you looked at in these pictures? What was the focus of your attention?

Client: Happy smiling faces. Happy smiling children's faces
              ... Oh, yes! I know what you are thinking. These chil-
              dren are being abused, how can they be happy? But
              there were many. You just had to search for them ...

Therapist: And when you saw a happy face, how did that make
              you feel?

Client: Not sexual. I was not sexually aroused. I was stimu-
              lated, curious, alive. It reminded me of the few times I
              was happy as a child.

When explaining their pornographic viewing history in therapy, men often talk of looking at faces as well as genital areas. Of course, these men were not *only* looking at faces, but their comments provide an indication of the facial orientation of the amygdala and how it contributes to the addictive process. Quayle and colleagues also noticed this when working with Internet offenders. They argued that men saying they were looking for happy children's faces were demonstrating a cognitive distortion, minimizing the impact of their offence (Quayle, Erooga, Wright, Taylor, & Harbinson, 2006). But looking at faces *is* a prime focus of the amygdala, and people will do it in all image viewing. Goffman (1976, p. 48) held that smiling served as a ritualistic mollifier "signalling that nothing antagonistic is intended or invited, that the meaning of the other's act has been understood and found acceptable, that, indeed, the other is approved and appreciated". Lanning (2005) points out that it is an uncomfortable truth for our society to know that children in pornography can be seen laughing or giggling through an abusive act. It is easier for us to categorize all offenders as completely "bad" and all victims as completely "good", with the victim playing no part in the maintenance of the offence, whereas that may not be the reality of the situation.

But why do Internet addicts not just stay with ordinary pictures? Why are they pornographic, and why do some men move on to viewing sexualized images of children? Recall that we talked about the trance-like state and the cognitions being switched off in the process as the SEEKING circuit is engaged. Siegel describes this process of using the "quick and dirty route" (LeDoux, 1996) of visual processing as "the lower mode", where behaviours become reflexive. He continues, "the mind becomes filled with deeply engrained, inflexible patterns of response. In such a condition, emotions may flood the mind and make rational thought and mindful behaviour quite impaired" (Siegel, 2003, p. 51).

This trance-like state means that the Internet viewer loses cognizance of what is he is looking at, but also of what is happening around him. Thus, children in the family may inadvertently come across the images stored on the computer, or inadvertently see the sexual behaviour of the adult in front of the computer in addition to what is on the screen.

Does looking lead to doing?

There is a great debate as to whether people who view erotic pictures of children, or even those who have a paedophilic interest but have no previous contact offences, will go on to commit sexual offences against children. In a meta-analysis of the literature, Hanson and Bussière (1998) suggested that sexual arousal to children (as measured through the penile plethysmograph (PPG)) and anti-social lifestyle were the strong predictors of sexual offence recidivism. However, their findings were based upon contact offenders who had actually acted upon their sexual interest and who were subsequently tracked for risk of future offending. Similarly, Seto and colleagues have looked at sexual arousal interests as predictive of future sexual behaviours, but here again, we are dealing with persons who have already crossed inhibitory barriers (Seto & Eke, 2005; Seto, Cantor, & Blanchard, 2006).

Thus, the viewing or possession of abusive images of children may show deviant sexual interests or an Internet addiction, but, without prior behaviours that show that inhibitory barriers have been set aside, it is not predictive of future contact offending and that these people will pose a risk to real children, either within their family or outside of it (Middleton, Beech, & Mandeville-Norden, 2005; Sheldon & Howitt, 2007)

So, the predictions cannot apply to those who view images of children undetected, or even may fantasize about sexual activity with children, but may actively choose not to act them out. This group, who may never come to the attention of law-enforcement authorities, or even psychological researchers, may well manage their feelings by finding more appropriate outlets for being with children, or may chose ways of managing that interest to keep themselves and the children safe. For the true paedophile, however, there is a persistent sexual interest in prepubescent children as well as a situational interest (to be discussed in more detail in the next chapter). Interestingly, in a large study of adult male paedophiles, only 19% had molested a member of their own family (Abel & Harlow, 2001), which means that 81% did not.

Other factors in a risk assessment of whether a person may act on his impulses also enter into the equation, such as impulse control, social support, ability to regulate their emotions and distress tolerance. These are discussed further in Chapter Thirteen. But we do need to determine whether the men who have viewed abusive images of children on the Internet would be an actual risk to children. Seto and colleagues argue that they are. Interestingly, in their study, they removed nearly 23% of their forensic sample of 887 men because they had no phallometric response; that is, no penile engorgement on viewing the pornographic material (Seto, Cantor, & Blanchard, 2006). Maybe this suggests that a considerable proportion of men may be viewing this material for reasons other than sexual arousal, as I have proposed.

Society has become so paranoid about the presumed increase of the predatory paedophile that we have now reached a situation where any pictures of children are presumed to be child pornography, whether they are abusive images of children or not. These may include pictures of children playing in parks, on beaches, or at the swimming pool. Parents are no longer allowed to take pictures of their own child acting in school plays, in case one member of the audience is a paedophile. Stapleton (2010) notes the tautologous nature of how child pornography has come to be understood. All images of children now have the potential to be labelled child pornography if they are discovered in a collection of a person labelled (whether correctly or incorrectly) as a paedophile, and the possession of images of children will contribute to the pejorative labelling. He continues:

Referring to "child pornography" as "abusive images" serves to obscure the range of materials that meet the legal definition of "child pornography", and makes it unclear who is abused, and in what way, through their production and distribution. Is the act of recording images of children an inherently abusive process? Is it only when the producer does so for the purposes of sexual gratification that it become abusive? [Stapleton, 2010, p. 42]

Prosections of individuals for looking at pictures of children in swimwear or playing naked on a beach are currently taking place, and the assumption is made that anyone choosing to look at such imagery is, *ipso facto*, a paedophile.

Yet, the viewing images of children, even when those images have been sexualized, does not mean that the viewer is a paedophile and, therefore, poses a risk to children (Jenkins, 2001; Sheldon & Howitt, 2007). The reasons why people view abusive images of children are complex, and they are not a homogenous group (Middleton, Beech, & Mandeville-Norden, 2005). Some do have a paedophile orientation and are at risk of contact offending, or may have already done so. But the larger proportions of Internet offenders are trawlers (Krone, 2004), collectors, or traders of pornography, or they may be viewing (re-enacting) their own abuse. As Tomak and colleagues pointed out, individuals arrested for Internet sexual offences appear to be different from imprisoned contact offenders; they are less deviant, less physically aggressive, and less impulsive. However, in psychometric assessments, Internet offenders showed no problems with intimacy or dealing with negative emotions, no distortions in sexual scripts, and no antisocial cognitions. The researchers, therefore, concluded that they were more similar to members of the general population than they had previously anticipated (Tomak, Weschler, Ghahramanlou-Holloway, Virden, & Nademin, 2009). They also agreed with Sheldon and Howitt (2007) that Internet offenders show an inverse relationship between their viewing and their behaviour: the more the individual indulges in sexual fantasy via the Net, the less likely he is to act them out.

The waters become even more muddied when one considers that most Internet offenders are not actually committing contact offences. They are voyeurs, on the outside looking in. Carr (2003), however, does not care. As far as he is concerned, a person viewing abusive images of children is a modern-day curse and is abusing by proxy. But Maddison argues that it is these attitudes that give child pornography so much power:

As a fetish it achieves power through its oxymoronic status: to see it, to know its existence is to be guilty; one can only remain free from its taint by being ignorant of its existence and vociferous in its denunciation. [Maddison, 2010, p. 32]

The issue becomes more complex in reference to the construction and viewing of pseudo-images, when no actual child is involved at all. A man may take an innocent photograph of a child, and make it indecent by adding images of genitalia; thus, the relationship is with a pseudo-photograph and not with a child. Taylor and Quayle (2003) point out that actually there is little congruence between pornographic content and behaviour, and suggest that what is more indicative of contact offending is whether the viewer identifies in some way with the material; that is, their perception of it.

Intellectually, one can argue that male Internet offenders show no victim empathy, and, by their behaviour, they collude and perpetuate the enormity of the sexual abuse of children. I agree. However, there is no evidence that their escalation will inevitably mean the actual abuse of a child (Marshall, 2000), either within their own family or outside of it. And even if there were evidence (e.g., through the use of penile plethysmography, which is discussed in Chapter Thirteen) that these men were aroused by the images of children, there is no evidence that they would actually act that out in reality. Indeed, some argue that the ability to view the pornography inhibits the impulse to commit contact offences (Carter, Prentky, Knight, Vanderveer, & Boucher, 1987). Cooper and colleagues discussed a study conducted by Hernandez, where twenty-nine men were in prison for Internet offences and eighteen of these later admitted to prior contact offences (Cooper, Golden, & Marshall, 2006). One does have to be cautious of studies of prisoners where admitting offences is part of a parole system. However, even if the proportion could be extrapolated from this small sample to the general population, there are still a considerable number of men who have been imprisoned for looking but not touching.

We also need to consider the size of the viewer's pornography collection. As O'Donnell and Milner argued when discussing the vast collections that some of these men have accumulated, it might take (if allowing one minute per picture) up to forty years of unbroken attention to view them all. Clearly, then, it is the collecting that is the compulsion (O'Donnell & Milner, 2007). As Quayle and colleagues have elaborated, how the individual deals with the collection in the way it is categorized and filed may provide the key to understanding the underlying motivation of the individual (Quayle, Erooga, Wright, Taylor, & Harbinson, 2006).

Looking at things that others do that we may never do ourselves is part of the human psyche, as Jones (2010) argues, situated between horror, amusement, desire, and morbid curiosity. Thus, people enjoying seeing the graphic images of murdered, decapitated, and tortured bodies in a movie entertainment. Motorists slow down on the opposite side of a motorway to where an accident has occurred, rubbernecking to catch a glimpse of injured drivers. Viewers watch endless television programmes showing forensic science post mortems, cosmetic surgery, and criminal activity. Internet pornography includes sites representing the body in excessive and gross ways, like "war-porn" or "atrocity-porn", designed equally to shock and to fascinate (Attwood, 2010a). This watching is tapping into the SEEKING circuit orientated by the amygdala and firing the dopamine pathways in a mixture of fascination and horror at viewing what other people might do. In no criminal activity do we make the leap of logic that says "seeing equals doing" other than with abusive images of children on the Internet. Without undermining the distress that this activity causes the majority of us, as therapists it is our professional responsibility to be more discerning with the people we work with, and not make assumptions without evidence.

In addition, our legal adversarial system distorts what is really happening with these men. I am not going to criticize the police, as they have a really difficult job to do, although it may be preferable for them to concentrate their limited resources and expertise on the distributors, rather than the viewers, of abusive images of children. The target-driven government has a considerable responsibility for encouraging this approach. As already mentioned, it is the role of the police to count all of the images of children being sexualized, and to provide this as evidence of offending. The courts will not be told of all the other images that the person has viewed in terms of bizarre or deviant sexual images (although recently a new offence of viewing "extreme pornography" has been placed on the UK statute book, which includes extreme violence and sex with animals). Other images, although offensive to many, are not illegal, and as such are irrelevant for the prosecution case, so are not discussed. However, the court then makes the assumption that the viewing of abusive images of children is all that the person had viewed and that this indicates that the man is a paedophile, and, therefore, a risk to children. Courts and probation services may, therefore, inappropriately label the men as paedophiles when they are actually demonstrating a voyeuristic paraphilia (Galbreath, Berlin, & Sawyer, 2002). No consideration is given to the fact that a man may be addicted to deviant pornography *per se*.

Then media forces come into play. The (tabloid) press report on the prosecution. The man is publicly labelled as a "paedo" and a "pervert". Journalists catastrophize from a man who has viewed Internet pornography to high profile cases of rape and murder of children. His relationship is placed under considerable pressure and may fail as a consequence of this public opinion, increasing his potential for recidivism. He loses his employment, as the employer cannot take the risk of employing the "lepers" of our society. The social services place his children on the "at risk register", or take them away completely. Wives are told to choose between staying with their husbands or losing their children. Many of my clients are told that they will never see their children again until they pass the age of eighteen, and no consideration is given to the damage that this removal is doing to the children *per se*, and the attachment injury this behaviour causes to his innocent children. He is hounded by his neighbours and dropped by his friends. Such alienation and isolation is more likely to produce recidivism than any other factors.

In summary

Not all sexual encounters on the Internet are negative. Some people have been able to develop sexually, buy sexual aids, and meet sexual partners via the computer. It is a positive outlet for the disenfranchised, such as the disabled, to explore their sexuality. Most people experience few problems with the use of their computer. However, there is an increasing prevalence of addiction to the Internet *per se*, for example, addiction to eBay, shopping, etc., and about 1% of Internet users spend more than forty hours per week in online sexual activities (Cooper, 1997).

The Internet has the ability to provide previously unseen visual information for the browser. He can learn of new experiences and a sexual repertoire previously unencountered in graphic detail. However, this creates such high levels of arousal that it invokes a conditioned physiological response and a psychological need for more. Those individuals who are already predisposed to addictions will find that exploring Internet pornography may lead them into sexual addiction. As Schneider and Weiss argued (2001), Internet pornography is the crack cocaine of porn.

Application in the therapy room

In the USA, the most common method of working with sexual and Internet addiction is the use of the twelve-step programme (Careaga, 2002; Carnes, 2001; Watters, 2001), which has been so successful in some areas when working with alcoholics. In the UK, the twelve-step programmes are less successful, partly due to our being a less Christian-based and more multi-cultural society, and partly, I feel, because we are more cynical about evangelical approaches such as giving oneself over to a higher power. In addition, as shame is so high in sexual addiction, perhaps more so than any other addiction because of the way society responds to those who sexually step out of line, group therapy is less effective.

In the UK, Quayle and colleagues have developed useful treatment protocols for working with Internet offenders, which are based on the cognitive–behavioural model of contemporary Sex Offenders Treatment Programmes (discussed further in the next chapter). However, despite their uncompromising stance, they acknowledge that the CBT approach is a necessary but not sufficient way of working with such individuals that has limited outcome success, so have introduced more compassionate components to their programme. They have introduced mindfulness ideas into their structure (discussed further in Chapter Fourteen), and have proposed that the client strive for positive goals of living a good life, and acceptance of the individual with a commitment to change, which may produce better outcomes than the current focus on the negatives of the individual and relapse prevention strategies (Quayle, Erooga, Wright, Taylor, & Harbinson, 2006). This is an

interesting move forward to a more collaborative and compassionate way of working with these individuals than hitherto has been
recommended. However, they still do not address, other than in
passing, the damaged history of the individual that may lead to the
acting out in the first place. And also, they make the assumption
that all offending is a cognitive decision and intention, thus requiring cognitive interventions related to offending pathways. Whereas
some men will purposefully search for images of sexualized children on the Internet, and that may lead to eventual contact offences,
that may not apply to all Internet offenders. As discussed in the last
chapter, some men get drawn into an escalation of their sexual
acting out when their SEEKIING system is attached to the
computer, and their cognitive system (long and accurate route—see
Figure 7, p. 34) is bypassed. Thus, when being challenged by a
cognitive therapist to account for their automatic thoughts leading
to the offending, the client may not be able to provide such information, as he was actually in a trance-like state. He may then be
accused of avoidance or minimization, which may later be used
against him to demonstrate his inability to face the responsibilities
of his own behaviour, and thus still be considered at high risk of
reoffending. It is vital that these clients feel safe and attached within
their therapy, rather than seeing it as an intellectual wrestling match
in which they have to think the thought and talk the talk approved
of by their therapist in order to "prove" they can walk the walk on
being released from their treatment. Otherwise, the therapy *per se*
will invoke ideas that the individual is incapable of change, and
invoke alienation, making recidivism most likely.

Delmonico and colleagues' therapeutic structure of first-order
and second-order changes provides a very useful protocol for
working with these Internet addicts, irrespective of the therapeutic
model involved (Delmonico, Griffin, & Carnes, 2002). First-order
changes are the crisis prevention method of dealing with the presenting issue, which works on the practicalities of preventing
offending and escalation. Breaking down denial, and reaching an
understanding that viewing sexualized images of children colludes
with their actual abuse, is essential here. Second-order changes are
the processes of more in-depth therapy, to work with the attachment insecurities, historical issues of abuse, and post trauma stress.
It is essential at this stage to work with childhood trauma, and

every subsequent developmental stage thereafter, as there is a ripple effect that happens through therapy in the same way as happens through life: each developmental stage must be resolved before moving on to the next. I also have a third component of introducing the partner into the work when the time is right, to help the couple rebuild their damaged relationship and sexual repertoire. Therapists do need to be mindful that the client who has an avoidant attachment style will act that out within the therapy: he will avoid, be late, sometimes not attend, and sometimes lie, both to others and to his therapist. Shame is very high in this client presentation.

If the predisposition to Internet addiction is hardwired into the brain, can it be changed? Most definitely, although it does need the individual to have a conscious awareness of his addiction and a strong motivation to change. I use the analogy of a road map with my clients, to provide knowledge and hope. Imagine that the blue motorway routes are neural pathways representing our automatic, addictive behaviours. We go down these paths automatically, as they are convenient, we are familiar with them, and they get us from point A to point B very rapidly. Change means consciously getting off the motorway at the next exit, and using the A roads and B roads to get to where a person wants to be. Yes, it will be a longer and a more diverse route, they will feel uncomfortable, as it is unfamiliar, and will be out of their comfort zone. Sometimes they will get lost. But if they persist with the different ways of being on these alternative routes, eventually the motorways will atrophy and die away. The "use it or lose it" process of neural firing and wiring. This mindfulness process is discussed further in Chapter Fourteen.

I realise that these proposals may arouse emotive contention. By suggesting hardwiring of the brain resulting in offending behaviour, I am implying an opportunity for the clients to diffuse some of the responsibility for their viewing of very emotive material. But, in therapy, I find that when the denial is broken down with many of these clients, they do accept personal responsibility, and are often appalled by their own behaviour, which may be described by others familiar to them as completely out of character. As therapists, we need to be compassionate and discerning in trying to develop a real understanding of the psychological and physical processes involved. Some of these men will be paedophiles, and may pose a very real risk to children, in a sexual orientation that cannot be changed. However, many men I have seen who have compulsively viewed Internet pornography, including sexualized images of children, do not necessarily have a paedophilic orientation. They have escalated their sexually addictive processes, and these are open to change. If therapists adopt a non-judgemental and respectful stance with these clients, they can learn secure attachments, appropriate victim empathy, and the ability to regulate their extreme emotions, especially shame and disgust. As Cooper and colleagues pointed out, these clients get enough anger, revulsion, and discomfort from others; it is, therefore, our role to be non-judgemental, experienced, and knowledgeable (Cooper, Golden, & Marshall, 2006), and I would also add compassionate. They may be sex offenders, but are still entitled to respect from their probation officers and from their therapists. Chapter Fourteen elaborates on this issue.

Therapeutic intervention needs to pay attention to the right hemisphere that is creating so much of this havoc. Rossi (2002) proposed that healing takes place via art, beauty, truth, and exercise; that the undertaking of these activities produces brain proteins, which, in turn, leads to neurogenesis. Neurogenesis promotes a large growth spurt of neural dendrites and supportive glial cells, to enhance new neural connections. These are right brain activities, and soothe the hyperactive HPA axis by invoking the parasympathetic nervous system. A fuller discussion of this takes place in Chapter Fourteen.

Gordon and Rachel's review

Rachel is pregnant. Gordon thinks it was an accident, but Rachel "accidentally" forgot to take her pill when she knew she would be at peak ovulation. She wanted a child because she felt so unloved. When she first met Gordon, he made her feel loved and wanted for the first time in her life. Now he is too absorbed with his car engines and his computer to give her much time. So she made up her mind that a baby was the answer. A baby will always love her and want to be with her. And if she and Gordon spilt up, she would still have the baby. Her mum had mental health problems, so could not be a good mum to Rachel, but she is going to be a good mum to her baby. She will give him or her all the things that she did not have as a child, and more besides. She is convinced that once Gordon is holding his own child, especially if it is a son, he will change his behaviour and become a good dad. Then they can be a proper family.

Gordon's narcissism is raging against a potential interloper—this baby. He knows the child will take Rachel's attention away from him, and he does not like the idea, even before it arrives. Gordon has already told Rachel, when he reluctantly agreed to let her keep the child, that she was not allowed to breast-feed, and that she will have to find a child-minder and go back to work because he could not afford to keep them both. Plus she keeps spending stupid amounts of money on equipment and clothes. He told her quite clearly that she had to get things from charity shops, but now she spends hours wandering from one shop to another looking for things for the baby, instead of things for him. Whenever Gordon starts to ruminate on the potential difficulties that are coming up with this "brat", he takes himself off to the computer and starts clicking on familiar and unfamiliar images. He has also "met" others on the computer, who swap pictures with him, and who commiserate with him about their future event. He feels more connected with these guys than he does with Rachel.

Both Gordon and Rachel's attachment systems have been activated at the prospect of a new addition to the family. Gordon's avoidant system is trying to push out the child so he can maintain control over the relationship between himself and Rachel, and keep her all to himself. Rachel's preoccupied system is filling the space she feels from Gordon's avoidance by introducing a new attachment that will never leave her: the child. Together, they repeat the attachment styles of Gordon's parents, Jenny and Joe.

CHAPTER TWELVE

Stalking and violence

Rachel absent-mindedly pulled open the net curtain of her first-floor bedroom and looked out on to the street below. She knew Gordon was down there, somewhere, although she could not see him. She looked back into the room that was now her living room and bedroom, still holding the net curtain in her hand. Two months earlier, she had given birth to a son, Conner, who was sleeping fitfully in a cot near her bed. She had had a diffi-cult birth, spanning thirty-six hours, and eventually required a Caesarean section as Conner had gone into foetal distress. He then spent the next week in the Special Care Baby Unit, as he had jaun-dice and they were worried about his heart. Conner proved to be a sickly child, rarely sleeping for more than three hours at a time, and was only quiet when Rachel held him close to her chest. But she is so tired, and Conner is more demanding than his father.

When Conner was less than a month old, Gordon had been out drinking heavily. He came home late in a foul temper. Conner sensed Rachel's fear and started to cry vehemently. Rachel could not pacify the child or his father. Gordon demanded that she put Conner in his cot and leave him alone. He wanted sex, even though the doctors had told her not to have sex yet. She had not taken any of her mood stabilizers throughout her pregnancy, which had completely destabilized her, and now she had post natal depression. Her hair was lank, her body unwashed, her face thin and wan with fatigue. Yet Gordon still wanted sex. Rachel had started to cry, and that triggered Gordon into a rage about how stupid, ugly, scarred, and pathetic she was. A blow, first with his fists and then with his feet, followed each criticism. Neighbours, hearing Rachel's' screams, Gordon's rants, and the baby screaming, called the police.

Rachel was hospitalized for a week with her baby, and then transferred by the social services to a safe house for battered women. She was informed by the duty social worker that if she returned to her relationship with Gordon, Conner would be placed into foster care, and he may subsequently be placed out for adoption. Rachel did not feel able to care for herself, but she desperately did not want to lose her son.

Gordon did not take the enforced separation from his woman and his child lightly. Despite being charged by the police with grievous bodily harm, he was determined to find where she was and force her to return to him. He stopped going to work and spent hours texting to her mobile phone, calling her friends, and visiting the places where she used to shop. Eventually, he discovered through subterfuge where the safe house was, phoned repetitively asking to speak to Rachel, and stayed outside the house for days on end. He knew she would have to come out sometime. And when she did, he would be waiting.

Rachel looked back out at the street below, and saw Gordon step out from a neighbour's garden gateway. He stared meaningfully at her window. She gave a gasp and stepped back from the window, letting the net curtain fall back into place. She felt trapped. She was trapped. There was no escape from Gordon. And also, she missed him.

What is stalking and what is its prevalence?

Stalking has been defined as "a constellation of behaviours in which one individual inflicts on another repeated unwanted intrusions and communications" (Pathé & Mullen, 1997, p. 12). These intrusions have been variously described as: following, loitering, maintaining surveillance, approaching, and communications via letter, telephone, texts, email, graffiti, or notes attached to the victim's car. The intrusions can also include unsolicited gifts, ordering (e.g., taxis, pizzas) or cancelling services (e.g., phone, electricity) on the victim's behalf (Mullen, Pathé, & Purcell, 2000b). In a computerized self-completion questionnaire attached to 1998 British Crime Survey, stalking, defined in this study as "persistent and unwanted attention", was found to have a prevalence rate of 11.8% in the UK population ((Budd, Mattinson, & Myhill, 2000); that is, 16.1% of women and 6.8% of men in the population experienced a situation of being stalked or harassed by another individual at some time in their lives. Eighty-one per cent of the incidents reported were perpetrated by men and accounted for 90% of the incidents against women and 57% of the incidents against men.

Meloy and Gothard (1995, p. 258) defined stalking as "an abnormal or long-term pattern of threat or harassment directed toward a specific individual". They elaborated that it has to be more than one act of unwanted pursuit and has to be perceived by the victim as harassing. One act of harassment would obviously not constitute a long-term pattern, but this definition does create the difficulty of where do you draw the line in how much behaviour one accepts, and what sort of behaviour constitutes harassment? Later in the paper, Meloy and Gothard further elaborate stalking as: "the wilful, malicious, and repeated following or harassing of another person that threatens his or her safety" (ibid.). This definition implies that the stalker's intention is to harass and to cause distress, yet in many cases of harassment, the stalker does not want to cause unhappiness, but is pursuing the victim in order to obtain, or regain, a loving relationship with the victim. It is the stalker's neediness and desire for a close attachment that creates persistent obsessive behaviour perceived by the receiver as harassing and fearful.

This is not to undermine the effect of the stalking on the victim, however. Victims of stalking often describe feelings of violation, a profound sense of loss of control over their lives and a pervasive mistrust of others (Mullen, Pathé, & Purcell, 2000a). In fact, Wilson, Emshar, and Welsh (2006) consider that the stalkers who deliberately leave signs of their presence or allow themselves to be seen stalking their victims are engaging in emotional sadism. "The sudden terror induced in the victims can provide sadistic gratification to the stalker and also maintain a paranoid bond, in which the victim's hypervigilance for further sightings serves as a perverse substitute for affection and attachment" (*ibid.*, p. 145). In Pathé and Mullen's study of 100 victims of stalkers, 24% had seriously considered or had attempted suicide, and 75% expressed overwhelming feelings of powerlessness. Eighty-three per cent reported increased levels of anxiety, 55% experienced flashbacks and intrusive recollections, with nightmares, appetite disturbances, and depressed mood being commonly reported (Pathé & Mullen, 1997). They use expressions like "emotional rape" and "psychological terrorism", the effects of which were felt long after the stalker had withdrawn.

Who are the people who stalk?

It is interesting to question why people do it. Kamphuis and Emmelkamp (2000) hypothesized that stalkers may form a very heterogeneous group with widely different motivations, and this view is consistent with those of Boon and Sheridan (2002). Mullen and colleagues used their considerable clinical experience of working therapeutically with stalkers to develop a pragmatic taxonomy of stalking (Mullen, Pathé, & Purcell, 2000a). They describe the following:

the rejected stalker—usually pursuing an ex-intimate either to obtain reconciliation or to exact revenge. Characterized by overdependence, poor social skills, and poor social network;

the resentful stalker—intending to cause fear and apprehension in their victim, their behaviour emerges in a desire for retribution. Two types: the vengeful and the resentful. The former is often the result of a short burst of anger and burns out fairly quickly, whereas the latter is persistent and calculating;

the predatory stalker—predominantly men who are preparing a sexual assault on the victim. Often surreptitious stalking occurs while in preparation for the planned attack;

intimacy seekers—in their desire for a relationship with their victim, they often feel that they are entitled to the relationship as a reward for their consistent loyalty;

incompetent suitors—they initiate persistent inept attempts to begin a relationship with the victim. These are different from intimacy seekers in that they need a relationship, whereas intimacy seekers are searching for love.

This appears to be a comprehensive typology trying to encapsulate the very different types of motivation that lead a person to obsess about another, although some of the differences are very subtle. For example, it may be very difficult to determine the difference between an intimacy seeker and an incompetent suitor. Both are searching for, or desiring, an intimate relationship with their victim, and they are both incompetent in how they go about it. Finding out the difference between whether they are searching for love or a relationship is likely to be a subtle distinction that only a therapist would be able to determine, and may, therefore, be an unnecessary distinction for a law enforcement agency. However, in reviewing the typology, each category can be viewed as a manifestation of feelings of rejection or abandonment; that is, insecure attachments.

Insecure attachments

To iterate what has been discussed in previous chapters, an infant's memories and emotional experiences of attachment are laid down in the right hemisphere of the brain in the first three years of life, and may be secure or insecure in her attachment. Insecure children demonstrate difficulties in social interaction and an inability to cope with stress, due to a failure of good enough attachment and bonding. They also manifest an inability to sustain a sense of self and a sense of relatedness with significant others during stressful moments. These extreme emotions are taken into adulthood, and form a working model of how an adult will respond to perceived or actual situations of rejection and abandonment. Some people who are insecurely attached may believe that they are so unlikely to be loved, as they have had little or unpredictable experience of it, that sex is the only way that they can get their intimacy needs met, so will obsessively do anything they can to get and maintain a relationship, even if that relationship does not make them happy.

Even minor threats to such a tenuous attachment bond in a relationship can be experienced as devastating and disequilibriating to such individuals (Holmes, 2001), yet they repeatedly behave in ways that provoke abandonment and rejection as the self-fulfilling paradox. Stalking, therefore, is simply a dysfunctional way of trying to regain connection with the attachment figure and prevent rejection and abandonment.

Meloy (1996) contended that the root of stalking lies in narcissistic fantasy; that when rejected, the stalker feels humiliation or shame that is defended against with rage. The desire to hurt, control or destroy restores the narcissistic fantasy. Meloy (1998) later developed his theory into an attachment pathology, as the majority of forensic stalkers have been shown to have a personality disorder, which again can be understood to be a disorder of attachment (Meloy & Gothard, 1995), as elaborated in Chapter Seven. Meloy (1996) reviewed ten empirical studies of stalking, which were predominantly case studies. He suggested that the typical stalker was a single or divorced man in his thirties, unemployed, of above-average intelligence, with a criminal and/or psychiatric history. When comparing stalkers with other offenders, Meloy and Gothard (1995) found the stalkers to be better educated, significantly older, and more intelligent (consistent with their resourcefulness and manipulativeness) and significantly more likely to have a personality disorder (other than antisocial personality disorder), and less likely to have antisocial personality disorder (as stalking behaviour is the antithesis of being antisocial). Substance abuse is common, and many have a mood disorder. Meloy's analysis, however, was taken purely from a very small forensic population, which did not include "domestic" stalkers. Also, this study was conducted in the very early days of legislation making stalking a criminal offence, therefore it was only the more severe cases that were likely to be prosecuted and consequently sampled within the study.

Wilson and colleagues proposed stalking as a model of paranoid attachment in which perpetrators of domestic violence and sexual offenders are of high risk (Wilson, Ermshar, & Welsh, 2006). They defined paranoid attachment as encompassing paranoid and obsessional ideas, underpinned by insecure attachment, and manifesting in aggression, fears of victimization and loss, grandiosity, or inferiority. The links to narcissism are clear here, as discussed in Chapter Six, as they suggest that when the grandiose defences fail, either because of rejection or abandonment (LOSS), the more primitive paranoid processes emerge (FEAR, RAGE).

Cyberstalking

In the previous chapter, I discussed how the Internet could reactivate insecure attachments, especially under conditions of stress or depression. One of the more perverse sides of an insecure attachment is cyberstalking, which may manifest from either a preoccupied or avoidant attachment style. Bocij (2004) argued that although cyberstalking uses harassing behaviours described above, the methods of doing so are very different. He describes:

- making threats via emails;
- making threats in chat rooms;
- accessing confidential information stored with the victim's computer;
- monitoring the victim's computer usage by installing Trojan horse software into the victim's computer system
- ordering goods in the victim's name, and paying for them online with the victim's credit card details;
- encouraging others to threaten or harass the victim through cyberspace;
- impersonating the victim in emails to friends, family, or colleagues;
- damaging the victim's computer by sending massive sized files or malicious viruses.

Harassment through cyberspace may commence at an early age, and may start as a form of bullying between children, either directly or through chatrooms. Delmonico and Griffin (2007) suggested that 40–60% of children either bully or are bullied via their computers or mobile phones.

Thus, cyberstalking may involve intentions of predatory harassment or emotional abuse, may escalate into violence, or it may be designed to be sexually coercive. Women are equally capable of cyberstalking, especially if it is from an unrequited love perspective (erotomania), and are more likely to be emotionally malevolent; for example, by sending multiple emails that blacken a person's character, threatening to reveal secrets, or making vexatious claims of sexual harassment or rape. Cyberstalking involving sexual coercion, however, tends to be perpetrated predominantly by men, whether it is towards adults or children (Spitzberg & Rhea, 1999).

Sexually coercive stalking describes predatory paedophiles who use the Internet as a means of grooming children to engage in sexual activity. Seto and colleagues classified these into five groups:

- stalkers who wish to gain physical access to children;
- cruisers who use the Internet for reciprocated sexual pleasure without the physical contact;
- masturbators who use the Internet for the pornography;
- networkers or swappers, who use the Internet to contact like-minded others and to swap or barter images to enhance their own collections;
- a combination of the above categories (Seto, Cantor, & Blanchard, 2006).

A definition and profile of paedophiles is discussed in the next chapter.

Stalking of therapists

In 2001, I conducted a study of the prevalence of stalking among therapists who worked in primary care settings. Mindful that a lot of colleagues had spoken of difficult stalking situations with former or current clients, I wondered whether the incidence of stalking in the mental health services would be higher than had been determined from the general population by Budd, Mattinson, and Myhill (2000). My sample was over a thousand counsellors, psychologists, and psychotherapists working in the UK, and I found that in comparison to the general population prevalence of 11.8%, the incidence of stalking of therapists was 23%, twice the national average (Hudson Allez, 2002). I found no gender differences in the harassers of the therapists, but the victims were predominantly female. What I did find, though, was that the stalkers fell into three broad groups:

- those clients who were needy and made early attachments to their therapists (preoccupied);
- those experiencing erotic transference (unrequited love);
- those with cluster C personality disorders.

As has been made clear throughout this book, these are all disorders of attachment. It also became clear that there was a level of denial on behalf of the therapists as to the seriousness of the harassment situations, some of which were very severe. Yet only 11% of the therapists who had been harassed felt it was a crime, and only 2% had contacted the police. This denial is very interesting in terms of the attachment style of the therapist, and how they relate to their client's needs but not their own. More is discussed on the therapists' attachment style in Chapter Fourteen.

Stalking and violence

It could be argued that there is a general tendency to over-focus on violent or sexual offending, as opposed to offending in general. Violent offences account for less than 10% of male prosecutions and less than 4% of female prosecutions (Blackburn, 1993). Similarly, Bradford, Bloomberg, and Boulet (1988) found that for sexual offences, only 17% of the younger offenders used violence, only 5% used extreme violence, and the number of older offenders who used violence was negligible. Yet, some violence can be considered so extreme that it promotes a huge public outcry, usually whipped up by the tabloid press. Thus, the public and politicians demand a theory of violent offending, as they seek to apportion blame.

English law divides crime into two categories: crimes that are *mala in se*, that is, treacherous, and those that are *mala prohibita*, or against the rules of society, although the boundaries between the two often become blurred. Violent offending falls under the former category, and because of this criminologists, lawyers, and psychologists tend to pay particular attention to it. Thus, in developing theories of general offending, notice is particularly taken of theories designed to predict, or elaborate on the reasons for, violent crime.

Henderson (1986) broke these down more specifically from her sample of male offenders, whose crimes tended to fall into four specific situations:

- violence committed with another crime, for example, armed robbery;
- violence within the family, as discussed in Chapter Eight;

- violence within a public place, such as a public house;
- violence within an institution, such as a prison.

However, as mentioned in Chapter Eight, the most common place for violence to occur is within the home (Godsi, 1999), and much of it goes unreported.

Are there any specific factors that can trigger violence? There are physical factors, such as heat (Anderson, 1989) and noise (Green & McCowan, 1984). There are social factors such as verbal provocation (Zillman, 1979), stress and anxiety (Novaco, 1975), third party instigation (Milgram, 1974), and breaking territorial boundaries (Lazarus, 1991). Biological factors may also be relevant, as men commit more crimes than women, and score higher on measures of direct aggression than women (Fossati et al., 2009). In 2004, male offenders in England and Wales outnumbered female offenders by more than four to one (Walker, Kershaw, & Nicholas, 2007). Violence by women amounts to less than 9% of convictions, and less than 1.5% of sex crimes. Youth and maleness seem to be the two ubiquitous factors that are indicative of violent behaviour. So, is it androgens such as testosterone? It is known that testosterone stimulates aggressive responses, just as oestrogen and progesterone inhibit them (Gilligan, 1996). Most men have testosterone, but not all men are violent. The neurotransmitter serotonin is known to be a biological inhibitor of violent behaviour, both homicidal and suicidal, and some men are thought to have low levels of serotonin. This may well relate to maternal and infant nutrition. Ridgway and House (2006) point out that we have only recently found compelling correlations between presentations of homicide, suicide, depression, and violence and a low consumption of fish.

Of course, social class is an inevitable factor in terms of crimes of violence. Gilligan (1996) argues that people who are in lower status groups are more likely to commit homicide, whereas those in higher status groups are more likely to commit suicide. He also highlights that for every 1% rise in unemployment in the USA, there is an increase in the mortality rate of 2%, an increase in the infant mortality rate of 5%, and an increase in homicides and imprisonment by 6%. Gilligan also agrees with Godsi's (1999) micro-level view of the damage of the individuals' psyche by childhood abuse and neglect. There is no doubt that aggression in adult life is correlated with neglect for the person as a child before they reached the age of two years (Dubowitz, 1999). But Gilligan goes into deeper psychoanalytical depth by proposing that the reason why these individuals create acts of violence is that as they become damaged, they develop an inner sense of shame and guilt. Meloy (1996) also agreed with this concept of aggression defending against shame. In discussing violent stalkers, he argued that they feel the rejection of their victims as a disturbance of their narcissistic fantasy, triggering feelings of shame and humiliation that are defended against with rage. However, Lake (1981) continues the argument for transgenerational transmission: "Some of the violence that lands people in prison may well be an offloading of the violence experienced in the womb" (p. 131).

Here, again, is the reprise of the insecure attachment template, and the individual building a working model triggered by FEAR and RAGE. Gilligan views violence, like de Zulueta (2006), as a defensive act and therefore preventable.

Other theorists take a reductionist approach to the concept of violent behaviour by looking at neuropsychological principles. Case studies like the classic case of Phineas Gage (Solms & Turnbull, 2002), who was a mild-mannered man until his brain injury, which changed him into a violent alcoholic, have led to the proposal that brain damage may cause irritability and disinhibition that can lead to violence. For example, Fred West was held to have suffered brain trauma as the result of a motorbike accident (Godsi, 1999). Berkowitz (1989) contended, however, that even if this is the case, the aggressive person still needs an environmental stimulus to trigger the violence. In defending the frustration-preceding-aggression hypothesis (Berkowitz, 1971), he experimentally demonstrated how more severe aggression can be triggered by environmentally aggressive cues, such as the sight of a gun (Berkowitz & LePage, 1967), although this proposal has been contended by Ellis, Weiner, and Miller (1971). Panskepp concurred that frustration may reflect the mild arousal of the RAGE circuitry, which then can eventually trigger full-blown anger. However, he pointed out that aggression is not a unitary concept. There is evidence for two types of aggression: predatory attack in the form of stalking, or affective rage that one sees in domestic violence and crimes of passion (Panskepp, 1998). Meloy agreed, and similarly distinguished between the violent attacks of stalkers as to whether they were affective or predatory, the former being the hot emotional consequence of rejection of an ex-lover where the victim is likely to be a private individual, and the latter being the cold, planned, purposeful hunting of a public individual. The latter stalker may be a man with an avoidant insecure attachment working on a RAGE circuit in response to some perceived slight against his entitlement, which he is defending against in narcissistic rage. The former stalker may be a man with a preoccupied attachment style working on a FEAR circuit in response to abandonment. To reprise the point in Chapter Eight, a fearful preoccupied man attacks externally to defend against what he perceives as belonging to him. A common comment of the preoccupied stalker is: "If I can't have you, then no one will."

Risk of stalking and violence

Kienlen (1998) highlighted two factors in risk assessment of stalking behaviour: that early attachment disturbance might predispose an individual to stalk, and that recent adult loss might precipitate it. Thus, the loss of a significant other can be a catalyst for obsessional behaviour if they are already predisposed by attachment disorder.

There is a growing literature on violence prediction research and actuarial predictors (Monahan & Steadman, 1994; Wilson & Hernstein, 1985). Some researchers maintain that stalkers, even after a year or more of pursuit, will not physically attack their victims (Zona, Sharma, & Lane, 1993) and the risk of actual physical harm posed by erotomaniacs (who have the delusion that the victim loves the perpetrator in return) may be less than for other categories of stalkers. However, Meloy (1996) found that half of obsessional followers made threats to person and property and a quarter of these acted on that threat. Violence in the past is considered an important factor for risk assessment, as is the abuse of substances or alcohol. But Meloy cautioned that the absence of violence in the past does not mean that someone could not be very dangerous in the present, and this caution is consistent with the findings of Dietz and colleagues (1991a,b) who found that threats were not positively associated with approaching the victim. In Meloy's view, the incidence of violence among stalkers is 25–40%, and 50% for ex-intimates, which can be seen as an extension of the domestic violence as discussed in Chapter Eight. This is confirmed by the British Crime Survey (Mirrlees-Black, 1999), which found that a large number of women reported being stalked by their ex-partner when there had been violence within the relationship. Meloy suggested that if one were conducting a risk assessment of the threat of violence to the victim, if the stalker is male, an ex-intimate, and the threat has been verbalized, then there is a high risk of it being carried out. If the victim is a public figure, the stalker is less likely to verbalize the intent but still carry it out. More is discussed regarding risk assessment in Chapter Thirteen.

So, can people with a predisposition to stalking be helped? Mullen and colleagues argued that only comprehensive treatment approaches that encapsulate both offence-specific and offence-related factors are likely to succeed in reducing recidivism (Mullen, Pathé, & Purcell, 2000b), and, as there is such a paucity of such programmes available, both nationally and internationally, that incarceration is the only realistic option for serious recidivist stalking offenders. Clearly, a stalker is demonstrating attachment dysfunctions, although currently there is no requirement for treatment within the UK forensic services, but any treatment that does not work on making the person secure as well as dealing with cognitive distortions is going to fall short. Clearly, when one considers that a child is preprogrammed to attach, and that stalking is an extreme form of attachment, therapeutic work in this area will not be easy.

Gordon's review

Gordon's world has fallen apart. He had a fantasy of a brilliant future: owning his own successful garage, driving a brand new BMW, a new house where he and Rachel would live comfortably and grow old together. Instead, Rachel rejected him in favour of a brat he did not want her to have, and now the state nosey-parkers have taken her away from him, and he feels totally abandoned. His normal coping strategy of hard work and perfectionism has failed him, and his addictions of smoking, drinking, and sex have completely taken him over. He ceased to be functional at work, and was eventually fired. He has no concept of remorse for his physical abuse of his girlfriend. He simply feels affronted at her absence and humiliated at being paraded in the police station and being charged with a criminal offence. What do they know anyway? She had it coming, didn't she? She belongs to him and no one, NO ONE, is going to get in the way of what belongs to him.

CHAPTER THIRTEEN

Paraphilias and sexual offending

G ordon sat on the side of the bench in the bare cell in the police station with his face buried in his hands. "How did I ever get to this?" he wondered to himself, and tears slowly seeped through his fingers. He had not seen Rachel or his son for nearly a year now. They had been moved into another house as soon as the authorities had realized Gordon knew where they were. He was also visited by the police at the time, and cautioned about further stalking or harassment behaviour. Ignoring this, at first he was frantic in his search for them. He searched all the places he thought Rachel might go to. He harassed all her friends, but they became angry and tight-lipped. He wandered the streets of the suburbs, and stood outside mother-and-toddler groups in the hope of stumbling across her, but he had no idea of where she might be. Then he began to realize that Rachel and Conner might have been sent to another city, and his hopes of finding them diminished.

Filled with the despair of abandonment, he turned back to his computer for comfort. As he was now unemployed, he would sleep until early afternoon, get up and sit at the computer to watch movies or view pornography through to the early hours of the next day. He had escalated his pornography viewing into any picture that might be outside of the norm: he laughed at pictures of people having sex with animals, was fascinated by all of the alternative methods of S&M, was aroused by swinging group sexual activity with women, particularly simultaneous vaginal and anal sex, salivated at sex with transsexuals, and was curious at the pictures of people having sex with children remembering his own experience as a child. Cigarette ash and butts piled up beside the keyboard, and the desk and floor were littered with empty beer cans and burger wrappers. He had run out of money while still searching for Rachel, and his job-seeker's allowance did not cover the cost of his addictions. He had stopped paying his rent several months before, was now being hassled by his landlord for the arrears, and was being threatened with eviction.

Last week there had been a knock at his front door. Two large men in black barged passed him, announcing they were bailiffs charged with the collection of goods equivalent to his rent arrears. Among items seized was Gordon's precious computer. Despite his protestations, all his electric equipment was taken away; his computer, his TV, his digital radio, his iPod, his HiFi, all gone. Without his usual method of self-soothing, Gordon slumped into a deep depression; he stopped eating, smoked and drank continuously, thought incessantly about killing himself, and slept round the clock.

He was woken in the early hours of that morning by a heavy thumping at the door. Unwashed, with several days of beard growth, a thumping head and mouth like a sand-pit, he stumbled half-awake–half-asleep to the door. When he released the catch, the door burst open and in charged four uniformed policemen and a detective in plain clothes, who looked Gordon up and down as if he was a piece of filth. The bailiffs, they told Gordon, had sold Gordon's computer, and the new owner discovered all of the pornography on the hard drive and notified the police. He was cautioned, handcuffed, taken roughly to the police station, and pushed into a cell to await further questioning. The police, however, were not in a hurry to sort out the situation of a paedophile.

Paraphilias

Unusual or bizarre sexual practices are called paraphilias, taken from the Greek: *para*: unusual, *philia*: love. There is a vast range of sexual activities that the incredible inventiveness of the human brain has devised. The late John Money created a typology, as follows.

- *Sacrificial and expiatory.* This requires a perception of sinful lust and consequent atonement in the behaviour. Sadism, masochism (S&M), and lustful murder fit in this category, as do coprophilia (love of excreta) and urophilia (love of urine: golden rain). There is a dark side to this group, which suggests it is all murky and unacceptable, whereas mild S&M may be part of many ordinary couples' sexual repertoire.
- *Marauding and predatory.* In this category, individuals take love by stealth without consent and sometimes with force. Rape, kleptophilia (stealing sexual objects) and necrophilia (sex with a corpse) are examples. One can determine from previous chapters that it suggests an avoidant attachment style that provides the sex without the intimacy.
- *Mercantile and venal.* In this category, sex is bartered, traded, or paid for; for example, the use of sex workers, prostitutes, rent boys, live sex shows, telephone sex (telephonicophilia), and Internet websites. In this group, sex is a commodity and not part of the loving, caring, secure template.
- *Fetishistic and talismanic.* Here a token, a fetish or a talisman, substitutes for the lover and creates the sexual arousal. The touch of fabrics like rubber or leather (hyphephilia), the smell (olfactophilia) of excreta, the touch of insects or animals in the genital areas (formicophilia), or the feel of enemas in the anal passages (klismaphilia). Transvestitism can also fall into this category if the person dresses to pass as a member of the opposite sex for sexual arousal. Many of these fetishes develop at the time of the development of the sexual template, and may link back in some way to feelings of security relating to the parent.
- *Stigmatic and eligibilic.* In this category, the partner must be stigmatized, ostracized as an outsider, or physically handicapped, such as amputees (acrotomophilia). Paedophilia and gerontophilia (sex with an elderly person) also fit into this category, as does bestiality and zoophilia (sex with animals). These are people who are not able to maintain relationships with similar

others, so are drawn into relationships with people of perceived lower status, or who have similar relationship difficulties.

- *Solicitational and allurative.* These behaviours involve displaying, watching, touching, or rubbing to elicit a sexual encounter.
Examples include exhibitionism (peodeiktophilia—flashing),
voyeurism (scoptophilia—"Peeping Tom"), providing live sex
shows (autagonistophilia), frottage (illicit massaging of
another's genitals in crowded places), promiscuity, and pornography. Stigmatophilia: being pierced, mutilated, or tattooed
is also considered allurative. These are people who either have
not learnt the boundaries of society, have been taught when
youngsters that society's boundaries do not have to apply to
them, or who are actively rebelling against such boundaries
when they have been enforced too rigidly or punitively.

As discussed in Chapter Four, Money (1986) believed that paraphilias are not generated at random, but fall into the categories
above due to a vandalized and redesigned lovemap (sexual template) caused by the neglect, traumatization, or suppression of the
normal heterosexual lovemap development. This vandalism creates
distortions, displacements, omissions, or inclusions in the individual's sexual repertoire, and becomes the only channel through
which sexual arousal and climax can take place. This lovemap
pathology manifests in full after puberty and is not subject to voluntary control. Each paraphilia has a dual existence: one in fantasy,
and one where the fantasy is played out in practice. It has also been
noticed that many individuals who demonstrate fetishes or paraphilias have more than one, suggesting there may be a biological
basis for them, or it may be that attachment insecurity makes a
person predisposed to search in more than one way, that is, sexual
way, for emotional security. Money believed that it is essentially a
developmental disability, and that boys are more predisposed to the
development of a paraphilia than girls. He argued that it is wrong
to call them sexual disorders, as they are really a disorder of pair-
bonding or attachment. Thus, they are disorders of love, not lust.
This proposal is consistent with the theory of an insecure attachment
I have discussed, predisposing a vulnerability to the vandalization
of the sexual template preparation for pubescent experimentation.

A child's concept of her own gender is said to be established firmly and irrevocably within the latter half of the practising period: that is, 18–24 months (Money & Ehrhardt, 1972). The process of upright posture and accompanied genital stimulation facilitates this. In particular, male toddlers at eighteen months of age become very interested in their genitals and the pleasure they experience in stimulating them, especially when in the presence of their mothers (Tabin, 1985). How the parent responds to this sexual display is imprinted within the child's right brain, and will have a direct influence later on sexual drive. Later, when the LUST circuit, or sexual template, comes online, as discussed in the preceding chapters, any vandalization at this vulnerable period of right-brain development can precipitate the development of sexual paraphilias, which often start to manifest themselves at the development of puberty. Any awareness of homosexuality or paedophilia may start emerging into conscious awareness this early. As Money (1986) proposed, vandalization by sexual molestation or abuse at this stage can have critical consequences in terms of the development of later paraphilias.

Solomon (1980) proposed that paraphilias were developed through an opponent process theory, where he viewed emotions coming in pairs, like fear–relief and pleasure–pain (Solomon, 1980). Solomon's model suggested a connection between the degree of pleasure a given state produces and its subsequent capacity to inspire withdrawal. It has been suggested that in the child/adolescent's mind, the pain experienced from an abusive act, such as being hit on a bare bottom with a cane, will be suppressed and eventuates in an opposite reaction, or opponent process, being erotized into pleasure from that experience in an adult fetish. Eventually, the opponent reaction comes to dominate the process of sex and becomes the individual's primary motivation for re-experiencing the stimulus. Solomon used the opponent process model to explain why some lovers cannot tolerate being apart. Yet, this separation anxiety seems less a measure of depth of emotion and more about an insecure attachment.

There are three common ways that a person develops a fetish or paraphilia following an incident, either at the time the sexual template was developed or later during adolescent neural pruning. First, the person may re-enact the incident subconsciously on a repetitive basis: for example, the girl who was sexually abused by her father goes on to become promiscuous with multiple casual sexual relationships, or moves into becoming a sex worker. Second, as suggested above, the man who is publicly beaten on his bare buttocks with a cane by a teacher at boarding school will develop a fetish for caning and will seek out a dominatrix for sexual arousal. Third, the aversive or abusive act may be eroticized towards another, so the girl who was abused may then abuse her own children, or the beaten man may want to beat others. If one considers the working model of an insecure template, then one could suggest that the girl who becomes a sex worker is operating on the "BAD-ME" circuit she had developed, because she does not consider herself worth protecting from the dangers that the profession may give her and that is all she deserves. As such, she will have overridden her social construction of shame, and, despite (or because of) feeling quite bad about herself, will sell her body as a piece of merchandise. To objectify herself in this way suggests she has already perfected the art of dissociation, so, as the punter takes her body, her self and her mind are elsewhere. Similarly, the man who enjoys being spanked with a cane has eroticized his FEAR circuit, making a close associative pathway between LUST and FEAR, whereas the man who likes to hit out at others has done the same with LUST and RAGE.

Can paraphilias be changed? It is useful to consider that fetishes are essentially conditioned behaviour and are, thus, open to deconditioning and to becoming extinguished, whereas sexual orientations, such as bisexuality, homosexuality, heterosexuality, and paedophilia, are imprinted into the person and therefore tend to be stable over time and almost impossible to change (Barbaree, Bogaert, & Seto, 1995). Thus, therapeutic help for the latter should be focused on management, self-acceptance, and ethical behaviour, rather than change.

Sexual offending

Janssen and colleagues have proposed a Dual Control Model of sexual arousal (Janssen, Vorst, Finn, & Bancroft, 2002). This proposed that there are two neurophysiological systems that contribute to sexual behaviour: a physiological excitation system and a psychological inhibitory system. Normal sexual activity requires that these systems are in balance. However, if the inhibitory system is too high and the excitation system is too low, sexual dysfunctions (such as erectile failure) occur; if the excitatory system is too high, and the inhibitory system is too low (and this can be shown by deactivation in the medial orbito-frontal cortex), sexual acting out (such as compulsive masturbation) or sexual offences may occur.

The literature on sexual offending tends to divide sexual offenders, *inter alia*, into two groups: those who use sexual violence with adults (i.e., rapists) and those who offend against children (i.e., paedophiles). Sometimes, researchers also divide child sexual offenders into intrafamilial offenders, or incest offenders, and predatory paedophiles. Comparisons are then made between the histories and behaviours of the groups and compared with other offenders and people who do not offend. Of course, these boundaries are blurred by reality, as there are offenders who both rape adults and molest children. There is also another group that is currently being investigated as a separate entity: those that look at, but do not touch, children. Thus, it could be argued that many of such Internet offenders would sit more comfortably with a group of voyeurs and exhibitionists rather than with predatory paedophiles.

As previously discussed in Chapter Eleven, attachment styles may predispose individuals to a trajectory of emotional disturbance and subsequent sexual offending. Ward, Hudson, and Marshall (1996) proposed three attachment styles that they viewed as being related to different forms of sexual offending:

- avoidant (dismissive) individuals would be hostile to others (especially women), would like sex without relationships, so may have a propensity to rape, or engage in incestuous offending. This would also suggest that they have reduced oxytocin levels;
- preoccupied individuals would want reassurance and love and may sexualize attachment relationships, so they may engage in sexual contact offences against children when they feel unable to make relationships with adults. This would also apply to incestuous relationships where the parent is manifesting abusive behaviour as an expression of their "love";

- disorganized individuals would seek intimacy through sexual encounters and may become coercive or sadistic, as was discussed in the previous chapter.

Offending against children

The construct of a paedophile is not unitary, so it is important for professionals working with offenders to be discerning of the differences.

- A paedophile is a person who is over sixteen years old who has a persistent sexual preference for prepubertal children (*ICD-10*), that is, less than thirteen years of age (Hall & Hall, 2007). This may be intrafamilial in incestuous sexual preference, or interfamilial, when it tends to be more predatory.
- A hebephile is a person over sixteen who has a persistent sexual attraction to early pubertal age girls.
- An infantophile is a person over sixteen years old who has a persistent sexual orientation towards children under five years old.
- An ephebophile is an adult who experiences a sexual preference for mid-to-late adolescents. There needs to be a minimum of five years difference between an adolescent with this sexual preference and the desired boy or girl to attract this classification (Hall & Hall, 2007).

There is a huge debate in the psychological literature about these respective classifications, especially the terms paedophilia and ephebophilia, so it would be valuable to adress each of these in turn.

Paedophilia

The appropriate psychopathological definition of a paedophile is a person who has a *persistent* sexual preference for prepubertal children. There is no such consistent definition within the legal system, or, indeed, within the forensic psychological literature.

Feelgood and Hoyer (2008) vociferously argued that the classification has been hijacked and generalised by the legal and sociolegal systems to include any person who molests a child, irrespective of the reason (Feelgood & Hoyer, 2008). Despite the *ICD-10* and *DSM-IV* classification criteria of persistent sexual preference, it is held that a paedophile's sexual orientation to children does not have to be exclusive, and many develop sexual relationships with adults to provide a cloak for their socially unacceptable predilection. More than 50% will marry at some point in their lives (Hall & Hall, 2007) and many are homosexual or bisexual in their orientation to children (Blanchard et al., 2000), that is, suggesting that any child will do. This blurring of the definition and classification boundaries has the implication of casting doubt over the construct validity of empirical research conducted into the area, and, as Okami and Goldberg (1992) argue, puts the whole understanding of child molestation and paedophilia into chaos.

From a neurological perspective, differences have been found in the structure of the brain between paedophiles and controls. In particular, changes have been found in the prefrontal cortex, the temporal lobe, and cerebellum (Cohen et al., 2002; Schiffer et al., 2006). Recall that in the development of the infant brain, it was the temporal lobe that was damaged in the neglected and abused orphans, and that the "volume control" of the extreme emotions of FEAR and RAGE develops in the prefrontal cortex. The temporal lobe has also been associated with the hypersexual behaviour found in temporal lobe epilepsy and Kluver–Bucy syndrome (Hall & Hall, 2007). Recall also that early childhood abuse changes the structure of the child's brain, which may account for some of this behaviour, and it has been suggested that when tracing the history of the most predatory offenders, very commonly it was the biological mother who was the abuser. What is even more interesting, in this light, is that Blanchard and colleagues found that a large proportion of their sample of paedophiles had experienced a head trauma leading to a loss of consciousness before the age of six years old (Blanchard et al., 2002) and were more likely to have had mothers who had received psychiatric care. They did not suggest that head injury lead to paedophilia, however. It might be that neurodevelopmental problems lead to accident proneness on the one hand and paedophilia on the other.

Another consistent finding in the literature is that is that a large majority of paedophiles were victims of abusive situations or trauma in their own childhoods (Howitt, 1995; Rich, 2006; Smallbone, 2005), which inevitably will affect their own attachment styles. This will manifest in inappropriate sexual behaviour from the age of eight or nine when the sexual template comes online, and for some of them, even years earlier. By the time they reach fifteen years old, 40% of paedophiles will have already molested a child (Abel & Harlow, 2001) (but see below in the section on ephebophilia, as the age of the child could be age-appropriate to the perpetrator, yet still invoke a prosecution).

Hall and Hall (2007) suggested a profile of a paedophile as a socially alienated person who is less emotionally stable than other people, with high incidence of anxiety disorders and depression. This is unsurprising for people considered by many to be the pariahs of society. It is also likely that these people will have other comorbid paraphilias, like frotteurism, exhibitionism, voyeurism, or sadism (Raymond, Coleman, Ohlerking, Christensen, & Miner, 1999). However, they also have a high incidence of cluster A and B personality disorders (see Chapter Seven), often with narcissistic, sociopathic, or antisocial personal traits. As such, they lack remorse, and the narcissistic style means that they lack the ability to have an empathic response to their victims. This is why treatment that focuses primarily on victim empathy is doomed to fail, demonstrated by the lack of empirical evidence as to the effectiveness of victim empathy (Hennessy, Walker, & Vess, 2002).

Cantor and colleages (2006) examined the school grades of sex offenders, comparing paedophiles with hebephiles, sex offenders aroused by adults, and non-sex offenders. The results showed that the hebephiles and paedophiles were twice as likely to be a grade behind in their education, or to being enrolled in special education, both before and after covarying for IQ. No significant differences were detected between the other sex offenders and the non-offenders groups. Blanchard agreed. He and his colleagues found that the lower the intelligence of the offender, the lower the age of the abused child (Blanchard et al., 1999). This suggests that people who develop an erotic preference for children do so as a result of developmental and social incompetence occurring early in life. Rich agreed with Hudson and Ward that the development of sexually abusive behaviour is driven by attachment difficulties and subsequent social deficits (Hudson & Ward, 2000; Rich, 2006), and that sexual offending is a "distorted attempt to build interpersonal closeness in the absence of the social and psychological skills required to build emotionally satisfying relationships" (Rich, 2006, p. 171).

Rich sees a pathway from attachment deficits predisposing children to becoming victims of sexual abuse that can precipitate a disorganized and fragmented attachment style. The memory of the abuse may become sexualized (opponent process) and can lead to re-enactment, so the victim becomes the perpetrator. The intervening and protective factor against this trajectory is a loving and supportive other, forming an attachment bond and a safe base (Kaufman & Zigler, 1987).

Re-enactment is a common theme with individuals looking at pictures on the Internet of children being abused, and it is common to find that the theme of the act the person is viewing is a repetition of events that occurred to the viewer when he was a child (again opponent process). Herman (1992) muses on the uncanny involuntariness of re-enactments, even when they are consciously chosen, and refers back to Freud's concept of repetition compulsion. The following is an account from one of my clients convicted of looking at abusive images of children:

Therapist: What were you looking for in these pictures?

Client: Faces. Strong arms, strong hands, and stern faces. Especially when they were looking directly back at me with an angry expression.

Therapist: Child faces or adult faces?

Client: No, adult faces. I was the child.

Therapist: What did that mean to you, when they were looking at you with a stern expression?

Client: It told me what a piece of shit I was and how I deserved to be punished. I know it sounds perverse, but it made me feel safe.

Repetition compulsion keeps people within the security of their insecure circuit in an attempt to master the overwhelming feelings of FEAR and RAGE. Herman (1992) opined: "The predominant unresolved feeling might be terror, helpless rage, or simply the undifferentiated 'adrenaline rush' of mortal danger" (p. 42).

The profile of an incest offender is different from that of an inter-familial paedophile, although, again, many will have experienced childhood abuse or family disruption in their own histories (Williams & Finkelhor, 1990). Ethrington highlighted this in her research of men who had been sexually abused:

> A conversation between an offender and journalist at a rehabilita-tion centre for sex offenders:
>
> "When did you start abusing?"
>
> Without hesitation, Ian replied, "When I was four."
>
> The journalist looked into Ian's bland small-boy-of-40 face and, keeping his voice level, asked:
>
> "And who did you abuse?"
>
> "My father." [Etherington, 2009]

Incestuous fathers are described as passive, dependent, and often suffer with depression and anxiety. They tend to be socially isolated and inept, have disorganized families, and describe dissat-isfaction with their adult relationships (Wakeling, Webster, Moul-den, & Marshall, 2007), the latter being considered as a significant risk factor (Black, Heyman, & Slep, 2001). Very often, the abuse of step-, foster-, and adopted children are treated in the literature in the same way as the abuse of a biological child, even though, etho-logically speaking, this is not incestuous. Again we have classifica-tion chaos, as the literature treats them as a homogenous group, and research into understanding the process of intrafamilial abuse that does not separate out these as different will be essentially empirically flawed.

It is more difficult to offer a profile of a female incestuous offender, as there is considerable underreporting of this occurring, and almost an unwillingness of society to accept that women are capable of such behaviour (Hudson, 2005). More is discussed on the issue of females who commit sexual offences later in this chapter.

Finally, it is vital to acknowledge that there is much about paedophilia we do not know, simply because many do not come to the attention of psychologists or the criminal justice system. Not all people with a paedophilic interest commit sexual offences against children and may well find other appropriate outlets for their feelings, or may choose ways of managing their interest to keep the children and themselves safe.

Ephebophilia

The term ephebophilia is used only to describe the *preference* for mid-to-late adolescent sexual partners, not the mere presence of some level of sexual attraction. It is defined as a sexual preference for girls generally 14–16 years old, and boys generally 14–18 years old. Because most late adolescents have physical characteristics near to that of full-grown adults, some level of sexual attraction to persons in the age group is common among adults of all sexual orientations. Therefore, such a distinct preference for individuals in mid- or late adolescence is not generally regarded by psychologists as a pathology when it does not interfere with other major areas of one's life. Few would want to label erotic interest in late or even mid-adolescents as a psychopathology, so ephebophilia is not listed by name as a mental disorder in the *ICD-10*, nor is it listed as a paraphilia.

Since the Sexual Offences Act of 2003, however, ephebophilia has become an illegal activity, and individuals have been prosecuted for thoughts (from viewing images), words (in text or email messages) and deeds (sexual activity), even when it is consenting and the "child" is over sixteen and is old enough to marry and capable of consenting to sexual activity. This includes under eighteen-year-old adolescents having peer relationships. As Stapleton (2010) pointed out, teenagers who record themselves in an erotic pose or engaged in acts of masturbation are actually engaged in the illegal act of producing child pornography, even though the act is not illegal *per se*. Gillespie (2008) argued that the law is now criminalizing adolescents for indulging in normal peer-related sexual activity. And the perverse side of the situation at present is that is is better for an adolescent to have penetrative sex with a peer adolescent under the age of consent, as he is only likely to get cautioned by the police, than to take a photograph of his topless adolescent girlfriend on his mobile phone, and end up on the Sexual Offenders' Register, a situation that will follow him for the rest of his life. Gillespie argued that given that adolescents are by their very nature sexually active and sexually explorative, it is unsurprising that they would search for sexual images on the Internet, and if they are age-approriate images, this necessarily falls foul of the law. As such, they are then (inappropriately) labelled as paedophiles because, as discussed above, the classification of paedophile has shifted to any sexual molestation offence, irrespective of the circumstances.

Offending against adults

Sexual offending against adults falls into two categories: contact and non-contact offences. For non-contact offences, the situations are predominantly voyeurism and exhibitionism. For contact offences, frotteurism, sexual assault (which may include when a negotiated sadomasochistic situation gets out of hand and the safe word is not respected), and rape. Both can be seen as a manifestation of an ambivalent attachment style, because the behaviours show approach regarding sex and avoidance in terms of intimacy in the situations.

Exhibitionists may manifest in the covert type of behaviour, where the person leaps out at an unsuspecting victim exposing gentialia, or the overt type where a person (or couple) advertise their intention to be sexual in a public arena ("dogging") or via a webcam on the Internet (CUSeeMe or ICUII). The latter will rarely produce a "victim" *per se*, unless someone stumbles across the situation inadvertently. However, the former covert "flasher" exhibitionist does so partly because he enjoys the feeling of the fresh air on his gentialia, which is a fetish developed during adolescence probably, and partly from the desire to shock the victim. This is not always in the male domain, as some women may exhibit sitting in public places or on public transport where they deliberately open their legs while not wearing any underwear. Unsurprisingly, however, there are few complaints about this behaviour, and men exposed to a woman's behaviour in this way rarely consider themselves to be victimized. Popovic (2007) quoted Short (1980) elucidating that, in law, women can be victims of exhibitionism but not perpetrators. Interestingly, exhibitionism has been decriminalized in Denmark.

There is a paucity of research into this phenomenon, especially the contribution that psychopathology has to play in it (Drake & Pathé, 2004), but it appears that the male exhibitionist who wants to shock is clearly using the FEAR and RAGE circuits in an insecure template; in the preoccupied style, he needs to keep approaching women to get his sexual needs met, with the self-fulfilling behaviour of rejection from the woman, leading to RAGE and subsequent repetition of behaviour with the next victim. Thus, exhibitionists have one of the highest recidivism rates, although they rarely show deviant sexual interest (Murphy & Page, 2008).

There is much ambivalence around the classification of the voyeur, as it is culturally sanctioned through the widespread use of pornography, and, thus, is neither illegal nor deviant. However, the voyeur is, by his very nature, covert, and part of the excitement for him is the seeing without those observed knowing, although there are the open voyeurs described in the dogging scenario above. There are debates as to whether there are victims in a "Peeping Tom" situation, as some have argued that if a person is being viewed as they are undressing, bathing, or having sex, and they have no knowledge of this, then they cannot be victimized. However, this is still sexual arousal and sexual activity by stealth without the consent of the person being viewed. Again, one can conceptualize the preoccupied style of the voyeur who roams the streets for hours searching for a suitable window to view through, the FEAR circuit impeding any form of intimacy, and the RAGE circuit that operates the ability to encroach on people's privacy without their consent.

Miner and Munns (2005) considered that masculine inadequacy was related to child offending, whereas masculine assertiveness was related to rape. Greenall and West conducted a study of men who had been convicted of raping strangers and were patients of high security hospitals in the UK. They found that the majority had experienced childhood, parental, and education problems, manifesting in adolescence through delinquency and sexual problems (Greenall & West, 2007). They divided offender histories into two types: men who had originated in antisocial childhoods that progressed into antisocial and criminal adulthoods, and men who had originated in families with psychiatric and substance abusing problems. With the former type, the offence tended to be characterized by violence; with the latter group, the offence was characterized by sexual deviancy. This is consistent with Groth (1978), who identified from his sample of convicted rapists that there were two predominant motives: anger and power, with a smaller proportion citing sexual gratification as a motive.

In considering violent sexual offences against adults, Panskepp (1998) pointed out that male sexuality requires an aggressive attitude and may be strongly linked to the SEEKING and RAGE circuits, although there are a high number of testosterone receptors that run from the amygdala through the hypothalamus to the periaqueductal grey, which is very different from the RAGE pathway. But with violent rapists, it seems that the LUST and RAGE circuits have become merged in some way. Relapse episodes of sexually aggressive individuals were reported by the protagonists to have been precipitated by a negative mood state, such as boredom, frustration, and anger (Serran & Marshall, 2006). Ninety-four per cent of rapists reported feeling anger immediately before offending, as reported by Pithers, Marques, Gibat, and Marlatt (1983), which are underpinned by themes of hostility and mistrust of women (Milner & Webster, 2005). Mann and Hollin (2007) agreed that anger, dominance, and humiliation are the primary motivators in a rapist, although they point out that many act because of a sense of grievance, so the anger is based on revenge and the punishment is to humiliate and degrade, with many using more force than is necessary (Christie, Marshall, & Lanthier, 1979). The narcissistic style discussed in Chapter Six is very apparent here, and, as Holmes (2007) pointed out, rape represents sex that is devoid of attachment. More recently, Jenkins (2009) proposed that

> Sexual assault requires an exaggerated sense of entitlement along with an abdication of responsibility for the feelings and well-being of the abused person who is in effect treated as an object to be conquered, possessed and used by the abusing person. [pp. 5–6]

Van der Kolk (2003) highlighted that women are more likely to be raped by someone they know, and that stranger rape is relatively rare, whereas men are more likely to be raped by a stranger.

Malamuth (1981) also noted a high (35%) "rape proclivity", defined as a self rating of the likelihood of raping if you could be assured of not being caught and punished. This rape proclivity is highlighted by Brownmiller (1975), who discussed the mass rape of women during times of war, mostly by men who presumably would not rape under normal circumstances. It was as if the war situation has a dehumanizing effect and rape is just an extension of other forms of violence used against the enemy.

Abel and colleagues contended that some rapists are "true paraphiliacs", in that their urges to rape go back to childhood, presumably to the eight or nine years of age threshold, and are linked with other paraphiliac activities such as voyeurism, sadism, and exhibitionism (Abel, Rouleau, & Coyne, 1987). Bancroft (1995) cautioned against this proposal, however, as he felt this could lead to the pathologizing of a rapist and treating him as if he were sick rather than criminal. He argued that rape should always be considered as a form of sexual assault. Bancroft (1995) and Abel, Barlow, Blanchard, and Guild (1977) agree, however, that rape needs to be viewed as *both* a sexual crime and an aggressive crime, not just one or the other, although contemporary thinking sees rape as a form of violence, domination, and humiliation, using sex as the mediating pathway.

Knight and Prentky (1990) have developed a typology of rapists based on their offending motivation (Knight & Prentky, 1990), which the researchers divided into four primary motivations of opportunistic, pervasively angry, sexual, and vindictive. These were further subdivided into nine subgroups, based on the social competency of the offender and the presence or absence of sadism in the offence. This has led to the development of an assessment tool called the MTC:R3 (Massachusetts Treatment Centre, Version 3). This breakdown provides a good insight into the motivations of the rapist for clinical interventions (Greenall & West, 2007).

There is little research looking at attachment styles and rapists (Gannon & Ward, 2008), although it clearly manifests an avoidant attachment style, wanting the gratification of sex without the relationship. The RAGE circuit fuels the avoidance, and if one adds narcissistic rage to the equation, then the predisposing factors become clearer.

Female offenders

Although most sexual offenders are men, there is evidence that females offending against children are on the increase (Davin, 1999). Home Office figures for 2008 suggest that 3% of those cautioned for, or found guilty of, a sexual offence are women. Greyston and DeLuca (1999) assessed that females account for approximately 5% of childhood sexual abuse, whereas Finkelhor and colleagues conducted a study of sexual abuse in day care and found that 40% of the perpetrators were women (Finkelhor, Willimans, & Burns, 1988). These offenders were ordinary women, well educated, well regarded in their communities, and with no history of offending behaviour. Finklehor highlighted how important it is not to overlook the capacity of women to offend, although their methodology has been severely criticized, as they included cases in their sample where the allegations had been denied, reversed, or where prosecutions had resulted in acquittals. Notwithstanding, women of all ages have abused both male and female children, and for female sexual offenders, their sexual offence is most likely to be their first offence (Tyman & Worthington, 2009).

Female sexual offenders tend to fall into four categories, although there may be some overlap between them.

- Those whose victims are prepubescent children. Often these abusers have a psychiatric diagnosis (O'Connor, 1987).
- Those who target adolescents, and tend to see their behaviour resulting from a love relationship (Mathews, Mathews, & Speltz, 1989). Very often the victims in these cases suggest it felt more like a "rite of passage" rather than abuse.
- Female offenders who abuse to get the approval or attention of their male lover, very similar to Myra Hindley or Rose West.
- Incestuous relationships. Ward (1988) discussed the concepts of mother–son incest, and noted that because clinical case studies are so rare, very few generalizations can be drawn from them. O'Connor (1987) found nine of his sample of eighty-one female offenders to be mothers or stepmothers (O'Connor, 1987), although I believe the psychological impact of being biological mother and stepmother to be very different and, thus, they should have been classified separately.

Many retrospective studies have been conducted to determine the impact of sexual abuse in children, particularly surveying college students (Fritz, Stoll, & Wagner, 1981; Fromuth & Burkart, 1987). Because the definition of "sexual abuse" varies so widely between the studies, it is difficult to pick up generalizations regarding predicative characteristics. Many of the adolescent boys reported a sexual experience, often with an adolescent babysitter, but considered the experience as positive rather than abusive (Risin & Koss, 1987). The profile of a female offender, therefore, tends to be young women in their twenties to early thirties, who have poor coping skills, may be depressed, or substance abusers, and may also meet the criteria for being personality disordered (Hall & Hall, 2007).

What causes a female to offend? My view is the same predispositions that cause men to offend, although, as discussed in Chapter Four, women may be protected somewhat by their higher levels of oxytocin and lower levels of testosterone. However, the insecure attachment, the vandalized sexual template, and adolescent trauma all have their part to play in the development of a female sexual offender. In Faller's (1987) study of seventy-two female sexual abusers, only 15% had no prior history of childhood trauma. Similarly, other studies have suggested that nearly all female sexual offenders experienced sexual assault when they were children (Vandiver & Kercher, 2004). Ford (2006) considered that it is an unpalatable truth that some women do experience sexual arousal to children without being coerced by men. And, as Peter (2006) argued, these women are labelled as mad, bad, or victims to explain behaviour that is considered outside of societal norm.

Transgenerational transmission makes it evident that some women do not know how to be maternal, will treat their children badly, will treat other women's children even worse, and pass this lack of caring and empathy on to their own children. When they did not learn boundaries as a child, they have no concept of boundaries with their own children. It needs the intervention of a significant caring attachment figure, and psychoeducation in understanding how to change, to break the cycle of abuse. Etherington (1997) found in her (albeit small) sample of men who had experienced childhood abuse by their mothers that all were first-born sons, and five out of seven were first-born children. This suggests that the mother was re-enacting her own abusive history with her first child, as that is how the memory works. Preparation for parenthood programmes could include a discussion about childhood sexuality to allow potential mothers to consider their own history, which may protect her children from her past.

Biological and behavioural models of treatment

In the early days of treatment of sex offenders, there was a predominance of biological and behavioural methodologies. If one takes a biological stance on their treatment, then the reduction of androgens in males may be seen as a way of reducing sexual interest, although there is no evidence that sexual arousal, even when it is reduced, is correlated with decreased recidivism of the sexual offender (Marshall & Barbaree, 1988; Quinsey, 1983). More recently, Beech and Mitchell (2005) have proposed the use of SSRIs (Specific Serotonin Reuptake Inhibitors prescribed as an antidepressant) as a treatment for offending. Their argument is that as many sex offenders have attachment disruptions and neglect in their histories, they will also have a reduction in oxytocin and vasopressin, the neuropeptides produced to make us CARE for one another. Oxytocin and vasopressin are found to be dependent on serotonin levels; thus, reducing the reuptake in serotonin might facilitate more appropriate attachment behaviours. As discussed in Chapter Eleven, stress, anxiety, and depression are often triggers for offending behaviour, so SSRIs may also have the effect of reducing the catalyst to the offence. In considering treatment, however, Finkelhor (1986) and Perkins (1989) maintained that negative blocks to deviant behaviour, such as being caught, being punished, feeling remorse, etc., will interrupt the offending cycle but will not prevent reoffending. They also highlight that offending has been an enormous, all-consuming part of the offender's life, and he has enjoyed it. If he is no longer going to do it, something powerful needs to take its place, and successful treatment programmes need to be cognizant of that (Garrison, 1992).

Sexual offender treatment programmes

The contemporary method of treatment of sexual offenders is the therapeutic relationship, conducted either with individuals or within groups. More recently, the move has been towards cognitive–behavioural treatment (CBT) methods that can shape the behaviour of the individual, and also focus on the cognitive distortions that allow the behaviour to occur. As Garrison (1992) contended, being motivated to rape or to abuse a child suggests something beyond the desire to abuse. It suggests intent. It also suggests a thought and behaviour cycle in which conscious fantasies, rehearsals, and planning takes place. "If to commit an offence, the perpetrator has to over-ride internal inhibitions, a deliberate decision must be made in which he justifies that judgement to himself, dismisses 'anti-motivations' and rationalises the proposed behaviour" (Garrison, 1992, p. 3).

It is on this premise that Garrison calls for cognitive-based behaviour programmes of treatment that will tap into this distorted thinking, called cognitive distortions, which include denial, minimization, normalization, justification, blame, and excuses (Powell, 2007). There are now psychometric scales available that will tap into the acceptance of rape myths and cognitive distortions about adult–child sex that enable therapists to assess the full extent of an offender's irrational beliefs (Salter, 1988). Cognitive skills training programmes (Ross & Fabiano, 1985) were devised to target the thinking styles that offenders develop which sustain criminal behaviour, and include working on impulse control, victim empathy, moral reasoning, problem-solving, and relapse prevention strategies. This is working on the presumed deficits of the individual and underestimates any propensity that the man may have to engage respectful or ethical improvements (Jenkins, 2009).

However, many research specialists have cautioned against this simplistic view that cognitive distortions and the abuse of children are actually related (Sheldon & Howitt, 2007). Laws and colleagues argued that it is a "received wisdom" to use these basic cognitive–behavioural methods of treatment of sex offenders, even though there is no substantial outcome evidence of their efficacy, predominantly because the model is insufficiently broad enough to encompass the wide variety of behaviours commonly found in sexual offending (Laws, Hudson, & Ward, 2000). Smallbone (2006) concurred, pointing out that cognitive distortions may emerge to rationalize the sexual offending, but they may not demonstrate why the offending behaviour occurred in the first place. Rich (2006) also agreed, and pointed out that although such cognitive interventions may be important aspects in helping recidivism, a thorough treatment has to involve attachment-informed therapy if one is looking for complete behavioural change. I agree with this. For a man who has committed an offence to be able to relax into his therapy, he needs to feel safe, so that he can integrate his current behaviour with his history. This ability to integrate is learnt behaviour that can only occur under conditions of safety. Confrontational or punitive methods of treatment can make them worse rather than better. It is alienation that will produce recidivism.

Offenders who externalize blame, or fail to take responsibility for their actions, are considered by many who work with sexual offenders to have a form of cognitive distortion that demonstrates the offenders' malevolence. Yet, it has been empirically established that externalization of blame is elicited through the process of shame (Tagney, Wagner, Fletcher, & Gramzow, 1992). It would seem more appropriate, therefore, to work on the shame, which is the underlying reason for the cognitive distortion, rather than simply trying to change a symptom. Maruna and Mann (2006) also argue that challenging these defensive cognitive distortions may actually be detrimental to desistance from offending behaviour, and may well damage the offender's mental health, presumably because the person is stripped bare of defences against shame. Lilienfeld (2007) also argued that some therapists pay too much attention to our psychotherapeutic dogma and ignore the fact that the wrong therapeutic method for the wrong person might actually cause him harm.

The Sex Offender Treatment Programme (SOTP) (Cowburn, Wilson, & Loewenstein, 1992) has been operating in a number of prisons in the UK in recent years. Depending on the circumstances of the offence and the history of the offender, prisoners undergo a core or extended programme, with a booster prior to release (Taylor, 1997). It used to be voluntary, although there were many consequences for not taking part, like loss of remission or parole. The ethical issue regarding this is self-evident, although one could argue that any form of treatment is preferable to basic incarceration. Yet, as any therapist is aware, a participant in a treatment programme who is not motivated to change will get nowhere, and will just waste time and resources. However, more contemporary sentencing for sex offenders *requires* that they undertake an SOTP, so long as they are in prison long enough, and so long as they admit their offence (Quayle, 2005). Individuals who commit sexual offences yet only receive short custodial sentences are not given the opportunity to undergo an SOTP (Halliday, 2001), and Gillespie (2005) questioned whether a short custodial sentence was of any use at all under these circumstances.

The SOTP is implemented by prison officers with basic training supervised by prison psychologists, and is largely cognitive–behavioural in approach, and aims to address anger management, fantasy modification, victim empathy, relationship skills, cognitive distortions and relapse prevention (Greenall & Jellicoe-Jones, 2007). The Probation Service also runs groups outside of the prison system in some areas of the country. Typically, in the UK, a sex offender group will operate for two- or three-hour sessions, once a week for six or twelve weeks. Yet, in the USA, residential treatment programmes range from eight to eighteen months, with an average length of stay of ten months (Heinz, Gargaro, & Kelly, 1987). As with all other treatment programmes in the UK, resources are cut down to the minimum, making efficacy of the programmes more doubtful.

The reason that a group model is so extensively used in work with sex offenders, Garrison (1992) contends, is to break down the secretive nature and denial regarding offending. Similarly, Lindsay, Olley, Jack, Morrison, and Smith (1998) hailed the efficacy of group work after empirical studies involving (two) sexual offenders with learning disabilities. They demonstrated the ability to highlight cognitive distortions, facilitate behavioural change, and develop interpersonal skills within a group context. But, here, the notion of treating all sexual offenders as if they are the same has to be questioned. There is evidence to suggest that the nature of the offence is similar for both handicapped and non-handicapped offenders (Griffiths, Hingsburger, & Christian, 1985), yet research shows that offenders with learning disability are more likely to become violent (Gilby, Wolf, & Goldberg, 1989) and are more likely to have male rather than female victims (Griffiths, Hingsburger, & Christian, 1985). Similarly, rapists are more likely to be aggressive within treatment than other sex offenders, and are more likely to drop out of treatment programmes. So, they are clearly not operating on the same profiles. Ward and Marshall (2004) argued that reliance on manual-based interventions in the standard treatment of offenders means that therapists fail to see the individual with whom they are working.

Welldon and van Velson (1997) highlighted the conflict in people's values when considering the treatment of sex offenders. They pointed out that everyone cares for victims as they rightly should, yet the offenders are treated as if they are products of "evil forces" and there is a cultural denial of the empirical evidence that demonstrates that a large proportion of victims become perpetrators (Welldon, 1997). Sheath (1990) agreed, and questioned the validity of the assumptions about sex offenders of many probation workers. He argued that every offender is unique, and that the only purpose of the group confrontational style is that it gives the workers the opportunity to vent their personal feelings of disgust against offenders and to break them down. "Hooray, I hear people cry—if he tops himself then good riddance" (ibid., p. 161).

Others agree that sex offenders are heartily disliked by general psychiatrists and by some forensic psychologists, and there is a debate about whether they come under the remit of psychiatry at all (Welldon & van Velsen, 1997). This seems to have been acted out with some of the Internet offender clients I have seen. Despite never having been convicted of a "contact" offence against a child, and despite not having a paedophile orientation and, therefore, not having a predominant sexual interest in children, they are instantly removed from their own children by the social and probation services and told they will not have a relationship with their children until each reaches eighteen. While in prison, they are told that they will not get parole or go out on licence (especially if they have been given an indeterminate sentence for public protection (IPP), which essentially holds them for life until such time as they are considered suitable for release from bi-annual parole review boards) until they have admitted their offence and completed an SOTP. However, many prisons do not have the facilities to undertake SOTPs, and many others have no spaces on their SOTP. And anyway, the offenders are told, they need to conduct an ETS (Effective Thinking Skills) course first. But if they do an ETS course, they are told that the course will enable them to manipulate their way through an SOTP, so they are not considered suitable for it. And if the offender is rich enough to be able to pay for their own privately-based SOTP, they are denied permission to attend, as it may not meet all the criteria that has been set. These perpetual double-binds demonstrate the antipathy that professional workers covertly reveal in their dealings with these offenders, and continue to persecute and punish the offender long after serving the actual sentence for their crime. Ward and Connelly (2008) point out that everyone is entitled to their Human Rights, except those who have committed sexual offences. They elaborate that the correctional policies and subsequent interventions have focused solely on community protection and risk management. As a consequence, this managerial perspective has produced harsh and dispropor-tionate punishments and the denial of basic human rights.

Outcome research

The one point upon which most writers concur when discussing treatment for sex offenders is the paucity of valid empirical research, both on the theoretical underpinning of treatment pro-grammes, and their outcome evaluation (Bancroft, 1995; Blackburn, 1993; Howitt, 1995), although Marshall and Moulden (2006) point out that one person in every ten will reoffend after completing an SOTP. The use of the penile plethysmograph (PPG), which records penile tumescence, is a commonly used laboratory method of in-vestigating sexual arousal, and many outcome evaluations have been undertaken using this methodological procedure (Bancroft, 1974). For example, Abel and colleagues devised a rape index using the degree of erectile response to depictions of rape divided by the response to scenes of consensual sex. They demonstrated that they could discriminate between rapists and non-rapists with this index (Abel, Barlow, Blanchard, & Guild, 1977). However, one needs to be cautious in how one interprets the responses of men in laboratory conditions. Quinsey, Chaplin, and Varney (1981) found that the penile responses of men increased if they were told beforehand that normal men did that. Similarly, Malamuth and Donnerstein (1982) found that men showed high arousal if it was apparent that a female rape victim was involuntarily sexually aroused. Flak and colleagues argue that the reliability studies using PPG have been way below the minimum level one would expect from a psychometric test, especially as the response can be faked, noting that 20–30% of data from PPG studies have had to be excluded from the studies because of the low level of response (Flak, Beech, & Fisher, 2007).

Despite the methodological integrity of some of the research discussed above, though, researchers are making fundamental assumptions about the role of sexual arousal in sexual offending that may have no empirical validation. Howitt (1995) argued that sexual arousal and subsequent orgasm is not necessarily the aim of many paedophiles when they are with children, as they may choose to have their climax later when masturbating to the fantasies of being with the children. Thus, Howitt contends, this places in doubt the whole role of phallometric assessment in order to test hypotheses about sexual arousal, where no causal link has been demonstrated between that arousal and offending or recidivism.

Beckett, Beech, Fisher, and Fordham (1994) evaluated the therapeutic impact on sexual offenders from seven probation programmes that were well established and represented the range of treatment programmes offered by the Probation Services in the UK, using a pre- and post-test design. They found, interestingly, that 70% of their sample had been victimized as children, which is higher than has been found in other studies. Beckett and colleagues (*ibid.*) criticized the programmes for failing to adequately assess their clients systematically, for not giving support following discharge from the programme, and for treating rapists with offenders who abused children. Fisher (1994), found that 54% of offenders showed improvements after treatment, although short-term therapy had no effect with highly deviant men. Some other studies have suggested low recidivism rates post therapy, only to find that the follow-up period after treatment has been a short period of less than five years (Hanson, Morton, & Harris, 2003; Vandiver, 2006). Reconviction rates for sexual offenders are thought to be low (Grubin, 1998), although Craig and Beech (2009) argue that long-term recidivism rates can be high: as much as 39% for rapists and 52% for child abusers. Falshaw and colleagues conducted an investigation into the Thames Valley Project for the treatment of sex offenders (Falshaw, Friendship, & Bates, 2003). They found that the reconviction rate of 173 offenders who had undergone the TVSOTP was only 6%. However, even the non-offending behaviour of the offenders was deemed by the researchers to be indicative of potential recidivism. So, their perceived sexual recidivism rate was 5.3 times higher, and they were, therefore, calling for reconviction rates to be multiplied by this factor for risk assessment. This seems to be use and abuse of statistical information. What this false positive prediction actually does is to put low-risk offenders in expensive and unnecessary treatment, or cause them to remain in prison when they have little risk of reoffending (Craig & Beech, 2009).

Outcome evaluations of psychotherapeutic techniques for the treatment of sex offenders are few in the literature, most commonly because the nature of psychotherapy does not lend itself to the classic methods of research analysis. For example, the considered gold standard of randomized control trials (RCTs) would compare, say, cognitive–behavioural therapy with psychodynamic therapy with a placebo or "no-treatment" condition. Offenders would be allocated at random to one of these three groups. However, one would need a sufficiently large sample of offenders to fit into each group, which may not be available in certain areas of the country. Then the randomization itself would present ethical difficulties. It would mean allocating offenders to a no-treatment group when they may desperately need or want therapy, and, similarly, allocating offenders to a treatment group when they may not want to participate in that sort of programme. In addition, the relationship between the therapist and the client is considered one of the most fundamental aspects of good outcome of therapy (van Balen, 1990), yet randomization does not allow individuals to make choices about whether they can work with a specific therapist or client. Thus, the research methodology *per se* can confound the data one is trying to collect, and just highlights the manifest difficulties of trying to use an objective method to analyse a subjective process.

The available research literature tends to use self-report questionnaires to measure outcome, yet sex offenders are (understandably) characteristic for under-reporting of their offences. Many studies use forensic populations of offenders who are either in prison or out on licence. The incidence of respondents therefore being circumspect with the truth for fear of the consequences is again going to be understandable. Similarly, physiological methods that offer a quick objective measurement are used irrespective of the invalid assumptions regarding sexual arousal, as previously discussed. The late probation officer-turned-therapist Ray Wyre wanted a more practicable model for working with sex offenders that could be translated directly from the empirical research into treatment programmes (Wyre, 1987). He argued that research shows that sex offenders commit many more offences than they admit to, so the therapist should assume the validity of that contention and encourage (challenge) the offender to disclose the full extent of his offending. Wyre's approach to the treatment of sex offenders at the Gracewell Clinic has reported that no offender attending his programme has been convicted of a sexual offence since its establishment in 1988, as far as he was aware (Wyre, 2003), although we need to reiterate that being economical with the truth is a facet of the offender's problem, because levels of shame are so high. However, Wyre's approach to treatment tended to be highly confrontational, and research has demonstrated that a confrontational approach made some offenders worse (Marshall & Moulden, 2006; Marshall, et al., 2002). Furby, Weinrott, and Blackshaw (1989) conducted an extensive review of recidivism studies, and they noted that untreated sex offenders had lower recidivism rates than treated sex offenders. This is not necessarily a statement about the ineffectiveness of the treatment, however, but may be a statement about the lack of rigorous research. Howitt (1995) points out that this is a warning shot against complacency about SOTPs, and quotes Wyre as saying, "It may be that I'm just creating very clever offenders" (Fitzherbert, 1993).

As discussed above, the literature on the treatment programmes of sex offenders is rife with fundamental methodological flaws, and produces very little evidence of efficacy or effectiveness. However, the common use of therapy groups within the UK for dealing with sex offenders has financial imperatives that appeal to the accountants who determine the budgets for the treatment programmes, even though groups do not necessarily meet the needs of the individual sexual offender. The point made earlier about every offender being unique is an important one, and may contribute to the lack of effectiveness of many treatment programmes. If one makes a comparison with violent crime, would it be appropriate to group together professional "hit" men, and armed robbers, with the man who kills his wife in a furious row after he discovers she has been having an affair? Despite all being crimes of violence, they are fundamentally different responses to life situations and need to be treated as such. Similarly, it is inappropriate to group all sexual offenders together and offer the same treatment for all. As I have highlighted, many rapists have the arousing effect of aggression and violence contributing to their deviant behaviour, whereas an incestuous child abuser may perceive his behaviour as an extension of his love for the child. Both need to learn appropriate victim empathy and the extent of both the physical and psychological damage they can do to their victims, but the underpinning of their crimes is essentially very different and some aspects of their treatment should not be dealt with in a group situation. Having said that, Davenport and Fisher (2007) argue that contemporary emphasis on victim empathy as a demonstration of progress in a person's treatment is inappropriate, as it is wrong to work with the offender on dealing with the feelings of the victim when no one has considered his feelings after his own abuse or trauma (Davenport & Fisher, 2007; Jenkins, 2009).

It is also necessary to distinguish between the types of persons who offend against children, as again this is not a unitary concept. As previously discussed, there are those who are sexually aroused by infants and toddlers (infantophilia), so the underpinning and treatment for this paraphilia will need to be very different than for those hebephiles or ephebophiles who are aroused by fourteen- or fifteen-year old boys or girls (Lolita syndrome). Likewise, there is a difference between a predatory paedophile who will stalk, abduct, abuse, and maybe harm someone else's child when compared to an incestuous relationship with a child where the abuse takes place as part of the family system, or where someone has looked at pictures of children on the Internet but has not committed any contact offence. Differences in offending have been shown empirically. For example, Radzinowicz (1957) discovered that, after four years, twice as many men reoffended against male children as did those who offended against female children. We also know that incest offenders have the lowest recidivism rates (Bartosh, Garby, Lewis, & Gray, 2003). And there are differences between those who undertake actual contact offences against children compared to those who look at pictures (as discussed in Chapter Eleven), which are essentially offences of voyeurism. These fundamental differences in offending are not only lost in any generic treatment programme, but the offender may psychologically opt out of active participation in group treatment if he felt that he was different from the others in some way. Of course, child protection agencies will argue that looking at pictures of abuse is as bad as doing it, as the viewers are colluding with the abuse of a child. This is an academic argument that has merit, which serves to elaborate the enormity of the offence, to break down denial, and to encourage greater victim empathy. However, as far as treatment is concerned, looking is *not* doing, and treating a man who views abusive images of children in the same way as a man who abducts and murders a child is both disproportionate and inappropriate.

Nearly thirty years ago, West (1980) argued for the decriminalization of some sex offences, including incest, to keep the police and social services out of people's lives. He contended that therapists should be allowed to work with the individual on condition that the therapy was undertaken, and he advocated the treatment to include self-restraint, social responsibility, and social skills training rather than pure erotic orientation (although sometimes all will be required). Contemporary society would not accept this view, as all sexual offenders have become *personae non gratae*, despite being a society where sexual prowess is thrust into the public face through every conceivable electronic and marketing medium. There would be a huge public backlash if it were thought that men who offended against children would be given clemency. However, what is very clear is that if the roots of paedophilia lie in childhood (Howitt, 1995), these issues need to be addressed therapeutically in order to prevent recidivism, and cognitive–behavioural methods are necessary but insufficient. The very specific, individual issues of attachments, childhood trauma, and abuse cannot be worked through in group situations where shame is so high and the damage so great. This does require long-term one-to-one intensive psychotherapy, where the offender can develop trust and attachment to a therapist to help heal and change the working models and behavioural pathways. Circles of support, volunteers who befriend offenders in the community after they are released from prison, are also valuable as a means of reintegrating the "pariahs of our society" back into community living. It does seem to me to be incredibly short-sighted to always be counting the fiscal cost of how much this individual therapeutic treatment would be for each individual offender, without counting the fiscal cost of repetitively imprisoning a person for repeat offences, or considering the psychological and emotional costs to their victims and the damage done to society.

Risk assessment

Fernandez (2006) has argued that over the past decade, the focus of people working with offenders has been dominated by a risk management model, which not only has numerous flaws in its process, but also gives little attention for improving the individual's quality of life, although, parenthetically, some may argue, as discussed above, that a sexual offender has no right to demand any quality of life. Therefore, I want to spend some time discussing risk, considering that the intellectual argument of reducing risk is such a compelling one.

Craig and colleagues argue that risk assessment is the cornerstone of effective offender management (Craig, Browne, Hogue, & Stringer, 2004). But first, we need to discuss what risk assessment actually is. Doren (2006) argued that there are fundamental misconceptions occurring over this important concept, and that people use the notion of risk assessment when they are actually looking for predictions. He pointed out that these are essentially different things. A risk assessment is an evaluation on a degree of possibility that is here and now, whereas a prediction is a forecast and something that may or may not occur in the future.

So, is undertaking a risk assessment looking at a prediction of reoffending? We cannot possibly know how many people actually reoffend; we can only know how many people get *convicted* of reoffending. Reconviction rates are, therefore, used as the indicator of recidivism.

Recidivism actually means falling back into crime; that is, repeating what you have done in the past. Yet, many professionals use actuarial methods of risk assessment, based on recidivism studies, to determine whether the person's behaviour will escalate into other offending behaviour: for example, whether a man convicted of viewing imagery of abusive images of children on the Internet will actually act out fantasies and be at risk of contact offences with children. This is a leap of logic that actuarial instruments cannot possibly provide. Actuarial methods of risk assessment also need a normalization process to make a comparison with. The norming procedure of such instruments makes comparison with the (so-called) normal population and the offending population that do not undertake sexual offending. As already mentioned, researchers often categorize sexual offenders into three groups: rapists, paedophiles, and incest offenders (Marshall, 2006). Internet offenders do not fit comfortably with any of these groups, and have been shown to be significantly different (Sheldon & Howitt, 2007). When considering the risk of Internet offenders, it is known from Operation Ore that their offending profile is completely different: white, middle-aged, professional-class men in full-time employment compared to the socially isolated, inadequate person, often unemployed, with a lower than average IQ, of a predatory paedophile. Interestingly, *inter alia*, Internet offenders do not support attitudes that explicitly endorse or condone the sexual abuse of children (Bates & Metcalf, 2007), as is common with contact offenders.

Thus, to conduct a forensic risk assessment on Internet offenders, it would not be appropriate to use the standard SACJ, Static-99 or the Risk Matrix 2000 instruments, all of which have been developed using a different offender profile. And, as Bates and Metcalf (2007) point out, the higher IQ of the Internet offender would give them the capacity to fake a good psychometric assessment anyway. It is also inappropriate to use these instruments for female offenders, sexual offenders with learning disabilities, and people with a paedophilic orientation over the age of sixty years (Doren, 2006). Despite there not being any empirical evidence on the trustworthiness of clinical judgement, contemporary thinking in working with Internet offenders is that "assessment instruments cannot replace the personal interaction and clinical judgement of a trained therapist" (Delmonico, Griffin, & Carnes, 2002, p. 150), because tests to evaluate Internet offenders are still in the early stages of development (Cooper, Golden, & Marshall, 2006; Foley, 2002).

There is a plethora of literature debating the use of psychometric and actuarial methods of risk assessment compared to clinical judgement. Hanson and Bussière (1998) conducted a meta-analysis of sixty-one studies to identify factors that most strongly related to recidivism in sexual offenders, and essentially found that the predominant risk factors were those who showed sexual deviancy, previous convictions for sexual offences, and those who failed to complete treatment. Completing treatment is an important factor, as analysis has shown that those who complete treatment are less likely to have a history of non-violent offences and less often diagnosed with a personality disorder (Beyko & Wong, 2005). Hanson and Bussière also suggested that offenders with deviant sexual interests are those who victimize strangers, use force, select male victims, or select victims much younger or much older than themselves. Hall and Hall agreed. They suggested:

> The more deviant the sexual practices of the offender, the younger the abused child: the more sociopathic or antisocial personality traits displayed, the greater the treatment noncompliance; and the greater the paraphilic interests reported by the offender, the higher the likelihood of reoffence. [Hall & Hall, 2007, p. 467]

Again, it is unclear where individuals who view abusive images of children on the Internet but who do not commit any contact offences would fit into this. Some of the imagery they look at may be extremely deviant or bizarre, yet their sexual activity in relationships may be vanilla sex. Hanson and Bussière produced a table of predictors in sexual recidivism, but the predictive accuracy of most of them was so small, no justification could be given for viewing them in isolation. And, despite the contemporary emphasis on cognitive distortions as the focus for treatment, Hanson and Bussière's meta-analysis did not find that cognitions that excuse, justify, or rationalize offending behaviour predicted recidivism. Predictive factors that were significant were whether the person attends and responds well in a treatment programme, showing good motivation and expressing remorse, and taking responsibility for their behaviour and the consequences of it. In addition, one needs to consider whether alcohol or drugs played a part in the offending, whether they have social support in a relationship or close-knit family (attachments), and what the offender has to say about their strategies for relapse prevention. These are the predictive factors that need clinical assessment rather than psychometric measures. Hanson and Bussière called for further research into the contribution of other factors as yet inadequately researched, such as unfulfilled intimacy needs, using sex as a coping mechanism (Cortoni &

Marshall, 2001), and developmental precursors of sexual offending, which are the factors that I have tried to address herewith.

Having said all that, clinicians do vary in their individual ability to assess risk, and the drive to find actuarial methods of risk assessment comes from the desire to bring some reliability into the approach. That is why the Criminal Justice Act of 1991 requires the assessment of risk to be determined by a validated actuarial risk instrument. In making such an assessment, there is a need to view static risk factors, like the number of previous convictions, and whether the person is married or single, compared to dynamic factors such as attendance at treatment programmes and the extent of cognitive distortions. The main criticism of actuarial methods is that they oversimplify a multi-factorial event (Craig & Beech, 2009) and rely predominantly on static factors. Therefore, they do not take into account a person's response to treatment or change over time. For example, the Static-99 (Hanson & Thornton, 1999) does not predict recidivism *per se*. It gives a prediction that over a five-year follow-up, 39% of a sample will be reconvicted (*ibid.*). However, other research has suggested that these recidivism rates are too high (Nunes, Firestone, Bradsford, Greenberg, & Broom, 2002). Doren (2006) emphasized that if predictive assessments are to have any meaning, they must be based on stable dynamic risk factors, such as whether a person has benefited from a treatment programme. He argued that even the worst sex offenders are not offending all the time, so assessments need to tap into the latent potentials and triggers.

More recent developments in assessment tools are trying to introduce both stable and acute dynamic factors into the equation. An example of a stable dynamic factor would be an individual's attitude to his offence, tolerance of sexual crimes, or holding rape myths. Acute dynamic factors would be whether the individual abused drugs or alcohol likely to precipitate offending. The Structured Anchored Clinical Judgement (SACJ) tries to avoid the overdependence on static factors by introducing a three-stage assessment of: (1) assessment of static factors, (2) analysis of additional aggravating factors, and (3) a monitoring of offender performance over time (Grubin, 1998). Again, the last two stages rely on clinical information, whereas researchers seem to be working hard to move away from clinical dependency, so that police officers, probation officers, social workers, etc., can monitor risk without needing therapeutic input. The SACJ was, therefore, enhanced into the Risk Matrix 2000 (Hanson & Thornton, 2000) and the Sex Offender Need Assessment Rating (SONAR) (Hanson & Harris, 2000) for risk management plans. Predictive accuracy of the Risk Matrix 2000 is above chance levels over an eleven-year period (Kingston, Yates, Firestone, Babchishin, & Bradford, 2008), although the Sex Offender Risk Appraisal Guide (SORAG) was found to be superior.

The biggest problem with many of these actuarial instruments is that they are designed for a specific subgroup of sexual offender, and translate poorly into other offending groups (Craig, Browne, & Beech, 2008). In practice, sexual offenders and violent offenders are linked together as people who need special treatment, even though many sexual offenders are not predatory and have not committed any contact offences (like those who view images on the Internet). Yet, many are treated in the same way as those who are violent and rape and murder their victims. The methodology of combining all these different sexual offenders and merging them with violent offender groups, as is commonly found in risk assessment outcome literature, produces mismatched validity and is consistently being criticized (Craig, Beech, & Browne, 2007).

As Craig, Browne, and Beech (2008) point out, actuarial risk measures only provide probabilistic estimates of the likelihood that certain specific behaviours in a specific group of sexual offenders is likely to occur within a specified period of time. Actuarials make a good job of being able to rank an individual's recidivism risk relative to another for a particular offence, and being able to separate offenders into groups that differ in their likelihood of offending, so long as they are used in the context they were designed for rather than for a broad sweep of a categorized group of offenders. As Power (2003, p. 83) argued, they should not be used as "a blunt instrument". But their ability to determine an absolute risk factor to a specific individual at this stage is impossible. And, as Craig and Beech (2009) point out, they are designed only to identify those who will reoffend. No consideration is given to any factors that might indicate that the individual will desist from offending. It must be reiterated that although these tools are developing in sophistication and accuracy, they are measures of the risk of recidivism in a previous offence, and not a measure or prediction of future escalation of offences, or a risk predictor of future harm. Ward and Marshall

(2004, p. 155) argued that it is time to stop "the perception of offenders as bundles of risk factors rather than integrated, complex beings who are seeking to give value and meaning to their lives".

Smallbone (2006) also expressed doubts about the over-emphasis in risk assessment on individual cognitive distortions, empathy deficits, and sexual preferences, without considering the interaction between the offender and the situation he is in. He iterated Cohen and Felson (1979), who pointed out that offences against children have three elements, not just one offender: there is the potential offender, a potential child victim, and an absent guardian of the child. Interestingly, again, this does not seem to be the case for Internet offenders, as the child victims and their subsequent images were often the result of the behaviour of another offender. However, together with Wortley, Smallbone argued that the problem lies in the contemporary focus on risk factors for the individual, rather than considering the situations that allow offending to occur (Wortley & Smallbone, 2006). While agreeing with this concept wholeheartedly, I am mindful that the current focus of treatment is on the offence as if it defines the offender. It would be preferable, therefore, if we could take a preventative approach by offering help and support for vulnerable families, whose children are at risk of being damaged sexually, physically, or emotionally. It would also be helpful if social service and probation workers regain the connection, in their determination to protect children, by remembering that the offenders were once damaged children themselves. By making that connection, maybe their treatment could be more compassionate, and, with less alienation, recidivism could be reduced. Currently, what many professionals are doing is assessing the person's offence outside of the context of his attachment and developmental history. I hope this book has illustrated that when working with sexual offenders, we ignore their attachment and developmental history to everyone's cost. Successful understanding and treatment of sexual offenders is a child protection issue.

Gordon's review

Gordon could not bring himself to accept that Rachel had rejected and abandoned him. His frantic searching for her was precipitated from "running around" his insecure template, bouncing between feelings of PANIC and LOSS, eliciting huge sympathetic responses of FEAR and RAGE. With Gordon's usual, although dysfunctional, method of self-soothing taken away from him, in the loss of his computer, Gordon slumped into a depressive state with strong suicidal ideation. No longer having the ability to regulate his strong emotions of FEAR and RAGE, he used nicotine and alcohol to precipitate long periods of sleep in order to anaesthetize his pain. Events took him over, however, and he was left sitting in a prison cell to contemplate his fate.

As Gordon's narcissism was compensatory, his depression and the critical life event he experienced would provide a critical window of opportunity to change, should he be motivated to do so, and should he be given the right help and support in order to facilitate it.

CHAPTER FOURTEEN

The neurobiological effect of psychotherapy

Gordon was sitting in the interview room of the police station with the duty solicitor. He looked across at a young man on the other side of the table shuffling and sorting papers. He was dressed in a brown, well-cut suit and amber-coloured tie, and had neatly trimmed hair and fingernails. Gordon assessed that he and this solicitor were roughly the same age. It made Gordon take an inward look at himself, with a week's growth of beard, unkempt, unwashed, filthy, broken fingernails, torn jeans, and an unironed, out of shape, black T-shirt. The comparison made him draw a deep breath. In an instant, he seemed to be at the other side of the room watching himself and the solicitor together. How had he got himself into this? He had such plans, such dreams for himself: owning a garage, driving a smart new BMW, beautiful wife and a couple of kids living in a nice, modern four-bedroomed detached house on the nearby Bovis estate. Now he was virtually destitute. He had no family, was going to be evicted from his flat, and was facing a prison sentence. Even his mother would have nothing to do with him. What had gone wrong?

The solicitor looked up with a kindly smile. He had just explained to Gordon the procedure of how Gordon would be bailed

274 INFANT LOSSES, ADULT SEARCHES

pending the police investigation of his computer, as well as his DVDs and videos, which might take several months. Then his criminal charges will be based on the number and categories of illegal images that they find.

"I'll be honest with you, Gordon," the solicitor said. "I am not sure at this stage whether you are facing a custodial sentence or not. But what I do know is that the Bench is more lenient with guys like you if they show some remorse and try to make some reparation for what they have done. The best thing you can do over the next few months is try to sort yourself out. You are already known to the police because of your violence to your ex-partner, so the judge will not look kindly at that."

Gordon felt a sudden flash of anger, and opened his mouth to make a cutting remark. Then he felt a flush of shame, his face reddened, and his eyes looked at the floor. He could hear a voice, as if from the other side of the room, saying, "Keep your trap shut. This guy is trying to help you. It's your big ideas and big mouth that has got you into this mess."

Gordon closed his mouth and nodded. Then looked up and said, "What do you think I should do?"

"Well, a shower wouldn't go amiss. You really have let yourself go, haven't you? When did you last eat?"

Gordon did not reply. The solicitor started putting all the papers into a brown leather briefcase. "Try and get back to work. There are always jobs for good mechanics, I should imagine. You needn't disclose the pending prosecution until you are actually charged with something. Smarten up your act, and if you really want to turn your life around, I suggest you see someone—get some therapy. We will need a psychological report when it comes to your sentencing anyway, so it will make life easier if it is someone who already knows you quite well."

Gordon's stomach turned over. "You think I'm mad, then?" The solicitor closed his briefcase with a snap and stopped and looked at Gordon earnestly.

"No, I do not think you are mad, Gordon. But you are messed up and you have a serious problem with anger. It seems to me you have two choices. You can carry on going on as you are, but your next step on that path looks like living on the streets, or you can try to turn things around by learning to understand why you do the things you do and change them."

This time Gordon could not suppress his narcissistic rage. "It's all right for you public school boys, with your fancy suit and your fancy money!" he spat. "What do you know about living in the real world? Everyone is out to get you, one way or another!"

The smile on the solicitor's face froze. "Listen, Gordon," he said coldly. "Life is what you make it with the skills and talents that you were born with. I didn't go to public school. I went to the same comprehensive school as you did. I remember you. You were a couple of years in front of me. You had an attitude then, and you have an attitude now. And look where it's got you."

Gordon's face again flushed with shame. "But where do I go? Who do I see? I don't know anything about these things."

The solicitor took a small pad out of his jacket pocket, and scribbled down a name and a number. He ripped off the page and handed to Gordon, some warmth returning to his face.

"Here. This woman specializes in your kind of offence, and she has done some really good work with some of my other clients." With that, the solicitor shook Gordon's hand, and left the room.

Changing behavioural templates

John Bowlby considered that internal working models of behaviour were changeable via consistent disconfirming evidence that contradicts the internal working models (Shorey & Snyder, 2006). He proposed that once people became aware of their working models, where they come from, and what they do, they could learn to abandon them in favour of behaving in different ways (Bowlby, 1988). Davila and Levy (2006) listed the five tasks for psychotherapy, using Bowlby's perspective:

1.   To establish a secure base between therapist and client.
2.   To explore the client's attachment history.
3.   To relate the therapeutic relationship, using it as a method of understanding a different way of relating.

4.   Making links between past experience and present behaviour.
5.   Revising internal working models into more functional ways
      of behaving.

The ability to examine life events afresh and reconceptualize painful times in a narrative process is vital in healing attachment wounds. As Main (1991) suggested, the individual needs to take a step back and examine his own cognitive processes at work, re-evaluating the story in the process of telling it. The client needs to re-experience the original trauma within the safe frame of the new therapeutic attachment figure (Eells, 2001). This facilitates the mentalization of the story while regulating the hyperarousal. This may, of course, produce other emotional reactions: for example, the client may start mourning as he realizes what his life could have been and his missed opportunities. Holmes (1998) agreed with this therapeutic process. He called it a process of story-making and story-breaking, as the person is helped to reframe and retell the story in a healing light.

Therapy with neural connection

It used to be considered that the brain was not capable of change in adulthood; that its plasticity ceased around the age of fourteen years, as that is when the development of new neurones ceased. Contemporary thinking has modified this view, however, because the multiple numbers of neural dendrite connections is so vast that new connections can always be made. Further, it is held that processes such as psychotherapy, which involves an affective relationship with a therapist, can prompt actual biological change in the right hemisphere (Barbas, 1995) and much research is currently being conducted evaluating psychotherapeutic techniques with brain scanning outcome measures (Linden, 2006; Roffman, Marci, Glick, Dougherty, & Rauchl, 2005; Siegle, Carter, & Thase, 2006).

Kumari (2006) reviewed the evidence that successful psychological therapies induce changes to brain function, often in a way comparable to drug treatments. In a study of people with depression, brain imaging found recovery was associated with decreased metabolism in the ventrolateral prefrontal cortex, both in clients who had improved after taking Seroxat, and in clients who had undergone cognitive–behavioural therapy (CBT). Moreover, CBT elicited brain changes not seen with Seroxat, including increased activity in the cingulate, frontal, and hippocampus regions of the brain. However, Panskepp (1998) pointed out that some long-lasting fears and anxieties leading to chronic psychological distress do not always respond well to standard cognitive therapies, because the subcortical networks that are overactivated in trauma become so sensitized that they operate independently of cognitive functions. Similarly, Liotti (1993) argued that mentalization stops when the attachment system (PANIC) is triggered. It is vital, therefore, that talking therapies operate on calming the physiological systems of the body as well as dealing with the irrational or distorted thought processes.

Schore (2001) emphasized that it is not our expertly learnt interventions that promote psychobiological change, but the intersubjective process of therapy as the client learns to find a new secure base. By making secure attachments within the security of a therapeutic alliance, interrupted developmental processes can finally be completed (Gedo, 1979).

Insights into the physiological benefits of psychotherapy come from the use of positron emission tomography (PET), functional magnetic resonance imaging (fMRI), diffusion tensor imaging (DTI) and other scanning techniques to see how psychotherapy itself affects the brain. The focus is usually around the limbic system, the centre for the integration of the preprogrammed emotional circuits, learnt emotional responses, and somatic and semantic memories. The prefrontal cortex, which supplies the capacity for long-term planning, judgement, and self-control is also involved, as it connects to the subcortical emotional centres and gives the thinking systems the opportunity to reduce or modify the expressions of emotion. Straube and colleagues demonstrated through fMRI scanning that when a person who fears snakes is confronted with one, there is an increase in blood flow and energy consumption in the amygdala (Straube, Glauer, Dilger, Mentzel, & Miltner, 2006), discussed in Chapter Two, and FEAR and RAGE are triggered, with contemporaneous increases in the insula, a region that registers disgust and pain (possibly also connected to a RAGE circuit). Treatment with talking therapies will access the limbic system via the prefrontal cortex. As the language of the therapy modifies and reduces the strength of the emotion, it creates new emotional and behavioural circuits. These changes in several parts of the pre-frontal cortex have been identified with the scanning. Figure 23 elaborates the secure and insecure templates discussed in the previous chapters. Two processes are required to help the person move from an insecure working model to a secure one.

First, the therapist is providing a warm and supportive therapeutic alliance, with good eye contact, and warm and supportive encouragement of the client's autonomous attempts to change. The therapist mimics the original attachment model, and helps develop a new pathway back to CARE. For the adult client in therapy, becoming aware of this default behavioural pathway helps him to change. However, the insecure attachment template feels safe to him, even though it has negative consequences. It is his comfort zone. So, to move away from it in order to create a new, more secure attachment template, the person is required to move out of his comfort zone, and this is likely promote anxiety, until he gets used to the new way of being. Carroll (2003) described this change in neural templates as disorganization to reorganization, using well-timed chaos in therapeutic emotional outpouring to provide the turning point for deeper insight or reframing of traumatic historical events. However, this also mirrors the misattunement and rapprochement that occurs in the infant attachment process. As the

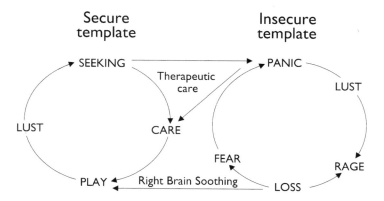

Figure 23. Therapy is designed to help the individual move from an insecure working model to a secure one, by providing therapeutic CARE and encouraging right brain soothing.

child tentatively but excitedly steps out of his comfort zone to explore new ways in the world, he checks back to mother for positive reinforcement, which attenuates the fear. So, too, with therapist and client: being the good enough therapist (mother or father), and providing positive reinforcement together with strong, clear boundaries for security. Cozolino (2002) argued that under these conditions of exploration of feelings without judgement and with good support, the stress produced in the client provides the right conditions for neural growth and integration. He highlighted the essential components of neurobiological therapeutic growth as:

- a secure attachment relationship with an attuned therapist;
- the activation of emotional arousal and cognitive systems;
- the construction of positive narratives to reflect a sense of self.

Above all, he emphasized the need for the attachment relationship with the therapist to activate the neuroplastic process (*ibid.*, p. 308).

In Figure 24, one can see a diagram of the brain viewed from the top. The emotional disturbance is in the limbic area of the right brain. The volume control to these emotions, called rationality, is in the prefrontal left brain. Good psychotherapy will create a new pathway between these two areas; first, by right brain soothing (to be discussed later in this chapter) to calm down some of the extreme emotions, and then, in therapy, using knowledge of the past to place the behaviour of the present into context, and then

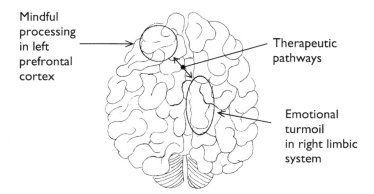

Mindful processing in left prefrontal cortex

Therapeutic pathways

Emotional turmoil in right limbic system

Figure 24. Therapy can establish a pathway between the two hemispheres.

visualizing and planning future changes. Here, we can see the parallels between Freudian ideas of making the unconscious conscious (Freud, 1915e) and neuroscientific ideas of reasserting the prefrontal cortex (or the slow and accurate route of analysis and response) over the limbic system (the quick and dirty route) (LeDoux, 1996). This reconnection of right and left brain processes are vital to the holistic long-term efficacy of therapeutic interventions, irrespective of the therapeutic model used. Integrating the processing of the two hemispheres enables traumatic memories to be processed in a new way, and to be saved in a new place in the brain, allowing resolution to occur (Siegel, 2003).

Indeed, one of the reasons that EMDR (eye movement desensitization and reprocessing) treatment is considered so effective for healing trauma is that it reactivates both hemispheres to allow emotional regulation and verbal cognition (Shapiro & Maxfield, 2003).

It has now been established that psychotherapy facilitates the alteration of emotional circuits, leading to changes in how socioemotional information is processed (Basch, 1988), particularly the connections between the limbic system and the prefrontal cortex (McKenna, 1994). Treatment with medication alone will reduce the activity of the limbic system, but will not make new circuitry changes in the prefrontal cortex. This demonstrates that the physiological effects of medication and psychotherapy are different.

Many clients are reassured to know that childhood memories are laid out neurally in the right brain at a preverbal level, and that they may evoke strong feelings, memories, or senses in the therapy, without the ability to explain why. It will also help to share with the client how some of their inner working models are dysfunctional, provoking the LOSS that they most fear from self-fulfilling behavioural repertoires. Clients who learn an understanding of the basis for their fears can subsequently learn how to moderate their emotions and construct appropriate emotional distances with their attachment figures.

Schore (2003c) highlighted that a good therapist needs to use both sides of her brain. The right side invokes her own intuitive, unconscious, subjective responses, while her left brain is using her objective, rational base in theory. Basch (1998) suggested that, in doing so, the therapist becomes the human corpus callosum of the client, helping to synchronize and communicate between the two sides of the client's brain, until the client is able to do it for himself. Transference and countertransference reactions between the client and the therapist occur at unconscious and preconscious levels as they are locked into right-brain-to-right-brain communication of emotional states. Attention also needs to be paid to the left side of the client's face, as it is this side that expresses the real emotional right hemisphere of the brain. False emotions are expressed in the left hemisphere and, therefore, show on the right side of the face. Which ear is the client offering to the therapist? Access to the real emotional pathways in the right hemisphere of the client is through the left ear. Access to impression management is via the right ear to the left hemisphere. In order to help the client learn better regulation of their painful emotions, the therapist needs to tap into this right hemisphere with his or own right hemisphere, to make a reconnection, preferably at visual and tonal levels, that re-enact the parent–infant attachment bond.

Attachments in the therapy room

McClusky (2005) highlighted how our infant attachment systems are repeated in the therapy room, as the client is SEEKING CARE, or, in her terms, care-seeking, from the therapist. She suggested that this takes two forms: seeking care and protection, and seeking support while exploring. Thus, in the former, it is SEEKING CARE, and the latter is CARE while SEEKING, and, it could be argued, introducing PLAY into the dynamic.

For the therapist, understanding the nature of neural development and the dynamics of attachment will inform the nature of the appropriate clinical intervention in therapy (Target & Fonagy, 1996). Attachment classifications provide metaphorical guidelines into the inner working models of the client, their expectations from relationships, how they may manage their emotional expression, and how they will cope with life events. The client's style of attachment will determine the treatment modality in the therapy room, as the client will act out his insecurity in the attachment with the therapist. McBride and colleagues highlighted that clients with a preoccupied style, who are over-focused on relationships and hypervigilant to cues of rejection, are going to respond best to inter-personal (psychodynamic) psychotherapeutic techniques, whereas clients with an avoidant style are more likely to respond to CBT techniques, because they deny the importance of relationships and value cognition over emotion (McBride, Atkinson, Quilty, & Bagby, 2006). But taking this approach may not provide the best outcomes, as, although people who are preoccupied will feel good pouring out their emotions in emotion-focused therapy, they need to access their left brain verbal reasoning to reach the "volume control" of emotion in the left prefrontal cortex and to be able to "turn it down". So, cognitive therapeutic styles may be preferable. Similarly, people with an avoidant style will be comfortable with CBT because they do not have to access their painful emotions and can apply ratio-nality to the process. But they actually need to open out and expe-rience the real pain in a calm and protected environment, rather than subconsciously acting on it in their day-to-day living.

Despite the method of therapy being used, however, incorpo-rating an understanding of an attachment style into your own way of working will enhance the process of the therapeutic work. Studies have shown that clinicians reliably are able to assess attach-ment styles within ongoing psychotherapy (Westen, Nakash, Thomas, & Bradley, 2006). There will be very clear identifiers to the client's style, without the need for specific attachment assessment instruments. For example, Slade (1999) highlighted how the preoc-cupied client will seek attention and reassurance, wanting to bring appointments forward by writing or phoning the therapist between sessions. Emotional outbursts within therapy may be common, with a long, confused, incoherent discourse, together with making threats of self-harm if the therapist resists demands for frequent attendance at therapy. He will test the therapist to the limits of her tolerance, and he may show hostility by criticizing her lack of help-fulness or availability. He may also show intolerance to being alone, and may rush from one person to the next in order to get emotional help and support. Fonagy and colleagues suggested that such people with a preoccupied style are particularly difficult to treat in therapy, as they jump from one issue to the next without any inter-nal consolidation or integration (Fonagy et al., 1996).

A client with an avoidant attachment style will feel nervous about a therapist who shows too much empathy too soon. So, he will "lock the therapist out as they themselves were locked out by their attachment figures" (Slade, 1999, p. 588). He will avoid the sessions by being late or not turning up. When he does attend, he will avoid or minimize the significant issues, or the emotional impact of traumatic events, within the room. Slade continued, "the therapist experiences what the patient cannot—the hopelessness of change and of attaining intimacy. And the therapist is left feeling much like the patient once felt as a child: angry, unacknowledged, silly and inept" (*ibid.*).

Working with a client with a disorganized style requires the focus of gently working through trauma without potentially retraumatizing, especially if the client uses a process of disassociation as a defence mechanism. A client with a disorganized attachment style is likely to be resistant, chaotic, or attacking within therapy. They have a deficit in mentalization, which may become acutely apparent within the therapy room in prolonged silences and confusion. These clients may present with stress or PTSD that has been kindled from a recent event. A mindful therapist will note that a minor life event has precipitated an extreme reaction in the client, out of proportion to the perceived significance of the event. This will suggest a rekindled trauma, and will require a sensitive approach not only to the presenting issue, but careful backtracking to previous traumatic incidents. Scaer (2001, p. 192) suggested that therapists should search for visual and olfactory triggers, as olfaction is the only primary sense that has access to the limbic system without the filter of the thalamus.

Schore (1994) pointed out that psychobiological attunement requires the therapist to use her countertransference visceral–somatic responses to read the client's internal state. In particular, the therapist needs to be attuned to the client's verbal and non-verbal expressions of shame within the therapy room. Hook and Andrews (2005) conducted a survey of people who had received therapy for depression and found that a half of the current clients and a third of former clients reported withholding some information about their depressive symptoms (e.g., low self-worth, suicidal thoughts) and behaviour (e.g., substance abuse, aggression) from their therapist because they felt ashamed. They also found that people who had concealed symptoms made less of a recovery on completion of therapy. Rarely will a client actually express feelings of shame to the therapist, but he may use self-deprecating expressions like "pathetic", "worthless", "ridiculous", or "foolish". In addition, there may be non-verbal expressions in gaze or eye contact aversion, covering the face or mouth with the hands, blushing, postural changes in slumping or shrinking into the chair. The Hook and Andrews' study suggested the effect that individual clients can have on their own therapeutic outcome. But it is also important for the therapist to consider how protective shame is, and that our very clever psychological interventions can strip a client bare of their defences before they have adopted new ones. Proeve and Howells (2006) highlighted that shame may also manifest in therapy through missing sessions, arriving late, saying little, or abruptly changing the subject, and one can identify the avoidant attachment style in these responses. The client with high levels of shame may also question the skills of the therapist or become hostile within the sessions, identifying the compensatory narcissistic form of defence. Tagney and Dearing (2002) suggested that this might reduce his motivation to change. Maruna (2001) agreed, pointing out that when working with people who have committed offences, forcing them to internalize their shame is neither necessary nor helpful in treatment. It is vital that good therapy provides a safe passage through shame (Jenkins, 2009). More will be discussed on this later in the chapter.

In therapy, the therapist will become the new attachment figure in a transferential process, so the (good enough) therapist needs to slowly support a client through his developing autonomy in the same way as a good enough parent supports the developing child. The work needs to be mediated by warm support, good eye contact between the therapist and the client to mimic the proto-conversation of the early years, and persistent non-judgemental encouragement. It is vital for the therapist to be clear in her own mind that what people do does not define who they are, while making clear statements regarding not condoning or colluding with offending behaviour, yet still supporting and respecting the person. Siegel (2003) proposed that this form of therapy can move people into a sense of "earned security", whereas Wilkinson (2006) preferred the concept of "learned security", to emphasize the positive outcome of change.

Attachment style of the therapist

An interesting study conducted by Dozier and colleagues tested the attachment base of both clients and their therapists (Dozier, Cue, & Barnett, 1994). They found that insecure clinicians were more likely to reinforce their client's insecure attachment styles, whereas secure therapists were more likely to address the issues. Preoccupied or enmeshed clients were seen by their insecure therapists as more needy and requiring greater therapeutic input than avoidant clients, while secure therapists had the reverse perception of their clients. The moral of this story is that psychotherapists need to pay very clear attention to their own attachment style, and not allow it to act out within the therapy room.

Therapists also need to work on their own inner critical parent and damaged child, in order to cope with the projective attacks of damaged clients. Epstein (1994) highlighted that therapists can project their own toxicity back on to the client by using defences such as sarcasm, teasing, and ridicule in order to control the person in some way.

Using the mind–body link

When I first trained in counselling in the 1980s, much emphasis was placed on the importance of steering clear of a medical model, and working only with the psyche. I think this emphasis came at a time when counselling was trying to make its mark on a cynical world, particularly in the UK, where there is a cultural stiff upper-lip regime. This separation of mind and body, which Damasio (1994) rightly called *Descartes' Error*, still prevails in the counselling world today. Only recently, I had an article on attachment and neuro-science rejected by a well-known UK counselling journal on the grounds that it was presenting a medical model.

But, over the years of working in a clinical context, I have been mindful that we ignore the mind–body link at our peril. As the previous chapters have demonstrated, there is an interaction between the physiological hardware and the psychological out-come. Shaw (2003) agreed that embodied experiences can be used within psychotherapy to enrich the co-constructed narrative between the client and the therapist. If we, as therapists, concentrate only on the mind, then we leave our job half done. This is especially important when working with current presentations of stress and post traumatic stress disorder. Scaer noticed this when working with clients presenting with serious psychological reactions to minor road traffic accidents (RTAs) producing whiplash injuries. Scaer looked for the meaning to the client of the precipitating RTA in relation to the injury, then found that the severity of the presenting symptoms was correlated to the cumulative load of traumatic events prior to the RTA. He argued that this accumulation of events leads to increased vulnerability and decreased resilience to further trauma (Scaer, 2001). He proposed, therefore, that it was not a case of a mind–body connection, but a mind–brain–body continuum. What this advocates is that therapists need to consider early life experiences, and attachment templates, even when one is dealing with issues that may be considered irrelevant to childhood.

Interaction between mind and body requires the therapist to consider the life-style of the client, which may be interfering with the processes of the mind, as some self-destructive processes can manifest in the way the person treats his body. It is not simply assessing whether the person over-uses substances like alcohol, nicotine, recreational drugs, or even caffeine, but whether he has sufficient self-regard to look after himself on a day-to-day level. For example, as discussed in Chapter Four, it has been shown that cannabis users have an avoidant attachment style and tend to underreport any problems as they do not tend to perceive problems appropriately, so do not ask for therapeutic support, even when it is necessary (Petersen & Thomasius, 2007).

It is vital to investigate food intake. Does he eat a healthy, nutritious diet little and often to maintain a stable blood sugar, as mood and food are inextricably linked? Does he exercise sufficiently to use up free-floating adrenaline from a stressful job, and to release endorphins and enkephalins, the body's natural antidepressants? Is he drinking sufficient fluid, as the first symptom of dehydration is often tiredness rather than thirst? Does he get sufficient rest and sleep, rather than pushing his body to extremes? Self-care has many levels, and if a client is very distressed from hyperactive right brain activity, encouraging practical lifestyle choices can provide the client with confidence that there are things he can do for himself to precipitate change. Vigilance over these choices can have a noticeable change in a short space of time to the client's subjective well-being, and can make the client feel he is getting control back into his life. In addition, encouraging physical skills, such as relaxation or meditation techniques, or parasympathetic breathing (I recommend the 4 × 7/11 technique: breathe in for a count of seven, out for a count of eleven, undertaken for four breaths) helps the client see for himself that calming the body helps to calm the mind.

Right-brain soothing

Throughout the lifespan, the right brain cycles into growth phases (Thatcher, 1994), allowing for the maturation of emotional responses and experience-dependent improvement of coping strategies to deal with adversity. To change old dysfunctional behaviour patterns into new adaptive ones, we need to invoke right-brain activity, which is involved in novelty and new learning, and to use the left brain to organize the new experiences into meaningful and coherent sequences.

Rossi (2002) proposed that novelty, enrichment, and exercise could precipitate neurogenesis. By combining with the brain-driven neurotrophic factor (BDNF) proteins (Rossi et al., 2006), these right-brain activities facilitate neurogenesis, which can precipitate change. Farley (2004) agreed. He pointed out that the shrunken hippocampus seen in childhood trauma and adult depression may not just be about cells dying, but also about a lack of cells being born, and, thus, the condition may be reversible.

Rossi (2002) had linked the theory of numinosum as a combination of fascination with the mysterious or tremendous to a tripartite model of body, mind, and spirit, as illustrated in Figure 25.

Rossi suggested that the combination of visual observation in numinosum and fascination (SEEKING) that elicits the implicit processing heuristics (unconscious processing) creates the environment for the development of new neuronal connections and pathways; that is, neurogenesis. He went on to propose that art, beauty, and truth (Figure 26) would be catalysts in this observational process, which, through a series of events, could promote healing.

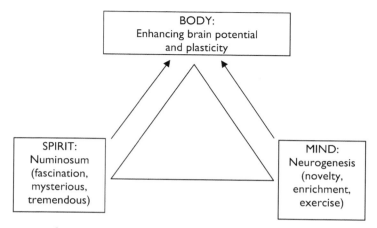

Figure 25.   The triad of body, spirit, and mind. After Rossi (2002).

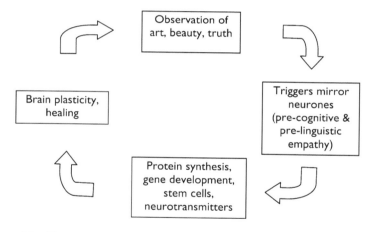

Figure 26.   Neurogenesis potential. After Rossi (2002).

Rossi's view has plausibility, and it fits with the theories of lateralization of the brain discussed in this book. We know from Sperry's (1966, 1982) split brain studies discussed in Chapter Two that when the two hemispheres of the brain are prevented from communicating with each other by the surgical division of the corpus callosum, such people can manifest two ways of being and, arguably, two forms of consciousness. As outlined in the earlier chapter, lateralization of the brain suggests that the left hemisphere is involved in logic, mathematics, and language, whereas the right hemisphere specializes more in art, music, colour, emotion, and spacial awareness. When a client presents with stress burnout from work overload, or if they have had a slight injury to the left hemisphere from, say, a minor RTA, often the left hemisphere seems to shut down, and people notice deficits in their cognitive functioning. This is the time that therapists need to encourage right-brain activities, allowing the left hemisphere some healing time.

So, what is right-brain soothing? It may be helpful to consider what soothes a child up to two years old, who only operates using right-brain processes. He loves touch and being held, nurturance and the enjoyment of food, rough and tumble play, bright colours, happy and relaxing music, singing nursery rhymes, splashing in water, being read stories, being outdoors, and laughter. There are adult versions of all of these that a therapist can discuss with the client.

- Touch is being held, massage, and sensate focus exercises.
- Food is preparing meals for your partner or family or friends: eating out in restaurants or having picnics, romantic evening dinners at the weekend when the children are in bed. Both touch and food access the CARE circuit.
- Rough and tumble play of the child is replicated through exercise and sport, especially in group and team sports, whether it is playing or watching/supporting.
- PLAY also involves arts and crafts, literature, poetry, theatre, and film.
- PLAY also needs humour, comedy, and laughter.
- Being outdoors, especially in the countryside, is especially soothing to the body and the spirit.
- Water is our first natural environment, and walking along rivers or beaches is soothing when a person feels stressed. Swimming and water-sports are invigorating. And for couples, taking spas, showers, or baths together is very connecting.
- Music and rhythm, whether playing an instrument, listening, or singing, access pathways in the brain between the cerebellum and the prefrontal cortex, thought to have developed preverbally (Levitin, 2006).

By calming the right brain with these right-brain soothing activities, the "volume control" in the left brain has a chance to take control. And if working with a couple, they need to do as much right-brain soothing together as possible. Soothing the body calms the mind and calms the couple.

Mindfulness

Mindfulness is intentionally paying attention to the present moment, allowing experience to unfold non-judgementally (Kabat-Zinn, 1994). In doing so, these meditative-related techniques are thought to produce serenity, heightened awareness, and other therapeutic effects. Physiologically, when the body is calmer through meditative right-brain soothing activities, the left brain can become more receptive to cognitive interventions. Some have suggested that the cerebral cortex becomes thicker than average in people who have had years of meditation experience (Cahn & Polich, 2006).

In Chapter Five, I discussed the Adult Attachment Interview, which was found to surprise unconscious processes (George, Kaplan, & Main, 1985), and how important the internal working models of an individual's attachment was in understanding emotional distress or psychopathology. I emphasized that it is not the childhood life event *per se* that causes the damage, but the script that the person develops to make sense of it, or, more importantly, the lack of a script if the event occurred during right-brain development. Consequently, by working therapeutically in a mindful way with the client, the therapist needs to attend less to the content of the story being told, and to focus more on the structure. How is the story being told? What can the person allow himself to think and feel? And what insight does that give the therapist to the person's attachment style, and, therefore, insight into his working model of expectations of life? A person with a preoccupied style will need to tell his story more dispassionately instead of being overwhelmed and tormented by his unregulated FEAR and PANIC systems. A person with an avoidant style needs to learn to be less rigid and inflexible with his story as inconsistencies become apparent, without defensively darting along his AVOID circuit, and to become more aware of, and regulate, negative affect. A person with a disorganized style will need gentle but strong support and strength to tell a coherent story of trauma, filling all of the hippocampal gaps as well as possible, without going into a freeze state and disassociating. So, the therapist needs to look for breaks, distortions, inconsistencies, and disruptions in the story, as this provides the window for the therapist to view how the client defends against the intrusion of unacceptable feelings or memories of traumatic events.

Fonagy and colleagues called the mindfulness process reflective self-functioning; the capacity to mentally perceive oneself and overview ones' behaviour in the context of, and in a dynamic with, others in terms of mental states (Fonagy, Steele, Moran, Steele, & Higgitt, 1992). This cognitive and verbal process allows the person to organize their thoughts and feelings more meaningfully by assessing situations, predicting outcomes, and to subsequently adapt his behaviour into more adaptive strategies than had been previously used with implicit automatic behavioural responses. In doing so, the individual will develop a stronger sense of self, and with it the ability to regulate the extremes of his emotional states. However, it is important to emphasize that these mindful cognitive processes need to be in play in contemporaneous emotional soothing. It is the balance between the two hemispheres that will promote emotional self-regulation and behavioural change.

The ultimate goal of understanding psychotherapy's effects on the brain is to influence the choice of treatments. Siegel (2003) found that certain brain activity patterns predicted whether depressed clients would or would not respond to cognitive–behavioural therapy. It has been hypothesized that eventually clients could be assigned to psychotherapy, medication, or other treatments on the basis of the information provided by their brain scans (Etkin, Pittenger, Polan, & Kandel, 2005), and monitoring the progress of their therapeutic treatment by tests of brain health, similar to the stress tests used by cardiologists to predict and oversee changes in heart health.

Assessment

Whether working with individuals or couples, a thorough assessment is essential before commencing therapeutic work. I start with a genogram as a preliminary information-gathering tool providing a snapshot of the client's family at that moment in time (DeMaria, Weeks, & Hof, 1999). I find it valuable to go back three generations to the grandparents, and further if the client has knowledge. This provides valuable information regarding the ripple effect of trans-generational transmission, and the predispositions of addictions or mental instability. It can also access family secrets, missing or adopted children, and deaths no longer discussed within a family. The construction of these diagrams, first by hand with the client, and later on computer (I use Genogram-Maker Millennium) helps to relax the client in preparation for what they sense is going to be a difficult time in disclosing their history.

I then take a full developmental history, again starting with the grandparents: what do they know of them and how did they affect their parents? What were their parents like, their personality, their relationship with each other, their parenting, and are there are any differences in their cultural or religious beliefs? What do they know about their own birth delivery? Were they planned children? What stressors were the parents under during the pregnancy? I move on to focus on early attachment years, especially, under five years old. What stories had they heard? Had they had any separations from mother or any losses during this time? What was their birth order, and what was their relationship with their siblings? Was their child-hood and schooling stable and secure or was there a lot of turbu-lence from the family moving repetitively (very common in Service families). Was the culture in which they were brought up safe, or were they surrounded by a society of turbulence or war? I then move on to the time of sexual template development. What hap-pened at eight–nine (boys) or six–seven (girls) after checking whether they developed earlier or later than their peers? Was their introduction into sex a natural development process, or were they vandalized (either by abuse, trauma or loss) during this time? (It is essential to stay very matter-of-fact during disclosure of abuse either to, or by, the client, and not make interjections of shock, sympathy, or blame. Even if the client's parent is the abuser, the client may be conflicted about how they feel about this, that is, both protective and betrayed. Therefore, I point out that parents are the product of their own parenting, so that blame is unhelpful at this stage.) How was life at school? Was there an attachment injury of boarding school, and what was that like? Did they have friends? Were they bullied, and if so, why? Moving on to adolescence, what did they think about themselves and what was their relationship with their peers? How did they achieve at school and what happened then? When did their sexual history commence? I then talk through significant relationships chronologically, looking for attachment styles and attachment injuries, sexual activities, conceptions, etc., until reaching the present day. I finish by asking about current stressors at home or at work, anxieties, depressive episodes through life, losses, past and present psychotropic medication, and past and present alcohol and recreational drug usage.

When all this information has been collected in a session that can last somewhere between one and two hours, I collate it into a formulation, which I write in the client's absence between sessions for the client to take away from the next session, after a thorough discussion of my views. This formulation essentially tells the client's story from someone else's perspective, and is enormously therapeutic even before therapy has formally started. Clients commonly find them incredibly moving and also very challenging. If the work is with a couple, I will have conducted a separate history for each partner in an individual session, but the formulation will be a single one as I move from one partner to the other throughout the history, comparing and contrasting their respective upbringings and value systems. If it is a heterosexual couple, I will add comments about classic gender differences that often are highlighted in the presentation of the couple, or gender differences in sexual arousal systems. If the couple are of the same sex, then I will look for any apparent internalized homophobia, and differences in how the families of origin respond to the relationship, or family, if they have children. Again, this is written down for the couple to take away, as these formulations may span five or six A4 pages of type, so it is impossible for the client to take in all the feedback during the course of one therapeutic session.

Working with couples

When a couple present for therapy, there have been many influences on each partner as to his or her inner working model, or neural template, of how that relationship should be. There is the original circuitry producing an attachment style, which may or may not match the style of the partner. There will be the style and behaviour of each partner's parents' relationship, which may be subconsciously mirrored, or consciously avoided. In addition, there will be the influences of previous failed relationships, which adapt each partner's perception of the other and expectations of the relationship. Often, as in systems theory, one partner may be singled out as being "the problem" in the pair bond, for putting it under threat by drinking too much, having an affair, spending too much, not wanting sex, wanting too much sex, working too much, using the Internet, or only being interested in the children. The list of perceived presenting "offences" can go on, but they are all merely symptoms of an underlying insecure process that is affecting the dynamic of the partnership. Recall from Chapter Eight that it is not the fights and the perceived offences that predict the prognosis of a damaged relationship, but how they repair their attachment injuries (Gottman, 1994; Solomon, 2003). The focus of working with couples, therefore, is to encourage each partner to work on the damaged SEEKING CARE circuit when PANIC is triggered. Many therapists will recount in supervision how a couple squabbled in therapy like children. And, in many respects, they are; they are adults still operating on a child's insecure attachment template. It is vital, therefore, that the therapist, in being "good-enough mother" or "good-enough father", treats each partner fairly in the therapy by not colluding with the "its all his/her fault" and "tell him/her off" routine, but emphasizing that the fault lies in the relationship dynamic contributed by both sides, and that healing involves them both moving towards one another in compromise.

When working with couples where domestic violence has been a chronic issue, the victim, who has been enduring long-term chronic stress, may experience atrophy in the dendrites of the neurons of the hippocampus of the brain (Siegel, 1999). This may lead to memory disturbances of actual violent incidents, yet the person may present with extreme somatic responses to the perception of anger in the partner. The fear responses when threat cues are perceived will readily trigger a hypersensitive HPA axis, and these FEAR signals may elicit the RAGE response in the aggressive partner, forming a self-fulfilling loop. Thus, drawing the attachment template for these couples who want to change the system, and getting them to suggest ways of breaking the chain of events, can be important in preventing the escalation of violence that so commonly occurs. Care needs to be taken, however, that the couple do not seek to bring the intensity of their fights into the therapy room. Scaer (2001) pointed out that such couples become so used to the activation of their endorphins to protect them from the repetitive abusive experiences that they unconsciously activate these systems, especially when the therapist encourages them to step out of the insecure template into a secure one. Taking a couple out of their comfort zone of what they are used to, even when that zone is a negative place, is hugely scary and activates default (maladaptive) protective mechanisms.

Insecure couples in heterosexual relationships regard classic male–female differences with suspicion, and their lack of empathy often means a misinterpretation of their partner's motives. A discussion in the therapy room regarding different approaches for dealing with communication, conflict, child-rearing, and sex can help to diffuse tense situations occurring outside of it. For example, a discussion about key conversational differences between men and women: many women may regard questions as a way of maintaining a conversation, whereas men tend to view them as requests for information. Women tend to view aggressiveness as an attack that disrupts the relationship, whereas men view it as a form of lively conversation. Women are mostly like to share feelings, problems, and secrets, whereas men tend to prefer less intimate topics, such as work, sport, or politics, and want to elicit solutions to problems. Of course, these are generalizations, but they are useful hypotheses in working with heterosexual couples, although these differences may also be found in gay relationships.

Intense emotional reactions within the couple dynamic may be based on incorrect perceptions of how the other "should" respond. Most overreactions could be alleviated if the partners would turn their attention away from their preoccupation with "injustice" or "impropriety" and focus on what Beck (1988) suggested was the underlying hurt or fear. If they could recognize that it is not what their partner does so much as what they are sensitive to that creates the conflict. It is the personal pain that loads the anger. The eye of the storm in a row is not the trivia that they complain of, like the inconvenience of having been kept waiting, or having to pick up dirty socks off the bedroom floor, but the *belief* that these events *"prove"* that the partner is irresponsible, insensitive, or disrespect- ful. It is the misinterpretations that people make that cause the problem. And it is these misinterpretations that trigger fears of rejection and abandonment. Thus, the primary focus for a therapist working with couples who manifest in a co-dependent relationship, which may or may not escalate into violence, is to focus on the inse- curity issues with each partner, their perceived inability to get their own needs met from the relationship, and their issues around inti- macy. They are both operating on a working model from a LOSS circuit; that they will be rejected or abandoned, and all they have to do is find the proof. Understanding that they are operating on old childhood survival systems that can be changed with adult cogni- tive and behavioural strategies is an enormously powerful way of breaking transgenerational transmission.

Having a partner with a pornography addiction can be very challenging, and spouses often feel responsible or blame them- selves for their partner's behaviour (Schneider, 2003). When men get addicted to porn on the Net, they tend to spend less time with their partners having real sex because the visual imagery is so intense and they have been aroused for so long that by the time they go to bed in the early hours they are exhausted. If they do want sex with their partners, however, they may often demand hard, aggressive, porn-like sex that hitherto had been outside their normal sexual repertoire: for example, anal sex. The female partner may feel humiliated and objectified by these demands, arguing that the loving and intimacy has disappeared from their love-making (Bridges, Bergner, & Hesson-McInnis, 2003). For the non-viewing partner, talking to a therapist separately first may provide him or her with a safe place to share frustrations and learn coping skills (Landau, Garrett, & Webb, 2008). It should be remembered, how- ever, that the pornography viewer should not be labelled as "the problem" in the relationship, and the therapist should not collude with the premise that "if he just stopped looking at pornography, everything would be all right". First, it is impossible to make others change; only they can choose to change. Second, as it is an addic- tion, that is easier said than done. If he is addicted, then honestly evaluating in therapy the impact of past pornography and possible future outcomes will help to strengthen his resolve to change. And third, it is vital to look at the other relationship dynamics so that the pornography viewer does not feel persecuted by everyone. Having said that, the porn-viewer needs to become aware and understand how pornography creates problems in his relationship, and the therapist needs to challenge any minimization and denial.

A woman who becomes addicted to the Internet chat room does so because she believes that the person she is having a cyber-relationship with understands her better than her real partner. She feels heard and understood. Clearly, communication is a vital component of this work in the therapy room (Zitzman & Butler, 2005). Couples need to have open conversations about the negative effects of the Internet on their relationship. Both should be encouraged to express how cyber-affairs made them feel, without interruption and judgement from the other person (Corley & Schneider, 2002). For a successful reconciliation of what essentially is an attachment injury, partners need to be encouraging and supportive of their partner's decision to change (providing CARE). Some of the areas that need to be addressed include issues of trust, gaining empathy, moving from anger to forgiveness, communication skills, and new ways of being intimate and recapturing their own way of being sexual, perhaps through a sensate focus programme. While the process of healing as a couple can be challenging, it is possible for couples to renew trust, improve communication, and repair the collateral damage. In particular, the therapist should encourage right-brain soothing activities in their partnership to boost their emotional and physical health and regain their confidence and self-esteem. Loving and compassionate partners can encourage change and help his or her spouse find positive methods of working through the addiction. When both partners are committed to working together in this way to have a healthy relationship, they can repair the damage in their relationship and even make it better.

Working with offenders

I discussed at great length in the previous chapter my view that sex offender treatment programmes that focus purely on cognitive–behavioural therapy (even though most of the behavioural part seems to have been lost *en route*) are necessary, but not sufficient methods of treatment. Working with cognitive distortions does not deal with the causes of offending when one considers that the vast majority of offenders were damaged children. Healing the attachment traumas, creating a new safe base, and learning to regulate the extremes of these overactivated or deactivated attachment systems are vital for the left brain–right brain balance required for psychological healing.

As with other clients, the works starts with a thorough assessment, as described above. In addition, for clients who have committed offences, the history-taking needs to acknowledge any forensic history. Often, this starts at puberty or adolescence, so greater focus needs to be placed on information gathering at this stage. For those who have committed sexual offences, check out the vandalization of the client's own sexual template. What methods of self-soothing did they use in their adolescence? Often, this is when compulsive masturbatory behaviours develop. Much of offending is compulsive repetition from their own childhood trauma. Once the client becomes mindful of that, they are more motivated into behavioural change. We also need full details of sexual practice: what, when, how long, with whom, at what costs, and what are the triggers? Many therapists are loath to go into the minutiae of this, but it is essential to keep asking, as the client is so used to, and so experienced at, withholding. (Withholding should not be interpreted as manipulative or malevolent. It is simply a defence strategy against shame.) For clients who are Internet addicts, questions should include current Internet viewing, how much, how long, what are they looking at, whether they have collections, and what other addictions or compulsions they have.

Key questions to ask if the client is presenting with a paraphilia are:

• do you do this to alter your mood?
• does this interfere with your daily living, your work, home, or family?
• is the sexual behaviour taking you away from real sexual relationships rather than enhancing them?
• what purpose does this paraphilia serve?

- what does not being able to be healthily sexual protect you from?
- what has led you to seek help?
- have you sought help before (counselling/psychiatric history)?
- why now?

Once the history is collected, I construct a time-line in five-year chunks from birth to present, and map sexual activity, sexual offences, and depressive/anxiety episodes on to it using different colour pens. This allows greater clarity for offence triggers. I also collect information using psychometric questionnaires to inform my view more thoroughly. The Sexual Excitation/Inhibition Questionnaire (SES/SIS) (Bancroft & Vukadinovic, 2004) measures the relationship between the sexual drives of excitation and inhibition, which, in healthy sexual behaviour, tend to be balanced with one another. If a person has too much excitation and too little inhibition, there tends to be sexually inappropriate acting out; too little excitation and too much inhibition tends to lead to sexual dysfunction. I have found a specific pattern that relates to Internet offenders that is very interesting: high inhibition and low arousal, the opposite of what one would anticipate finding from this measure. I also give the Mood and Sexuality Questionnaire (Bancroft et al., 2003), Hanson Sex Attitude Questionnaire (Hanson, Gizzarelli, & Scott, 1994), Bumby Cognitive Distortions Scale (Carich & Adkerson, 2003), and the Carich–Adkerson Victim Empathy and Self Report Inventory (*ibid.*). I also have some additional questionnaires that encourage the client to be more honest about their Internet usage. All this information forms the basis of the forensic formulation I will undertake, which may also form part of a legal report, if required. Again, the client gets a written copy of the formulation or the report. I feel it is disrespectful to write about people without discussing the situation with them and giving them a full copy of the account.

Once the information is collected, you will be in a position to collaborate with the client to determine what, if any, therapeutic work should be undertaken. If the client presents with a genuine desire for change, rather than just attending because his solicitor, wife, or employer demands that he must, then the process of first order–second order changes discussed in Chapter Eleven can commence. Davenport and Fisher proposed that therapy should include

Finkelhor's work, to understand the person's offending in relation to their life experiences (Davenport & Fisher, 2007; Finkelhor & Araji, 1986). Finkelhor's model involves working with four themes of abusive histories: feelings of powerlessness, betrayal, stigmatization, and traumatic sexualization. Finkelhor and Araji (1986) also proposed a four-factor model of examining the client's narrative as to why he wanted to offend, how he could justify his behaviour to himself, how he created the opportunity to offend, and how he overcame resistance of the victim. Marshall and Moulden (2006) suggested that this model provides the pathway for developing an offence pathway analysis, which can be worked through collaboratively with the client. In an interesting twist to risk assessment, Shingler and Mann (2006) suggested further that the use of risk assessment actuarials should be shared with the client throughout the therapy in a collaborative way, so that they both can use the assessment tool as a means of guiding them as to what needs to be worked on throughout the therapy. This would mean that the client would feel that his opinion would be validated, and he would be empowered to work on his own recovery, rather than waiting to be "done to" by the therapist. It is only when the client thoroughly understands why he does the things he does that he is ever going to use any strategies for change.

It is vital in this work that the therapist focuses on the individual's strengths and capacity to change, rather than his weaknesses or perceived deficiencies (Marshall, Anderson, & Fernandez, 1999). In a non-judgemental style of collaboration (Shingler & Mann, 2006), which conveys to the individual that the client is capable of change, the therapist builds up the client's damaged self-esteem by becoming a sensitive and attuned attachment figure. Marshall and colleagues have noted that the characteristics of the therapist that promoted the most positive treatment changes in sexual offenders were warmth, empathy, rewardingness and directiveness (Marshall et al., 2003). This way of being, which conveys mutual respect, trust, and honesty, is not colluding with inappropriate behaviour, but sets clear and safe boundaries, and differentiates between what people do and who they are. Notably, Marshall and Moulden (2006) pointed out that clients should be encouraged to describe themselves as someone who has committed a sexual offence, rather than a sexual offender.

Jenkins (2009) moves this process on by suggesting that in order to be congruent with ourselves in the light of the behaviour of our client, we need to work ethically with our client without losing our sense of outrage regarding his behaviour. Sometimes, the damage that has been done by the client to another is irreparable, and this needs to be clearly identified and understood. But we must not let our moral imperatives get in the way of the work we need to do. So, through encouraging the client to take a similar ethical stance, and reach out into the world of the other, rather than staying trapped within his own abusive state, he can then focus on the kind of person that he wants to be (Jenkins, 1990). To go through this process requires several stages, but particularly important is the process of feeling and being remorseful in order to move into restorative practice. Remorse has many layers: first there is a realization of the consequences of the behaviour undertaken. The client has to acknowledge the full nature of the abuse, without mitigation, and face the shame of its consequences. It is important at this stage, as discussed above, that the therapist allows the client to acknowledge the shame without inducing further shaming, which would trigger defensive responses. Jenkins elaborates that therapy provides a safe passage through shame, which, in turn, provides the window for behavioural change. Second, there needs to be restitution. What reparation can he make? What can he put back into the person or into society to make good what he has taken? Restitution means more than just an apology, involving also atonement in opening the client's eyes and seeing the world and the damage that surrounds it. Third, remorse involves restoration: acceptance without strings of the judgement and the punishment of others, and a determination that things will be different in the future.

Healing

Siegel (2003) emphasized that healing damaged or traumatized individuals occurs when overwhelming historical events and suboptimal developmental experiences that are trapped in a person's memory are freed from their restrictive or chaotic pathways, thus, freeing the person's vitality and creativity into a new way of being. Hence, working with clients and their attachments systems is an integrative process involving body, brain, and mind. To quote Chien-chih Seng-ts'an:

> To deny the reality of things
> is to miss their reality;
> To assert the emptiness of things
> is to miss their reality.
> The more you talk and think about it,
> the further astray you wander from the truth.
> Stop talking and thinking,
> and there is nothing you will not be able to know.
> To return to the root is to find the meaning,
> but to pursue appearances is to miss the source.
> [*Hsin Hsin Ming: (Inscribed on the Believing Mind)*]

People can learn new ways of being in their attachments systems by developing appropriate emotional responses, and learning to judge whether it is right to love or hate, trust or distrust, connect or abandon. They need to learn appropriate emotional distances; the preoccupied need to learn to let others go, the avoidants need to learn to let others in, the ambivalents need to become more stable, and the disorganized to resolve their losses and become less fragmented. Change will not be linear, but will roller-coaster through processes of organization, disorganization and reorganization. The therapist needs to encourage pleasurable activities: arts and crafts, exercise, culture, spirituality, and social connectedness. In the therapy room, the work has to be conducted with security, humour (laughing with people and not laughing at them), imagination, the joy of intellect, challenge, and the ongoing courage of the client. In allowing the client to develop a secure attachment with the therapist, the client will develop adult confidence in dealing with the pressures of life in adaptive ways. Maladaptive coping strategies to allow intense feelings of FEAR and RAGE will disappear in favour of self- and partner-soothing processes. No longer will the adult client search for what he lost as a child. He will launch himself into the world with confidence and good nature, and will be able to contribute to the well-being of himself, his family, and his society.

Gordon's ending or beginning?

The solicitor's firm but kindly words had had an effect on Gordon, and broke through his compensatory narcissism during a window of opportunity through Gordon's depression at a critical life event. Gordon went back to his flat, cleaned himself up, and then cleaned the flat. He went back to his old boss and told him the whole story. His boss took pity on him, and gave him his job back, more because Gordon was such a good mechanic than because he liked him, but he knew what potential Gordon had. The boss gave him an advance on his salary so he could pay off the arrears of rent and keep his home. However, his boss made it very clear that he was not going put up with the behaviours that Gordon had shown before. Gordon had to change.

Gordon kept his head down and worked hard. He stopped going to the pub, although he could not stop smoking. Working overtime helped him pay off his other debts. He still compulsively masturbated, but only used images from top-shelf magazines he had bought. He was desperately lonely, he had no friends, and he still missed Rachel. He wondered what Conner looked like, and whether the child knew about his father.

It was six months before Gordon took himself for his appointment with a therapist, a week after he had been charged with ten counts of making indecent images of children. He was nervous of the middle-aged woman who sat before him, and he felt too ashamed to tell her everything. But she seemed kind and gentle, and did not seem to be shocked at the story he had told her. He had come this far, and was starting to feel better about himself. He felt it was worth giving it a try.

REFERENCES

Abel, G. G., & Harlow, N. (2001). The Abel and Harlow child molestation prevention study. In: G. G. Abel & N. Harlow (Eds.), *The Stop Child Molestation Book* (pp. 301–324). Philadelphia, PA: Xlibris.

Abel, G. G., & Osborn, C. (1992). The paraphilias: the extent and nature of sexually deviant and criminal behavior. *Clinical Forensic Psychiatry*, 15(3): 675–687.

Abel, G. G., Barlow, D. H., Blanchard, E. B., & Guild, D. (1977). The components of the rapist's sexual arousal. *Archives of General Psychiatry*, 34(4): 395–403.

Abel, G. G., Rouleau, J.-L., & Coyne, B. J. (1987). Are some rapists paraphiliacs? Paper presented to the 13th Annual Meeting of International Academy of Sex Research, Tutzing, West Germany.

Abelin, E. (1971). The role of the father in the separation–individuation process. In: J. B. McDevitt & C. F. Settlage (Eds.), *Separation–Individuation* (pp. 229–252). New York: International Universities Press.

Abrams, J. L., & Spring, M. (1989). The flip-flop factor. *International Cognitive Therapy Newsletter*, 5(1): 7–8.

Abrams, L. S., & Stormer, C. C. (2002). Sociocultural variations in the body image perceptions of urban adolescent females. *Journal of Youth and Adolescence*, 31: 443–450.

Adams, M. J. (2003). Victim issues are key to sex offender treatment. *Sexual Addiction and Compulsivity: The Journal of Treatment and Prevention, 10*(1): 79–87.

Adolphs, R., Tranel, D., & Damasio, A. (1998). The human amygdala in social judgment. *Nature, 393*(6684): 470–474.

Ahmad, S. (2006). Adult psychosexual dysfunction as a sequela of child sexual abuse. *Sexual & Relationship Therapy, 21*(4): 405–418.

Ainsworth, M. D. S., Blehar, M. C., Waters, E., & Wall, S. (1978). *Patterns of Attachment: A Psychological Study of the Strange Situation*. Hillsdale, NJ: Erlbaum.

Akdeniz, Y. (1997). Governance of pornography and child pornography on the global internet: a multi-layered approach. In: L. Edwards & C. Waelde (Eds.), *Law and the Internet: Regulating Cyberspace* (pp. 223–241). London: Hart.

Akiskal, H. S. (1983). The bipolar spectrum: new concepts in classification and diagnosis. In: L. Grinspoon (Ed.), *Psychiatry Update: The American Psychiatric Association Annual Review* (Vol. 2, pp. 271–292). Washington DC: American Psychiatric Press.

Akiskal, H. S. (2003). Validating "hard" and "soft" phenotypes within the bipolar spectrum: continuity or discontinuity? *Journal of Affective Disorder, 73*(1–2): 1–5.

Alexander, P. C. (2003). Understanding the effects of child sexual abuse history on current couple relationships. In: S. M. Johnson & W. E. Whiffen (Eds.), *Attachment Processes in Couple and Family Therapy* (pp. 342–365). New York: Guilford Press.

Allen, J. G., Coyne, L., & Huntoon, J. (1998). Complex posttraumatic stress disorder in women from a psychometric perspective. *Journal of Personality Assessment, 70*(2): 277–298.

Ames, E. W. (1997). *The Development of Romanian Orphanage Children Adopted to Canada*. Burnaby, BC: Simon Frasier University Press.

Anderson, C. A. (1989). Temperature and aggression: ubiquitous effects of heat on occurrence of human violence. *Psychological Bulletin, 106*(1): 74–96.

Andreason, N. C., & Glick, I. D. (1988). Bipolar affective disorder and creativity: implications and clinical management. *Comprehensive Psychiatry, 29*(3): 207–217.

Aou, S., Oomura, Y., Nishino, H., Inokuchi, A., & Mizuno, Y. (1983). Influence of catecholamines on reward-related neuronal activity in monkey orbitofrontal cortex. *Brain Research, 267*(1): 165–170.

Appleby, L., Kapur, N., Shaw, J., & Robinson, J. (2003). Suicide and self-harm *The British Journal of Psychiatry*, *183*: 561–562.

Atkinson, B. J. (2005). *Emotional Intelligence in Couples Therapy*. New York: Norton.

Attwood, F. (2010a). Introduction: porn studies from social problem to cultural practice. In: F. Attwood (Ed.), *Porn.Com. Making Sense of Online Pornography* (pp. 1–16). New York: Peter Lang.

Attwood, F. (2010b). Younger, paler, decidely less straight: the new porn professionals. In: F. Attwood (Ed.), *Porn.Com. Making Sense of Online Pornography* (pp. 88–103). New York: David Lang.

Awad, G., Saunders, E., & Levene, J. (1984). A clinical study of male adolescent sexual offenders. *International Journal of Offender and Comparative Criminology*, *28*(2): 105–116.

Bach-y-Rita, G. (1974). Habitual violence and self-mutilation. *American Journal of Psychiatry*, *131*(9): 1018–1020.

Bagley, C. (1991). The prevalence and mental health sequels of child sexual abuse in a community sample of women aged 18 to 27. *Canadian Journal of Community Mental Health*, *10*(1): 103–116.

Bagley, C., Wood, M., & Young, L. (1994). Victim to abuser: mental health and behavioural sequels of child sexual abuse in a community survey of young adult males. *Child Abuse and Neglect*, *18*(8): 683–697.

Bak, M., Krabbendam, L., Janssen, I., de Graaf, R., Vollebergh, W., & van Os, J. (2005). Early trauma may increase the risk for psychotic experiences by impacting on emotional response and perception of control. *Acta Psychiatrica Scandinavia*, *112*(5): 360–366.

Bancroft, J. (1974). *Deviant Sexual Behaviour: Modification and Assessment*. Oxford: Clarendon Press.

Bancroft, J. (1995). *Human Sexuality and Its Problems* (2nd edn). New York: Churchill Livingstone.

Bancroft, J., & Vukadinovic, Z. (2004). Sexual addiction, sexual compulsivity, sexual impulsivity, or what? *Journal of Sex Research*, *41*(3): 225–234.

Bancroft, J., Janssen, E., Strong, D., & Vukadinovic, Z. (2003). The relation between mood and sexuality in gay men. *Archives of Sexual Behavior*, *32*(3): 231–242.

Bancroft, J., Janssen, E., Strong, D., Carnes, L., Vukadinovic, Z., & Scott Long, J. (2003). The relation between mood and sexuality in heterosexual men. *Archives of Sexual Behavior*, *32*(3): 217–230.

Bandura, A. (1973). *Aggression: A Social-Learning Analysis*. Englewood Cliffs, NJ: Prentice-Hall.

Barbaree, H. E., Bogaert, A. F., & Seto, M. C. (1995). Sexual reorientation therapy: Practices and controversies. In: L. Diamant & R. D. McAnulty (Eds.), *The Psychology of Sexual Orientation, Behavior, and Identity: A Handbook* (pp. 357–383). Westport, CT: Greenwood.

Barbas, H. (1995). Anatomic basis of cognitive–emotional interactions in the primate prefrontal cortex. *Neuroscience and Biobehavioral Reviews, 19*(3): 499–510.

Barone, L., & Guiducci, V. (2009). Mental representations of attachment in eating disorders: a pilot study using the Adult Attachment Interview. *Attachment and Human Development, 11*(4): 405–417.

Barron, M., & Kimmel, M. (2000). Sexual violence in three pornographic media: toward a sociological explanation. *The Journal of Sex Research, 37*(2): 161–168.

Bartels, A., & Zeki, S. (2004). The neural correlates of maternal and romantic love. *Neuroimage, 21*(3): 1155–1166.

Bartholomew, K. (1990). Avoidance of intimacy: an attachment perspective. *Journal of Social & Personal Relationships, 7*(2): 147–178.

Bartholomew, K., Henderson, A., & Dutton, D. G. (2001). Insecure attachment and partner abuse. In: C. Clulow (Ed.), *Adult Attachment and Couple Psychotherapy. The 'Secure Base' in Practice and Research* (pp. 43–61). London: Routledge.

Bartosh, D. L., Garby, T., Lewis, D., & Gray, S. (2003). Differences in the predictive validity of actuarial risk assessments in relation to sex offender type. *International Journal of Offender Therapy and Comparative Criminology, 47*(4): 422–438.

Basch, M. F. (1988). *Understanding Psychotherapy*. New York: Basic Books.

Bateman, A. W., & Fonagy, P. (2006). *Mentalization-Based Treatment for Borderline Personality Disorder*. Oxford: Oxford University Press.

Bateman, A. W., & Tyrer, P. (2004). Psychological treatment for personality disorders. *Royal College of Psychiatrists: Advances in Psychiatric Treatment, 10*(5): 378–388.

Bates, A., & Metcalf, C. (2007). A psychometric comparison of internet and non-internet sex offenders from a community treatment sample. *Journal of Sexual Aggression, 13*(1): 11–20.

Bechara, A., Tranel, D., & Damasio, H. (2000). Characterization of the decision-making deficit of patients with ventromedial prefrontal cortex lesions. *Brain, 123*(11): 2189–2202.

Beck, A. T. (1988). *Love is Never Enough*. New York: Penguin.

Beck, A. T., & Freeman, A. (Eds.) (1990). *Cognitive Therapy of Personality Disorders*. New York: Guilford Press.

Beckett, R., Beech, A., Fisher, D., & Fordham, A. S. (1994). *Community-Based Treatment for Sex Offenders: An Evaluation of Seven Treatment Programmes*. London: Home Office.

Beech, A. R., & Mitchell, I. J. (2005). A neurobiological perspective on attachment problems in sexual offenders and the role of selective serotonin reuptake inhibitors in the treatment of such problems. *Clinical Psychology Review, 25*(2): 153–182.

Belsky, J. (2006). Early child care and early child development. Major findings of the NICHD Study of Early Child Care. *European Journal of Developmental Psychology, 3*(1): 95–110.

Belsky, J., Steinberg, L., & Draper, P. (1991). Childhood experience, interpersonal development, and reproductive strategy: an evolutionary theory of socialization. *Child Development, 62*(3): 647–670.

Benazzi, F., & Akiskal, H. S. (2005). Irritable–hostile depression: further validation as a bipolar depressive mixed state. *Journal of Affective Disorder, 84*(2–3): 197–207.

Bench, C. J., Frackowiak, R. S., & Dolan, R. J. (1995). Changes in regional cerebral blood flow on recovery from depression. *Psychological Medicine, 25*(2): 247–251.

Beniart, S., Anderson, B., Lee, S., & Utting, D. (2002). *Youth at risk?: A national survey of risk factors and problem behaviour among young people in England, Scotland and Wales*. London: Joseph Rowntree Foundation.

Benoit, D., & Parker, K. C. H. (1994). Stability and transmission of attachment across three generations. *Child Development, 65*(5): 1444–1456.

Bentall, R. (2003). *Madness Explained*. London: Allen Lane/Penguin.

Berkowitz, L. (1971). The contagion of violence: an S-R mediational analysis of some effects of observed aggression. In: W. Arnold & M. Page (Eds.), *Nebraska Symposium on Motivation*, Volume 18 (pp. 95–135). Lincoln: University of Nebraska Press.

Berkowitz, L. (1989). Frustration–aggression hypothesis: examination and reformulation. *Psychological Bulletin, 106*(1): 59–73.

Berkowitz, L., & LePage, A. (1967). Weapons as aggression-eliciting stimuli. *Journal of Personality and Social Psychology, 7*(2): 202–207.

Berne, E. (1964). *Games People Play*. New York: Grove Press.

Beyko, M., & Wong, S. (2005). Predictors of attrition as indicators for program improvement not offender shortcomings: a study of sex offender treatment attrition. *Sexual Abuse: A Journal of Research and Treatment, 17*(4): 375–395.

Birnbaum, G. E. (2007). Attachment orientations, sexual functioning and relationship satisfaction in a community sample of women. *Journal of Social & Personal Relationships, 24*(1): 21–35.

Black, D. A., Heyman, R. E., & Slep, A. M. (2001). Risk factors for child sexual abuse. *Aggression and Violent Behavior, 6*(2): 203–229.

Blackburn, R. (1993). *The Psychology of Criminal Conduct*. Chichester: Wiley.

Blanchard, R., Barbaree, H. E., Bogaert, A. F., Dickey, R., Klassen, P. E., Kuban, M. E., & Zucker, K. J. (2000). Fraternal birth order and sexual orientation in pedophiles. *Archives of Sexual Behavior, 29*(5): 463–478.

Blanchard, R., Christensen, B. K., Strong, S. M., Cantor, J. M., Kuban, M. E., Klassen, P. E., Dickey, R., & Blak, T. (2002). Retrospective self-reports of childhood accidents causing unconsciousness in phallometrically diagnosed pedophiles. *Archives of Sexual Behavior, 31*(6): 511–526.

Blanchard, R., Watson, M. S., Choy, A., Dickey, R., Klassen, P. E., Kuban, M. E., & Ferren, D. J. (1999). Pedophiles: mental retardation, maternal age, and sexual orientation. *Archives of Sexual Behavior, 28*(2): 111–127.

Blos, P. (1984). Sons and fathers. *Psychoanalytic Study of the Child, 32*: 301–324.

Boardman, M., & Davies, M. (2009). Asymptomatic victims of child sexual abuse. A critical review. *Forensic Update, 99*: 6–12.

Bocij, P. (2004). *Cyberstalking: Harassment in the Internet Age and How to Protect your Family*. Westport, Connecticut: Greenwood Press.

Bohus, M., Limberger, M., Ebner, U., Glocker, F. X., Scwartz, B., Wernz, M., & Lieb, K. (2000). Pain perception during self-reported distress and calmness in patients with borderline personality disorder and self-mutilating behavior. *Psychiatry Research, 95*(3): 251–260.

Boon, J. C. W., & Sheridan, L. (2002). Conclusions. In: J. C. W. Boon & L. Sheridan (Eds.), *Stalking and Psychosexual Obsession* (pp. 237–239). Chichester: Wiley.

Borysenko, J., & Borysenko, M. (1994). *The Power of the Mind to Heal*. Carson, CA: Hay House.

Bow, J., & Boxer, P. (2003). Assessing allegations of domestic violence in child custody. *Journal of Interpersonal Violence, 18*(12): 1394–1410.

Bowlby, J. (1944). Forty-four juvenile thieves: their characters and home-life. *International Journal of Psycho-Analysis, 25*: 107–128.

Bowlby, J. (1951). *Child Care and the Growth of Love*. Harmondsworth: Penguin.

Bowlby, J. (1973). *Attachment and Loss, Volume 2. Separation: Anxiety and Anger*. London: Hogarth Press.

Bowlby, J. (1984). Violence in the family as a disorder of the attachment and caregiving systems. *American Journal of Psychoanalysis, 44*(1): 9–27.

Bowlby, J. (1988). *A Secure Base: Parent–Child Attachment and Healthy Human Development*. New York: Basic Books.

Bowlby, R. (2006). Personal communication.

Bowlby, R. (2007). Babies and toddlers in non-parental daycare can avoid stress and anxiety if they develop a lasting secondary attachment bond with one carer who is consistently accessible to them. *Attachment and Human Development, 9*(4): 307–319.

Bradford, J. M. W., Bloomberg, D., & Boulet, J. R. (1988). The heterogeneity/homogeneity of paedophilia. *Psychiatric Journal of the University of Ottawa, 13*(4): 217–226.

Braeutigam, S., Bailey, A. J., & Swithenby, S. J. (2001). Task-dependent early latency (30–60 ms) visual processing of human faces and other objects. *Neuroreport, 12*(7): 1531–1536.

Brazelton, T. B., & Cramer, B. G. (1990). *The Earliest Relationship*. New York: Addison-Wesley.

Bremner, J. D., & Narayan, M. (1998). The effects of stress on memory and the hippocampus throughout the life cycle: implications for childhood development and aging. *Development and Psychopathology, 10*(4): 871–888.

Brennan, K. A., & Shaver, P. R. (1995). Dimensions of adult attachment, affect regulation, and romantic relationship functioning. *Personality & Social Psychology Bulletin, 21*(3): 267–283.

Bridges, A., Bergner, R., & Hesson-McInnis, M. (2003). Romantic partners' use of pornography: its significance for women. *Journal of Sex & Marital Therapy, 29*(1): 1–14.

Brisch, K. H. (1999). *Treating Attachment Disorders*. New York: Guilford Press.

Broucek, F. J. (1982). Shame and its relationship to early narcissistic developments. *International Journal of Psychoanalysis, 63*: 369–378.

Broucek, F. J. (1991). *Shame and the Self.* New York: Guilford Press.

Brown, N. W. (2001). *Children of the Self Absorbed. A Grownup's Guide to Getting over Narcissistic Parents.* Oakland, CA: New Harbinger.

Brown, R., & Kulik, J. (1977). Flashbulb memories. *Cognition, 5:* 73–79.

Browne, C. J., & Shlosberg, E. (2005). Attachment behaviours and parent fixation in people with dementia: the role of cognitive functioning and pre-morbid attachment style. *Aging and Mental Health, 9*(2): 153–161.

Brownmiller, S. (1975). *Against Our Will: Men, Women and Rape.* New York: Bantam.

Buck, R. (1994). The neuropsychology of communication: spontaneous and symbolic aspects. *Journal of Pragmatics, 22*(3–4): 265–278.

Budd, T., Mattinson, J., & Myhill, A. (2000). *The Extent and Nature of Stalking: Findings from the 1998 British Crime Survey.* London: Home Office Research, Development and Statistics Directorate.

Bunclarke, J. (1999). Personal communication.

Byng-Hall, J. (1999). Family and couple therapy. Toward greater security. In: J. Cassidy & P. Shaver (Eds.), *Handbook of Attachment. Theory, Research, and Clinical Applications* (pp. 625–645). New York: Guilford Press.

Cahn, B. R., & Polich, J. (2006). Meditation states and traits: EEG, ERP, and neuroimaging studies. *Psychological Bulletin, 132*(2): 180–211.

Cantor, J. M., Kuban, M. E., Blak, T., Klassen, P. E., Dickey, R., & Blanchard, R. (2006). Grade failure and special education placement in sexual offenders' educational histories. *Archives of Sexual Behavior, 35*(6): 743–751.

Carden, S. W., & Hofer, M. A. (1990). Independence of benzodiazepine and opiate actions in the suppression of isolation distress in rat pups. *Behavioral Neuroscience, 104*(3): 160–166.

Careaga, A. (2002). *Hooked on the Net. How to say "Goodnight" when the Party Never Ends.* Grand Rapids, MI: Kregel.

Carich, M. S., & Adkerson, D. L. (2003). *Adult Sexual Offender Assessment Report.* Vermont: Safer Society Press.

Carlson, E. A. (1998). A prospective longitudinal study of attachment disorganization/disorientation. *Child Development, 69*(4): 1107–1128.

Carlson, V. J., & Harwood, R. L. (2003). Alternate pathways to competence. In: S.M. Johnson & W.E. Whiffen (Eds.), *Attachment Processes in Couple and Family Therapy* (pp. 85–99). New York: Guilford Press.

Carlson, V. J., Cicchetti, D., Barnett, D., & Braunwald, K. G. (1989). Finding order in disorganization. In: D. Chicchetti & V. Carlson (Eds.), *Child Maltreatment: Theory and Research on the Causes and Consequences of Child Abuse and Neglect* (pp. 484–528). New York: Cambridge University Press.

Carmen, E. H., Reiker, P. P., & Mills, T. (1984). Victims of violence and psychiatric illness. *American Journal of Psychiatry, 141*(3): 378–383.

Carnes, P. (2001). *Out of the Shadows. Understanding Sexual Addiction* (3rd edn). Minnesota, MS: Hazeldon.

Carnes, P. (2002). The sexual addiction assessment process. In: P. J. Carnes & K. M. Adams (Eds.), *Clinical Management of Sex Addiction* (pp. 3–19). New York: Brunner-Routledge.

Carnes, P., Delmonico, D. L., & Griffin, E. (2001). *In the Shadows of the Net. Breaking Free of Compulsive Online Sexual Behavior.* Minnesota, MS: Hazelden.

Carr, J. (2003). *Child Abuse, Child Pornography and the Internet.* London: National Children's Homes.

Carroll, R. (2003). "At the border between chaos and order". What psychotherapy and neuroscience have in common. In: J. Corrigall & H. Wilkinson (Eds.), *Revolutionary Connections. Psychotherapy and Neuroscience* (pp. 191–211). London: Karnac.

Carter, D., Prentky, R., Knight, R., Vanderveer, P., & Boucher, R. (1987). Use of pornography in criminal and developmental histories of sexual offenders. *Journal of Interpersonal Violence, 2*(2): 196–211.

Cassidy, J. (1994). Emotion regulation: influences of attachment relationships. In: N. A. Fox (Ed.), *The Development of Emotion Regulation: Biological and Behavioural Foundations, 59*(2–3), No. 240 (pp. 228–250). Monographs of the Society for Research in Child Development.

Cavanagh Johnson, T. (2002). *Understanding Your Child's Sexual Behavior: What's Natural and Healthy.* Oakland, CA: New Harbinger.

Chamberlain, D. (1998). *The Mind of your Newborn Baby.* Berkeley, CA: North Atlantic Books.

Charlton, B. (2000). Review of *The Feeling of What Happens: Body, Emotion and the Making of Consciousness,* Antonio Damasio, London: Heinemann, 1999. *Journal of the Royal Society of Medicine, 93*(2): 99–101.

Chiron, C., Jambaque, I., Nabbout, R., Lounes, R., Syrota, A., & Dulac, O. (1997). The right brain hemisphere is dominant in human infants. *Brain, 120*(6): 1057–1065.

Chisholm, K. A. (2000). Attachment in children adopted from Romanian orphanages: two case studies. In: P. M. Crittenden & A. H. Claussen (Eds.), *The Organization of Attachment Relationships: Maturation, Culture, and Context* (pp. 171–189). Cambridge: Cambridge University Press.

Christie, M. M., Marshall, W. L., & Lanthier, R. D. (1979). *A Descriptive Study of Incarcerated Rapists.* Ottawa: Report to the Solicitor General of Canada.

Chugani, H., Behen, M., Muczik, O., Juhasz, C., Nagy, F., & Chugani, D. (2001). Local brain function activity following early deprivation: a study of post-institutionalized Romanian orphans. *Neuroimage, 14*(6): 1290–1301.

Clulow, C. (2001). *Adult Attachment and Couple Psychotherapy.* Hove: Routledge.

Cobb, R. J., & Bradbury, T. N. (2003). Implications of adult attachment for preventing adverse marital outcomes. In: S. M. Johnson & W. E. Whiffen (Eds.), *Attachment Processes in Couple and Family Therapy* (pp. 258–280). New York: Guilford Press.

Cohen, L. E., & Felson, M. (1979). Social change and crime rate trends: a routine activity approach. *American Sociological Review, 44*(4): 588–608.

Cohen, L. J., Nikiforov, K., Gans, S., Poznansky, O., McGeoch, P., Weaver, C., King, E. G., Cullen, K., & Galynker, I. (2002). Heterosexual male perpetrators of sexual abuse: a preliminary neuropsychiatric model. *Psychiatric Quarterly, 73*(4): 313–336.

Cole-Detke, H., & Kobak, R. (1996). Attachment processes in eating disorder and depression. *Journal of Consulting and Clinical Psychology, 64*(2): 282–290.

Coley, R. L., & Medeiros, B. L. (2007). Reciprocal longitudinal relations between non-resident father involvement and adolescent delinquency. *Child Development, 78*: 132–147.

Constantine, L., & Martinson, F. (1981). Child sexuality: here there be dragons. In: L. Constantine & F. Martinson (Eds.), *Children and Sex. New Findings. New Perspectives* (pp. 3–8). Boston: Little, Brown.

Cookston, J. T. (1999). Parental supervisions and family structure. Effect on adolescent problem behaviors. *Journal of Divorce and Remarriage, 32*(1/2): 107–122.

Cooper, A. (1997). Sexuality and the internet: surfing its way to the new millennium. *Cyberpsychology and Behavior, 1*(2): 24–28.

Cooper, A. (1998). Sexuality and the internet: surfing into the new millennium. *Cyberpsychology and Behavior, 1*(2): 187–193.

Cooper, A. (2002). *Sex and the Internet. A Guidebook for Clinicians.* New York: Brunner-Routledge.

Cooper, A., Boies, S., Maheu, M., & Greenfield, D. (1999). Sexuality and the internet: the next sexual revolution. In: F. Muscarella & L. Szuchman (Eds.), *The Psychological Science of Sexuality: A Research Based Approach* (pp. 519–545). New York: Wiley.

Cooper, A., Golden, G., & Marshall, W. L. (2006). Online sexuality and online sexual problems: skating on thin ice. In: W. L. Marshall, Y. M. Fernandez, L. E. Marshall, & G. A. Serran (Eds.), *Sexual Offender Treatment: Controversial Issues* (pp. 79–91). Chichester: Wiley.

Cooper, A., Månsson, S-A., Daneback, K., Tikkanen, R., & Ross, M. W. (2003). Predicting the future of internet sex: online sexual activities in Sweden. *Sexual & Relationship Therapy, 18*(3): 277–291.

Cooper, A., Putnam, D., Planchon, L., & Boies, S. (1999). On-line sexual compulsivity: getting tangled in the net. *Sexual Addiction and Compulsivity, 7*(2): 5–29.

Cooper, P. J. (1995). Eating disorders and their relationship to mood and anxiety disorders. In: K. D. Brownell & C. G. Fairburn (Eds.), *Eating Disorders and Obesity* (pp. 159–164). New York: Guilford Press.

Corley, M., & Schneider, J. (2002). Disclosing secrets: guidelines for therapists working with sex-addicts and co-addicts. *Sexual Addiction & Compulsivity, 9*(1): 43–67.

Corodimas, K. P., LeDoux, J. E., Gold, P. W., & Schulkin, J. (1994). Corticosterone potential of learned fear. *Annals of the New York Academy of Sciences, 746*: 392–393.

Cortoni, F., & Marshall, W. L. (2001). Sex as a coping strategy and its relationship to juvenile sexual history and intimacy in sexual offenders. *Sexual Abuse: A Journal of Research and Treatment, 13*(1): 27–43.

Cosford, P. (2009). Personal communication.

Cowan, P., & Cowan, C. P. (2001). Transmission of attachment patterns. In: C. Clulow (Ed.), *Adult Attachment and Couple Psychotherapy* (pp. 62–82). Hove: Brunner-Routledge.

Cowburn, M., Wilson, C., & Loewenstein, P. (1992). *Changing Men. A Practice Guide to Working with Adult Male Sex Offenders.* Nottingham: Nottinghamshire Probation Service.

Cozolino, L. (2002). *The Neuroscience of Psychotherapy*. New York: Norton.

Cozolino, L. (2006). *The Neuroscience of Human Relationships*. New York: Norton.

Craig, L. A., & Beech, A. (2009). Best practice in conducting actuarial risk assessments with adult sex offenders. *Journal of Sexual Aggression, 15*(2): 193–211.

Craig, L. A., Beech, A., & Browne, K. (2007). The importance of cross-validating actuarial measures. *Forensic Update, 90*: 34–39.

Craig, L. A., Browne, K., & Beech, A. R. (Eds.) (2008). *Assessing Risk in Sex Offenders. A Practitioners Guide*. Chichester: Wiley.

Craig, L. A., Browne, K. D., Hogue, T. E., & Stringer, I. (2004). New directions in assessing risk for sexual offenders. In: G. Macpherson & L. Jones (Eds.) *Issues in Forensic Psychology: Risk Assessment and Management* (pp. 81–99. Leicester: British Psychological Society.

Crittenden, P. M. (1995). Attachment and psychopathology. In: S. Goldberg, R. Muir, & J. Kerr (Eds.), *Attachment Theory: Social, Developmental and Clinical Perspectives* (pp. 367–406). Hillsdale, NJ: Analytic Press.

Crittenden, P. M. (2007). Personal communication.

Crittenden, P. M. (2008). *Raising Parents. Attachment, Parenting and Child Safety*. Cullompton, Devon: Willan.

Crowe, M., & Bunclark, J. (2000). Self injury: a struggle. *International Review of Psychiatry, 12*(1): 48–53.

Crowell, J., & Treboux, D. (2001). Attachment security in adult partnerships. In: C. Clulow (Ed.), *Adult Attachment and Couple Psychotherapy. The "Secure Base" in Practice and Research* (pp. 28–42). London: Routledge.

Csikszentmihalyi, M. (1990). *Flow: The Psychology of Optimal Experience*. New York: Norton.

Cudmore, L., & Judd, D. (2001). Traumatic loss and the couple. In: C. Clulow (Ed.), *Adult Attachment and Couple Psychotherapy* (pp. 152–170). Hove: Brunner-Routledge.

Dabbs, J. M. J., & Hargrove, M. F. (1997). Age, testosterone, and behavior among female prison inmates. *Psychosomatic Medicine, 59*(5): 477–480.

Damasio, A. (1994). *Descartes' Error*. New York: Grosset/Putnam.

Damasio, A. (2003). *Looking for Spinoza. Joy, Sorrow and the Feeling Brain*. London: Vintage.

Damasio, A., Tranel, D., & Damasio, H. (1990). Individuals with sociopathic behaviour caused by frontal damage fail to respond autonomically to social stimuli. *Behavioral Brain Research, 41*(2): 81–94.

Davenport, R., & Fisher, D. (2007). Trauma related symptoms in men and women who commit sexual offences. *NotaNews, 55*: 14–16.

Davies, P. T., & Cummings, E. M. (1995). Marital conflict and child adjustment: an emotional security hypothesis. *Psychological Bulletin,* 116(3): 387–411.

Davis, R. A. (2001). A cognitive–behavioural model of pathological internet use. *Computers in Human Behavior, 17*(2): 187–195.

Davila, J. (2003). Attachment processes in couple therapy. Informing behavioral models. In: S. M. Johnson & W. E. Whiffen (Eds.), *Attachment Processes in Couple and Family Therapy* (pp. 124–143). New York: Guilford Press.

Davila, J., & Levy, K. N. (2006). Introduction to the special section on attachment theory and psychotherapy. *Journal of Consulting and Clinical Psychology, 74*(6): 989–993.

Davin, P. A. (1999). Secrets revealed: a study of female sex offenders. In: P. A. Davin, J. C. R. Hislop, & T. Dunbar (Eds.), *The Female Sexual Abuser: Three Views* (pp. 9–134). Brandon, VT: Safer Society Press.

Dear, G. E. (2002). The relationship between codependency and femininity and masculinity. *Sex Roles, 46*(5–6): 159–165.

DeBellis, M. D. (2002). Developmental traumatology: a contributory mechanism for alcohol and substance use disorders. *Psychoneuroendochrinology, 27*(1–2): 155–170.

DeBellis, M., Keshavan, M., Clark, D., Casey, B., Giedd, J., Boring, A., Frustaci, K., & Ryan, N. (1999). Developmental traumatology Part II: brain development. *Biological Psychiatry, 45*(10): 1271–1284.

Delmonico, D. L. (2004). Cybersex: a form/forum of sex addiction. Paper presented to the European Federation of Sexology 7th Congress, Brighton, May.

Delmonico, D. L., & Griffin, E. (2007). Prevention beyond the cyberpredator: a comprehensive internet safety plan for children and adolescents. *NotaNews, 55*: 4–7.

Delmonico, D. L., Griffin, E., & Carnes, P. (2002). Treating online compulsive sexual behaviour: when cybersex is the drug of choice. In: A. Cooper (Ed.), *Sex and the Internet. A Guidebook for Clinicians* (pp. 147–168). New York: Brunner-Routledge.

DeMaria, R., Weeks, G., & Hof, L. (1999). *Focused Genograms. Intergenerational Assessment of Individuals, Couples and Families.* Philadelphia, PA: Taylor & Francis.

Dennis, W. (1973). *Children of the Crèche.* New York: Appleton-Century-Crofts.

de Zulueta, F. (1996). Theories of aggression and violence. In: C. Cordess & M. Cox (Eds.), *Forensic Psychotherapy. Crime, Psychodynamics and the Offender Patient* (pp. 175–186). London: Jessica Kingsley.

de Zulueta, F. (2006). *From Pain to Violence. The Traumatic Roots of Destructiveness.* London: Whurr.

Diamond, G. S., & Stern, R., S. (2003). Attachment-based family therapy for depressed adolescents. In: S. M. Johnson & W. E. Whiffen (Eds.), *Attachment Processes in Couple and Family Therapy* (pp. 191–212). New York: Guilford Press.

Diehl, M., Elnick, A. B., Bourbeau, L. S., & Labouvie-Vief, G. (1998). Adult attachment styles: their relations to family context and personality. *Journal of Personality and Social Psychology, 74*(6): 1656–1669.

Dietz, P. E., Matthews, D. B., Martell, D. A., Stewart, T. M., Hrouda, D. R., & Warren, J. (1991a). Threatening and otherwise inappropriate letters to members of the United States Congress. *Journal of Forensic Sciences, 36*: 1145–1468.

Dietz, P. E., Matthews, D. B., Van Duyne, C., Martell, D. A., Parry, C. D., Stewart, T., Warren, J., & Crowder, J. D. (1991b). Threatening and otherwise inappropriate letters to Hollywood celebrities. *Journal of Forensic Sciences, 36*: 185–209.

Dixon, L., & Browne, K. D. (2003). Heterogeneity of spouse abuse: a review. *Aggression and Violent Behaviour, 8*(1): 107–130.

Dixon, L., & Browne, K. (2007). The heterogeneity of family violence and its implications for practice. *Issues in Forensic Psychology, 6*: 116–124.

Dobbing, J., & Sands, J. (1973). Quantitative growth and development of human brain. *Archives of Diseases of Childhood, 48*(10): 757–767.

Dolan, R. J., Fletcher, P., Morris, J., Kapur, N., Deakin, J. F., & Frith, C. D. (1996). Neural activation during covert processing of positive emotion facial expressions. *Neuroimage, 4*(3, Part 1): 194–200.

Donegan, N. H., Sanislow, C. A., Blumberg, H. P., Fulbright, R. K., Lacadie, C., Skudlarski, P., Gore, J. C., Olson, I. R., McGlashan, T. H.,

& Wexler, B. E. (2003). Amygdala hyperreactivity in borderline personality disorder: implications for emotional dysregulation. *Biological Psychiatry, 54*(11): 1284–1293.

Doren, D. M. (2006). Recidivism risk assessments: making sense of controversies. In: W. L. Marshall, Y. M. Fernandez, L. E. Marshall, & G. A. Serran (Eds.), *Sexual Offender Treatment: Controversial Issues* (pp. 3–15). Chichester: Wiley.

Dozier, M., Cue, K., & Barnett, L. (1994). Clinicians as caregivers: role of attachment organization as treatment. *Journal of Consulting and Clinical Psychology, 62*(4): 793–800.

Drake, C. R., & Pathé, M. (2004). Understanding sexual offending in schizophrenia. *Criminal Behaviour and Mental Health, 14*(2): 108–120.

Dubowitz, H. (1999). *Neglected Children. Research, Practice and Policy.* Thousand Oaks, CA: Sage.

Dutton, D. G. (1995). *The Domestic Assault of Women: Psychological and Criminal Justice Perspectives.* Boston: Allyn & Bacon.

Dutton, D. G. (1999). The traumatic origins of intimate rage. *Aggression and Violent Behavior, 4*(4): 431–448.

Dutton, D. G., & Nicholls, T. (2005). A critical review of the gender paradigm in domestic violence research and theory: Part 1: theory and data. *Aggression & Violent Behavior, 10*(6): 680–714.

Edwards, P., Harvey, C., & Whitehead, P. C. (1973). Wives of alcoholics: a critical review and analysis. *Quarterly Journal of Studies on Alcohol, 34*: 112–132.

Eells, T. D. (2001). Attachment theory and psychotherapy research. *Journal of Psychotherapy Practice and Research, 10*(2): 132–135.

Egeland, B., & Sroufe, L. A. (1981). Attachment and early maltreatment. *Child Development, 52*: 44–52.

Ellis, D. P., Weiner, P., & Miller, L. (1971). Does the trigger pull the finger? An experimental test of weapons as aggression-eliciting stimuli. *Sociometry, 34*(4): 453–456.

Epstein, R. S. (1994). *Keeping Boundaries: Maintaining Safety and Integrity in the Psychotherapeutic Process.* Washington, DC: American Psychiatric Press.

Erikson, E. (1963). *Childhood and Society.* New York: Norton.

Eron, L. D. (1987). The development of aggressive behavior from the perspective of a developing behaviorism. *American Psychologist, 42*(5): 435–443.

Essex, M., Klein, M., Cho, E., & Kalin, N. (2002). Maternal stress beginning in infancy may sensitize children to later stress exposure: effects of cortisol and behavior. *Biological Psychiatry*, 52(8): 776–784.

Etherington, K. (1997). Maternal abuse of males. *Child Abuse Review*, 6: 107–117.

Etherington, K. (2009). The impact of trauma and abuse on a man's sense of self and identity. Paper presented to the Working with Trauma and Sexuality in the Consulting Room Conference, British Association of Sexual and Relationship Therapy, June, Warwick.

Etkin, A., Pittenger, C., Polan, H. J., & Kandel, E. R. (2005). Toward a neurobiology of psychotherapy: basic science and clinical applications. *Journal of Neuropsychiatry and Clinical Neuroscience*, 17(2): 145–158.

Faller, K. C. (1987). Women who sexually abuse children. *Violence and Victims*, 2(4): 263–276.

Falshaw, L., Friendship, C., & Bates, A. (2003). *Sexual Offenders—Measuring Reconviction, Reoffending and Recidivism* (183). London: Home Office Research, Development and Statistics Directorate.

Farley, P. (2004). The anatomy of despair. *New Scientist*, 182(2445): 43–45.

Farrington, D. (1978). The family backgrounds of aggressive youths. In: L. Hersov, M. Berger, & D. Shaffer (Eds.), *Aggression and Anti-social Behaviour in Childhood and Adolescence* (pp. 73–93). Oxford: Pergamon.

Farrington, D. P. (1995). The development of offending and antisocial behaviour from childhood. *Journal of Child Psychology and Psychiatry*, 36(6): 929–964.

Favazza, A. R., & Rosenthal, R. J. (1993). Diagnostic issues in self-mutilation. *Hospital and Community Psychiatry*, 44(2): 134–140.

Federici, R. S. (1999). Neuropsychological evaluation and rehabilitation of the post institutionalized child. Paper presented at the *Children and Residential Care Conference*, 3 May, 1999, Stockholm, Sweden.

Feelgood, S., & Hoyer, J. (2008). Child molester or paedophile? Socio-legal versus psychopathological classification of sexual offenders against children. *Journal of Sexual Aggression*, 14(1): 33–43.

Feeney, J., & Noller, P. (1996). *Adult Attachment*. London: Sage.

Feher, L. (1980). *The Psychology of Birth: The Foundation of Human Personality*. London: Souvenir Press.

Feldman, L. B. (1982). Dysfunctional marital conflict: an integrative interpersonal intrapsychic model. *Journal of Marital and Family Therapy, 8*(4): 417–428.

Felitti, V. L., Anda, R. F., Nordenberg, D., Williamson, D. F., Spitz, A. M., Edwards, V., Koss, M. P., & Marks, J. S. (1998). Relationship of childhood abuse and household dysfunction to many of the leading causes of death in adults. Impact on children. *American Journal of Preventative Medicine, 14*(4): 245–258.

Fernandez, Y. M. (2006). Focusing on the positive and avoiding negativity in sexual offender treatment. In: W. L. Marshall, Y. M. Fernandez, L. E. Marshall, & G. A. Serran (Eds.), *Sexual Offender Treatment. Controversial Issues* (pp. 187–197). Chichester: Wiley.

Ferree, M. (2003). Women and the web: cybersex activity and implications. *Sexual & Relationship Therapy, 18*(3): 385–393.

Few, A. L., & Rosen, K. H. (2005). Victims of chronic dating violence: how women's vulnerabilities link to their decisions to stay. *Family Relations, 54*(22): 265–279.

Field, T. (1985). Attachment as psychobiological attunement: being on the same wavelength. In: M. Reite & T. Field (Eds.), *The Psychobiology of Attachment and Separation* (pp. 415–454). Orlando, FL: Academic Press.

Fields, R. D. (2004). The other half of the brain. *Scientific American, 290*(4): 54–61.

Fincham, F. D., Bradbury, T. N., & Scott, C. K. (1990). Cognition in marriage. In: F. D. Fincham & T. N. Bradbury (Eds.), *The Psychology of Marriage* (pp. 118–148). New York: Guilford Press.

Finkelhor, D. (1986). *A Sourcebook on Child Sexual Abuse*. Beverly Hills, CA: Sage.

Finkelhor, D., & Araji, S. (1986). Explanations of pedophilia: a four factor model. *Journal of Sex Research, 22*(1): 145–161.

Finkelhor, D., Willimans, L. M., & Burns, N. (1988). *Nursery Crimes: Sexual Abuse in Day Care*. Newbury Park, CA: Sage.

Fischer, K. W., & Pipp, S. L. (1984). Development of the structures of unconscious thought. In: K. S. Bowers & D. Meichenbaum (Eds.), *The Unconscious Reconsidered* (pp. 88–148). New York: Wiley.

Fisher, D. (1994). Sex offenders: who are they? Why are they? In: T. Morrison, M. Erooga, & R. C. Beckett (Eds.), *Sexual Offenders Against Children: Management and Policy*. London: Routledge.

Fisher, J., & Crandell, L. (2001). Patterns of relating in the couple. In: C. Clulow (Ed.), *Adult Attachment and Couple Psychotherapy. The 'Secure Base' in Practice and Research* (pp. 15–27). London: Routledge.

Fitzherbert, C. (1993). Inside the mind of the sex beast. *Sunday Telegraph*, 27 June.

Flak, V., Beech, A., & Fisher, D. (2007). Forensic assessment of deviant sexual interests: the current position. *Issues in Forensic Psychology, 6*: 70–83.

Fletcher, J. M., & Woolfe, R. (2009). Long-term consequences of childhood ADHD and criminal activities. *Journal of Mental Health Policy and Economics, 12*(3): 119–138.

Foley, T. P. (2002). Forensic assessment of internet child pornography offenders. In: B. Schwartz (Ed.), *The Sex Offender: Current Treatment Modalities and System Issues*, Volume IV (pp. 26.21–26.18). Kingston, NJ: Civic Research Institute.

Fonagy, P. (2001). *Attachment Theory and Psychoanalysis*. New York: Other Press.

Fonagy, P., Leigh, T., Steele, M., Steele, H., Kennedy, R., Mattoon, G., Target, M., & Gerber, A. (1996). The relationship of attachment status, psychiatric classification and response to psychotherapy. *Journal of Consulting and Clinical Psychology, 64*(1): 22–31.

Fonagy, P., Steele, H., & Steele, M. (1991). Maternal representations of attachment during pregnancy predict the organization of infant–mother attachment at one year of age. *Child Development, 62*(5): 891–905.

Fonagy, P., Steele, M., Moran, G. S., Steele, H., & Higgitt, A. (1992). The integration of psychoanalytic theory and work on attachment: the issue of intergenerational psychic processes. In: D. Stern & M. Ammaniti (Eds.), *Attaccamento e Psiconalis* (pp. 19–30). Bari, Italy: Laterza.

Ford, H. (2006). *Women Who Sexually Abuse Children*. Chichester: Wiley.

Fossati, A., Acquarini, E., Feeney, J., Borroni, S., Grazioli, F., Giarolli, L. E., Franciosi, G., & Maffei, C. (2009). Alexithymia and attachment insecurities in impulsive aggression. *Attachment & Human Development, 11*(2): 165–182.

Fraiberg, S., Adelson, E., & Shapiro, V. (1975). Ghosts in the nursery: a psychoanalytic approach to impaired infant–mother relationships. *Journal of the American Academy of Child Psychiatry, 14*(3): 387–421.

Fraley, R. C., & Waller, N. G. (1998). Adult attachment patterns: a test of the typological model. In: J. A. Simpson & W. S. Rhodes (Eds.), *Attachment Theory and Close Relationships* (pp. 77–114). New York: Guilford Press.

Frei, A., Erenay, N., Dittman, V., & Graf, M. (2005). Paedophilia on the internet: a study of 33 convicted offenders in the Canton of Lucerne. *Swiss Medical Weekly*, *135*(33–34): 488–494.

Freud, S. (1901b). The psychopathology of everyday life. *S.E.*, *6*. London: Hogarth.

Freud, S. (1914c). On narcissism: an introduction. *S.E.*, *14*: 67–102. London: Hogarth.

Freud, S. (1915e). The unconscious. *S.E.*, *14*: 159–204. London: Hogarth.

Friedman, A., & Poulson, M. C. (1981). The hemispheres as independent resource systems: limited-capacity processing and cerebral specialization. *Journal of Experimental Psychology: Human Perception and Performance*, *7*(5): 1031–1058.

Friedman, J. I., Temporini, H., & Davis, K. L. (1999). Pharmacological strategies for augmenting cognitive performance in schizophrenia. *Biological Psychiatry*, *45*(1): 1–16.

Friedrich, W., Davies, W., Feher, E., & Wright, J. (2003). Sexual behavior problems in preteen children: developmental, ecological and behavioral correlates. *Annals of the New York Academy of Sciences*, *989*: 95–104.

Fritz, G., Stoll, K., & Wagner, N. (1981). A comparison of males and females who were sexually molested as children. *Journal of Sex & Marital Therapy*, *7*(1): 54–58.

Fromuth, M. E., & Burkart, B. R. (1987). Childhood sexual victimization among college men: definitional and methodological issues. *Violence and Victims*, *2*(4): 241–253.

Furby, L., Weinrott, M. R., & Blackshaw, L. (1989). Sex offender recidivism: a review. *Psychological Bulletin*, *105*(1): 3–30.

Gaensbauer, T. J., Harmon, R. J., Cytryn, L., & McKnew, D. H. (1984). Differences in the patterning of affective expression in infants. *Journal of the American Academy of Child Psychiatry*, *141*(2): 223–229.

Galbreath, N. W., Berlin, F. S., & Sawyer, D. (2002). Paraphilias and the internet. In: A. Cooper (Ed.), *Sex and the Internet. A Guidebook for Clinicians* (pp. 187–205). New York: Brunner-Routledge.

Gallagher, B. (2007). Internet-initiated incitement and conspiracy to commit child sexual abuse (CSA): the typology, extent and nature of known cases. *Journal of Sexual Aggression*, *13*(2): 101–119.

Gannon, T. A., & Ward, T. (2008). Rape. Psychopathology and theory. In: D. R. Laws & W. T. O'Donohue (Eds.), *Sexual Deviance. Theory, Assessment, and Treatment* (pp. 336–355). New York: Guilford Press.

Garrison, K. (1992). *Working with Sex Offenders. A Practice Guide.* Norwich: Social Work Monographs.

Gazzaniga, M. (1995). *The Cognitive Neurosciences.* Cambridge, MA: MIT Press.

Gedo, J. (1979). *Beyond Interpretation.* New York: International Universities Press.

George, C., Kaplan, N., & Main, M. (1985). *The Adult Attachment Interview.* Berkeley: University of California.

George, N., Dolan, R. J., Fink, G., Baylis, G. C., Russell, C., & Driver, J. (1999). Human fusiform gyrus extracts shape-from-shading to recognize familiar faces. *Nature Neuroscience, 2*(6): 574–580.

Gergely, G., & Watson, J. (1996). The social biofeedback model of parental affect-mirroring. *International Journal of Psychoanalysis, 77*(6): 1181–1207.

Gerhardt, S. (2004). *Why Love Matters. How Affection Shapes a Baby's Brain.* Hove: Brunner-Routledge.

Gerhardt, S. (2007). Making a person: the lasting impact of babyhood. *Counselling Psychology Review, 22*(3): 37–44.

Ghaemi, S. N., Ko, J. Y., & Goodwin, F. K. (2001). The bipolar spectrum and the antidepressant view of the world. *Journal of Psychiatric Practice, 7*(5): 287–297.

Gilby, R., Wolf, L., & Goldberg, B. (1989). Mentally retarded adolescent sex offenders, a survey and pilot study. *Canadian Journal of Psychiatry, 34*(6): 542–548.

Gillespie, A. A. (2005). Tackling child pornography: the approach in England and Wales. In: E. Quayle & M. Taylor (Eds.), *Viewing Child Pornography on the Internet* (pp. 1–16). Lyme Regis: Russell House Publishing.

Gillespie, A. A. (2008). Adolescents accessing indecent images of children. *Journal of Sexual Aggression, 14*(2): 111–122.

Gilligan, J. (1996). *Violence. Reflections on our Deadliest Epidemic.* Philadelphia, PA: Jessica Kingsley.

Glaser, D. (2003). Early experience, attachment and the brain. In: J. Corrigall & H. Wilkinson (Eds.), *Revolutionary Connections. Psychotherapy and Neuroscience* (pp. 117–133). London: Karnac.

Glueck, E. T., & Glueck, S. (1966). Identification of potential delinquents at 2–3 years of age. *International Journal of Social Psychiatry, 12*(1): 5–16.

Godsi, E. (1999). *Violence in Society. The Reality Behind Violent Crime.* London: Constable.

Goffman, E. (1976). *Gender Advertisements*. New York: Harper Colophon.

Goldberg, S., Corter, C., Lojkasek, M., & Minde, K. (1990). Prediction of behavior problems in four-year-olds born prematurely. *Development and Psychopathology, 2*(1): 15–30.

Goldberger, L. (1982). Sensory deprivation and overload. In: L. Goldberger & S. Breznitz (Eds.), *Handbook of Stress: Theoretical and Clinical Aspects* (pp. 410–418). New York: Free Press.

Goldstein, A. P., Glick, B., Irwin, M. J., Pask-McCartney, C., & Rabama, I. (1989). *Reducing Delinquency: Intervention in the Community*. New York: Pergamon.

Goleman, D. (1995). *Emotional Intelligence*. London: Bloomsbury.

Goodman, A. (1992). Diagnosis and treatment of sexual addiction. *Journal of Sex & Marital Therapy, 18*(4): 551–572.

Goodman, L. A., Rosenberg, S. D., Mueser, K., & Drake, R. E. (1997). Physical and sexual assault history in women with serious mental illness: prevalence, correlates, treatment, and future research directions. *Schizophrenia Bulletin, 23*(4): 685–696.

Gordon, H. W. (2002). Early environmental stress and biological vulnerability to drug abuse. *Psychoneuroendochrinology, 27*(1/2): 115–126.

Gottman, J. (1994). *Why Marriages Succeed or Fail*. New York: Simon & Schuster.

Graham-Kevan, N. (2007). Johnson's control-based domestic violence typology: Implications for research and treatment. *Issues in Forensic Psychology, 6*: 109–115.

Green, A. H. (1980). *Child Maltreatment*. New York: Jason Aronson.

Green, R. G., & McCowan, E. J. (1984). Effects of noise and attack on aggression and physiological arousal. *Motivation and Emotion, 8*(3): 231–241.

Greenall, P. V., & Jellicoe-Jones, L. (2007). Themes and risk of sexual violence among the mentally ill: implications for understanding and treatment. *Sexual & Relationship Therapy, 22*(3): 323–337.

Greenall, P. V., & West, A. G. (2007). A study of stranger rapists from the English high security hospitals. *Journal of Sexual Aggression, 13*(2): 151–167.

Greenberger, D., & Padesky, C. (1995). *Mind Over Mood. Change How You Feel by Changing the Way that You Think*. New York: Guilford Press.

Greenfield, D. (1999). *Virtual Addiction: Help for Netheads, Cyberfreaks and Those Who Love Them*. Oakland, CA: New Harbinger.

Greenspan, S. I. (1981). *Psychopathology and Adaptation in Infancy and Early Childhood*. New York: International Universities Press.

Gregory, E. (1975). Comparison of postnatal CNS development between male and female rats. *Brain Research, 99*: 152–156.

Greyston, A. D., & DeLuca, R. V. (1999). Female perpetrators of childhood sexual abuse: a review of the clinical and empirical literature. *Aggression & Violent Behavior, 4*(1): 93–106.

Griffiths, D., Hingsburger, D., & Christian, R. (1985). Treating developmentally handicapped sexual offenders: the York behavior management services treatment program. *Psychiatric Aspects in Mental Retardation Review, 4*: 49–53.

Groth, A. N. (1978). Patterns of sexual assault against children and adolescents. In: A. W. Burgess, A. N. Groth, L. L. Holstrom, & M. Groi (Eds.), *Sexual Assault of Children and Adolescents* (pp. 3–24). Boston, MA: Heath.

Grubin, D. (1998). *Sex Offending against Children: Understanding the Risk* (Police Research Series Paper 99). London: Home Office.

Gundel, H., Lopez-Sala, A., Ceballos-Baumann, A. O., Deus, J., Cardoner, N., & Martin-Mittage, B. (2004). Alexithymia correlates with the size of the right anterior cingulate. *Psychosomatic Medicine, 66*(1): 132–140.

Hagan, L. K., & Kuebli, J. (2007). Mothers' and fathers' socialization of preschoolers' physical risk taking. *Journal of Applied Developmental Psychology, 28*(1): 2–14.

Hall, R. C. W., & Hall, R. C. W. (2007). A profile of pedophilia: definition, characteristics of offenders, recidivism, treatment outcomes, and forensic issues. *Mayo Clinic Proceedings, 82*(4): 457–471.

Halliday, R. (2001). *Making Punishment Work*. London: Home Office.

Hanson, R. K., & Bussière, M. T. (1998). Predicting relapse: a meta-analysis of sexual offender recidivism studies. *Journal of Consulting & Clinical Psychology, 66*(2): 348–362.

Hanson, R. K., & Harris, A. J. R. (2000). Where should we intervene? Dynamic predictors of sexual assault recidivism. *Criminal Justice Behaviour, 27*(1): 6–35.

Hanson, R. K., & Thornton, D. (1999). *Static-99: Improving Actuarial Assessment of Sex Offenders*. Corrections Research, Ministry of the Solicitor General of Canada.

Hanson, R. K., & Thornton, D. (2000). Improving risk assessments for sex offenders: a comparison of three actuarial scales. *Law and Human Behavior, 24*(1): 119–136.

Hanson, R. K., Gizzarelli, R., & Scott, H. (1994). The attitudes of incest offenders. *Criminal Justice and Behavior, 21*(2): 187–202.

Hanson, R. K., Morton, K. E., & Harris, A. J. (2003). Sexual offender recidivism risk: what we know and what we need to know. *Annals of the New York Academy of Sciences, 989* (Part III: Risk Assessment): 154–166.

Harrington, A. (1985). Nineteenth-century ideas on hemisphere differences and "duality of mind". *Behavioral and Brain Sciences, 8*: 617–634.

Harris, L. J., Almergi, J. B., & Kirsch, E. A. (2000). Side preference in adults for holding infants: contributions of sex and handedness in a test of imagination. *Brain & Cognition, 43*(1–3): 246–252.

Harter, S., Marold, D. B., Whitesell, N. R., & Cobbs, G. (1996). A model of the effects of perceived parent and peer support on adolescent false self behavior. *Child Development, 67*(2): 360–374.

Hartmann, E., Russ, D., Oldfield, M., Falke, R., & Skoff, B. (1980). Dream content: effects of L-DOPA. *Sleep Research, 9*: 153.

Hawton, K., Fagg, J., Simkin, S., & Bond, A. (1997). Trends in deliberate self-harm in Oxford, 1985–1995. *British Journal of Psychiatry, 171*: 556–560.

Hawton, K., Haw, C., Houston, K., & Townsend, E. (2002). Family history of suicidal behaviour: prevalence and significance in deliberate self harm. *Acta Psychiatrica Scandinavia, 106*(5): 387–393.

Hazan, C. (2003). The essential nature of couple relationships. In: S. M. Johnson & W. E. Whiffen (Eds.), *Attachment Processes in Couple and Family Therapy* (pp. 43–63). New York: Guilford.

Hazan, C., & Shaver, P. R. (1987). Romantic love conceptualized as an attachment process. *Journal of Personality and Social Psychology, 52*(1): 511–534.

Hazan, C., & Zeifman, D. (1999). Pair bonds as attachment: evaluating the evidence. In: J. Cassidy & P. Shaver (Eds.), *Handbook of Attachment. Theory, Research and Clinical Implications* (pp. 336–354). New York: Guilford Press.

Heard, D. H., & Lake, B. (1997). *The Challenge of Attachment for Caregiving*. London: Routledge.

Heard, D. H., Lake, B., & McClusky, U. (2009). *Attachment Therapy with Adolescents and Adults*. London: Karnac.

Heath, L., Kruttschnitt, C., & Ward, D. (1986). Television and violent criminal behavior: beyond the Bobo doll. *Violence and Victims, 1*(3): 177–190.

Hebb, D. O. (1949). *The Organization of Behavior*. New York: Wiley.

Heilbrun, A. B. (1982). Cognitive models of criminal violence based on intelligence and psychopathy levels. *Journal of Consulting and Clinical Psychology, 50*(4): 546–557.

Heinz, J. W., Gargaro, S., & Kelly, K. F. (1987). *A Model Residential Juvenile Sex Offender Treatment Program — The Hennapin County Home School*. Brandon, VT: Safer Society Press.

Henderson, M. (1986). An empirical typology of violent incidents reported by prison inmates with convictions for violence. *Aggressive Behavior, 12*(1): 21–32.

Hennessy, M., Walker, J., & Vess, J. (2002). An evaluation of the empathy as a measure of victim empathy with civilly committed sexual offenders. *Sexual Abuse: A Journal of Research and Treatment, 14*(3): 241–252.

Herman, B. A., & Panskepp, J. (1978). Effects of morphine and naloxone on separation distress and approach attachment: evidence for opiate mediation of social effect. *Pharmacology, Biochemistry and Behavior, 9*(2): 213–220.

Herman, J. L. (1992). *Trauma and Recovery. From Domestic Abuse to Political Terror*. London: Pandora.

Herzog, J. M. (2001). *Father Hunger. Explorations with Adults and Children*. Hillsdale, NJ: Analytic Press.

Hess, E. H. (1975). The role of pupil size in communication. *Scientific American, 233*(5): 110–119.

Hesse, E., Main, M., Abrams, K. Y., & Rifkin, A. (2003). Un-resolved states regarding loss or abuse can have "second-generation" effects: disorganization, role inversion, and frightening ideation of the offspring of traumatized non-maltreating parents. In: M. F. Solomon & D. J. Siegel (Eds.), *Healing Trauma. Attachment, Mind, Body, and Brain* (pp. 57–106). New York: W. W. Norton.

Hicks, D. (1968). Short- and long-term retention of affectively-varied modeled behavior. *Psychonomic Science, 11*: 369–370.

Hildyard, K. L., & Wolfe, D. (2002). Child neglect: developmental issues and outcomes. *Child Abuse and Neglect, 26*(6–7): 679–695.

Hiller, J. (2004). Feelings, sex and neurochemistry. Paper presented to the European Federation of Sexology Congress, Brighton.

Hinde, R. (1989). Relations between levels of complexity in the behavioral sciences. *Journal of Nervous and Mental Disease, 177*(11): 655–667.

Hofer, M. A. (1994). Hidden regulators in attachment, separation, and loss. *Monographs of the Society for Research in Child Development*, 59: 192–207.

Holmes, J. (1996). *Attachment, Intimacy, Autonomy: Using Attachment Theory in Adult Psychotherapy*. Northvale, NJ: Jason Aronson.

Holmes, J. (1998). Defensive and creative uses of narrative in psychotherapy: an attachment perspective. In: G. Roberts & J. Holmes (Eds.), *Narrative in Psychotherapy and Psychiatry* (pp. 49–68). Oxford: Oxford University Press.

Holmes, J. (2001). *The Search for a Secure Base*. Hove: Brunner Routledge.

Holmes, J. (2007). Sex, couples, and attachment: the role of hedonic intersubjectivity. *Attachment: New Directions in Psychotherapy and Relational Psychoanalysis*, 1(1): 18–29.

Holtzworth-Munroe, A., & Meehan, J. C. (2004). Typlogies of men who are maritally violent: scientific and clinical implications. *Interpersonal Violence*, 19(12): 1369–1389.

Holtzworth-Munroe, A., & Stuart, G. L. (1994). Typologies of male batterers: three sub-types and the differences among them. *Psychological Bulletin*, 116(3): 476–497.

Home Office (2008). *British Crime Survey; Criminal Statistics, England and Wales 2007–8*. London: Home Office.

Hook, A., & Andrews, B. (2005). The relationship of non-disclosure in therapy to shame and depression. *British Journal of Clinical Psychology*, 44(3): 425–438.

Hook, E. B. (1973). Behavioral implications of the human XYY genotype. *Science*, 179(69): 139–150.

Howard, J. (2000). Working with child abuse and neglect issues. *CSAT Treatment Improvement Series*, 36: 1–9.

Howitt, D. (1995). *Paedophiles and Sexual Offences Against Children*. Chichester: Wiley.

Hudson, K. (2005). *Offending Identities: Sex Offenders' Perspectives on their Treatment and Management*. Cullompton, Devon: Willan.

Hudson, S. M., & Ward, T. (2000). Interpersonal competency of sex offenders. *Behavior Modification*, 24(4): 233–242.

Hudson-Allez, G. (2002). The prevalence of stalking of psychological therapists working in primary care by current or former clients. *Counselling and Psychotherapy Research*, 2(2): 139–146.

Hutton, L., & Whyte, B. (2006). Children and young people with harmful sexual behaviours: first analysis of data from a Scottish sample. *Journal of Sexual Aggression*, 12(2): 115–125.

ICD-10 (1994). *ICD-10 Classification of Mental and Behavioural Disorders.* Geneva: World Health Organisation.

Insel, T. R. (2000). Toward a neurobiology of attachment. *Review of General Psychiatry*, 4(2): 176–185.

Izard, C. E. (1991). *The Psychology of Emotions.* New York: Plenum Press.

Jaffe, P., Wolfe, D., & Wilson, S. (1990). *Children of Battered Women.* Newbury Park, CA: Sage.

Jamil, O. B., Harper, G. W., & Fernandez, W. I. (2009). Adolescent trials network for HIV/AIDs interventions. *Cultural Diversity and Ethnic Minority Psychology*, 15(3): 203–214.

Janssen, E., Vorst, H., Finn, P., & Bancroft, J. (2002). The Sexual Inhibition (SIS) and Sexual Excitation (SES) Scales: measuring individual differences in the propensity for sexual inhibition and sexual excitation in men. *Journal of Sex Research*, 39(2): 127–132.

Jenkins, A. (1990). *Invitations to Responsibility. The Therapeutic Engagement of Men Who Are Violent and Abusive.* Adelaide: Dulwich Centre Publications.

Jenkins, A. (2009). *Becoming Ethical. A Parallel, Political Journey with Men Who Have Abused.* Lyme Regis: Russell House Publishing.

Jenkins, P. (2001). *Beyond Tolerance. Child Pornography on the Internet.* New York: New York University Press.

Johnson, P. A., Hurley, R. A., Benkelfat, C., Herpertz, S. C., & Taber, K. H. (2003). Understanding emotional regulation in borderline personality disorder: Contributions of neuroimaging. *Journal of Neuropsychiatry and Clinical Neuroscience*, 15(4): 397–402.

Johnson, S. M. (1987). *Humanizing the Narcissistic Style.* New York: W. W. Norton.

Johnson, S. M. (2002). *Emotionally Focused Couple Therapy with Trauma Survivors: Strengthening Attachment Bonds.* New York: Guilford Press.

Johnson, S. M. (2003). Attachment theory. A guide for couple therapy. In: S. M. Johnson & W. E. Whiffen (Eds.), *Attachment Processes in Couple and Family Therapy* (pp. 103–123). New York: Guilford Press.

Johnson, S. M., Makinen, J., & Millikin, J. (2001). Attachment injuries in couple relationships: a new perspective on impasses in couples therapy. *Journal of Marital and Family Therapy*, 27(2): 145–155.

Jones, S. (2010). Horrorporn/Pornhorror: the problematic communities and contexts of online shock imagery. In: F. Attwood (Ed.), *Porn.Com. Making Sense of Online Pornography* (pp. 123–137). New York: David Lang.

Josephson, G. J. (2003). Using attachment-based intervention with same-sex couples. In: S. M. Johnson & W. E. Whiffen (Eds.), *Attachment Processes in Couple and Family Therapy* (pp. 300–317). New York: Guilford Press.

Kabat-Zinn, J. (1994). *Wherever You Go, There You Are. Mindfulness Meditation for Everyday Life*. London: Piatkus.

Kahr, B. (2007a). The infanticidal origins of psychosis: the role of trauma in schizophrenia. In: *The John Bowlby Memorial Conference. Shattered States: Disorganized Attachment and its Repair*. London: Karnac.

Kahr, B. (2007b). Infanticidal attachment. *Attachment: New Directions in Psychotherapy and Relational Psychoanalysis, 1*(2): 117–132.

Kalin, N. H. (1993). The neurobiology of fear. *Scientific American, 268*(5): 54–60.

Kalishian, M. M. (1959). Working with the wives of alcoholics in an outpatient clinic setting. *Marriage and Family, 21*(2): 130–133.

Kamphuis, J. H., & Emmelkamp, P. M. G. (2000). Stalking—a contemporary challenge for forensic and clinical psychiatry. *British Journal of Psychiatry, 176*: 206–209.

Karama, S., Roch Lecours, A., Leroux, J-M., Bourgouin, P., Beaudoin, G., Joubert, S., & Beauregard, M. (2002). Areas of the brain in males and females during viewing of erotic film excerpts. *Human Brain Mapping, 16*(1): 1–13.

Karpman, S. (1968). Fairy tales and script drama analysis. *Transactional Analysis Bulletin, 7*(26): 39–43.

Kaufman, J., & Zigler, E. (1987). Do abused children become abusive parents? *American Journal of Orthopsychiatry, 57*(2): 186–192.

Kernberg, O. (1975). *Borderline Conditions and Pathological Narcissism*. New York: Jason Aronson.

Kienlen, K. K. (1998). Developmental and social antecedents of stalking. In: J. R. Meloy (Ed.), *The Psychology of Stalking. Clinical & Forensic Perspectives*. San Diego: Academic Press.

Killgore, W. D., Oki, M., & Yurgelun-Todd, D. A. (2001). Sex-specific developmental changes in amygdala responses to affective faces. *Neuroreport, 12*(2): 427–433.

Kingston, D. A., Yates, P. M., Firestone, P., Babchishin, K., & Bradford, J. M. (2008). Long-term predictive validity of the Risk Matrix 2000. *Sexual Abuse: A Journal of Research and Treatment, 20*(4): 466–484.

Kinzl, J. F., & Mangweth, B. (1996). Sexual dysfunction in males: significance of adverse childhood experiences. *Childhood Abuse & Neglect, 20*(4): 759–766.

Kirkpatrick, L. A., & Davis, K. E. (1994). Attachment style, gender and relationship stability: a longitudinal analysis. *Journal of Personality and Social Psychology, 66*(3): 502–512.

Klein, M. (1957). *The Writings of Melanie Klein*. London: Hogarth Press.

Knight, R. A., & Prentky, R. (1990). Classifying sexual offenders: the development and corroboration of taxonomic models. In: W. L. Marshall, D. R. Laws, & H. E. Barbaree (Eds.), *Handbook of Sexual Assault: Issues, Theories, and Treatment of the Offender* (pp. 23–52). New York: Plenum Press.

Kobak, R., & Hazan, C. (1991). Attachment in marriage: effects of security and accuracy of working models. *Journal of Personality and Social Psychology, 60*(6): 861–869.

Kobak, R., & Mandelbaum, T. (2003). Caring for the caregiver. An attachment approach to assessment and treatment of child problems. In: S. M. Johnson & W. E. Whiffen (Eds.), *Attachment Processes in Couple and Family Therapy* (pp. 144–164). New York: Guilford Press.

Kobak, R., Ferenz-Gillies, R., Everhart, E., & Seabrook, L. (1994). Maternal attachment strategies and emotion regulation with adolescent offspring. *Journal of Research on Adolescence, 4*(4): 553–566.

Kochman, F. J., Hantouche, E. G., Ferrari, P., Lancrenon, S., Bayart, D., & Akiskal, H. S. (2005). Cyclothymic temperament as a prospective predictor of bipolarity and suicidality in children and adolescents with major depressive disorder. *Journal of Affective Disorder, 85*(1–2): 181–189.

Kohut, H. (1972). Thoughts on narcissism and narcissistic rage. *Psychoanalytic Study of the Child, 27*: 360–400.

Kolb, L. C. (1987). Neurophysiological hypothesis explaining post-traumatic stress disorder. *American Journal of Psychiatry, 144*: 989–995.

Koukkou, M., & Lehmann, D. (1983). Dreaming: the functional state-shift hypothesis. *British Journal of Psychiatry, 142*: 221–231.

Krone, T. (2004). *A Typology of Online Child Pornography Offending*. Canberra: Australian Institute of Criminology.

Krone, T. (2005). Developing measures of prevention and enforcement against the backdrop of international difference: protecting children from online sexual exploitation: in search of a standard. Paper presented to the Safety and Security in a Networked World: Balancing Cyber-Rights & Responsibilities Conference, 8–10 September, University of Oxford.

Krystal, H. (1988). *Integration and Self-Healing. Affect–Trauma–Alexithymia.* Hillsdale, NJ: Analytic Press.

Krystal, J., Bennett, A., Bremner, J., Southwick, S., & Charney, D. (1995). Toward a cognitive neuroscience of dissociation and altered memory functions in post-traumatic stress disorder. In: M. J. Friedman, D. S. Charney, & A. Y. Deutch (Eds.), *Neurobiological and Clinical Consequences of Stress* (pp. 244–245). Philadelphia, PA: Lippincott-Raven.

Kumari, V. (2006). Do psychotherapies produce neurobiological effects? *Acta Neuropsychiatrica, 18*(2): 61–70.

Lake, F. (1981). *Tight Corners in Pastoral Counselling.* London: Darton, Londman & Todd.

Lancker, V. (2006). *Speaker Recognition.* New York: Wiley.

Landau, J., Garrett, J., & Webb, R. (2008). Assisting a concerned person to motivate someone experiencing cybersex into treatment. *Journal of Marital & Family Therapy, 34*(4): 498–511.

Landolt, M. A., & Dutton, D. G. (1998). Power and personality: an analysis of gay male intimate abuse. *Sex Roles, 37*(5–6): 335–358.

Lanning, K. V. (2005). Compliant child victims: confronting an uncomfortable reality. In: E. Quayle & M. Taylor (Eds.), *Viewing Child Pornography on the Internet* (pp. 49–60). Lyme Regis: Russell House Publishing.

Lara, D. R., Pinto, O., Akiskal, K., & Akiskal, H. S. (2006). Toward an integrative model of the spectrum of mood, behavioral and personality disorders based on fear and anger traits: 1. Clinical implications. *Journal of Affective Disorders, 94*(1–3): 67–87.

Laws, D. R., Hudson, S. M., & Ward, T. (2000). The original model of relapse prevention with sexual offenders: promises unfulfilled. In: D. R. Laws, S. M. Hudson, & T. Ward (Eds.), *Remaking Relapse Prevention with Sexual Offenders: A Sourcebook* (pp. 3–24). Thousand Oaks, CA: Sage.

Layden, M. A., Newman, C. F., Freeman, A., & Morse, S. B. (1993). *Cognitive Therapy of Borderline Personality Disorder.* Needham Heights, MA: Allyn & Bacon.

Lazarus, R. S. (1991). *Emotion and Adaptation.* Oxford: Oxford University Press.

LeDoux, J. E. (1996). *The Emotional Brain.* London: Weidenfeld & Nicolson.

LeDoux, J. E. (2002). *Synaptic Self. How Our Brains Become Who We Are.* New York: Penguin.

Lerner, H. (1985). *The Dance of Anger*. New York: Harper & Row.

Levine, P. (1997). *Waking the Tiger. Healing Trauma*. Berkeley, CA: North Atlantic Books.

Levitin, D. J. (2006). *This is Your Brain on Music: Understanding a Human Obsession*. London: Atlantic Books.

Levy, T. M., & Orlans, M. (2000). Attachment disorder and the adoptive family. In: T. Levy (Ed.), *Handbook of Attachment Interventions* (pp. 243–259). San Diego, CA: Academic Press.

Levy, T. M., & Orlans, M. (2003). Creating and repairing attachments in biological, foster and adoptive families. In: S. M. Johnson & W. E. Whiffen (Eds.), *Attachment Processes in Couple and Family Therapy* (pp. 165–190). New York: Guilford Press.

Lifton, R. J. (1973). *Home From the War: Vietnam Veterans: Neither Victims nor Executioners*. New York: Simon & Schuster.

Lilienfeld, S. O. (2007). Psychological treatments that cause harm. *Perspectives on Psychological Science, 2*(1): 53–70.

Lindemann, E. (1944). Symptomatology and management of acute grief. *American Journal of Psychiatry, 101*(3): 141–149.

Linden, D. E. J. (2006). How psychotherapy changes the brain—the contribution of functional neuroimaging. *Molecular Psychiatry, 11*(2): 528–538.

Lindsay, W. R., Olley, S., Jack, C., Morrison, F., & Smith, A. H. W. (1998). The treatment of two stalkers with intellectual disabilities. *Journal of Applied Research in Intellectual Disabilities, 11*(4): 333–344.

Lindgren, S. (2010). Widening the glory hole: the discourse of online fandom. In: F. Attwood (Ed.), *Porn.Com. Making Sense of Online Pornography* (pp. 171–185). New York: David Lang.

Lingford-Hughes, A., Potokar, J., & Nutt, D. (2002). Treating anxiety complicated by substance abuse. *British Journal of Psychiatry, Advances in Psychiatric Treatment, 8*(2): 107–116.

Liotti, G. (1993). Disorganized attachment and dissociative experiences: an illustration of the developmental ethological approach to cognitive therapy. In: H. Rosen & K. T. Kuehlvein (Eds.), *Cognitive Therapy in Action* (pp. 213–239). San Francisco, CA: Jossey Bass.

Loeb, T., Williams, J., Carmona, J., Rivkin, I., Wyatt, G., Chin, D., & Asuan-O'Brien, A. (2002). Child sexual abuse: associations with sexual functioning of adolescents and adults. *Annual Review of Sex Research, 13*: 346–389.

Lyons-Ruth, K., & Jacobvitz, D. (1999). Attachment disorganization. Unresolved loss, relational violence, and lapses in behavioral attentional strategies. In: J. Cassidy & P. R. Shaver (Eds.), *Handbook of Attachment. Theory, Research, and Clinical Applications* (pp. 520–554). New York: Guilford Press.

Lyons-Ruth, K., Alpern, L., & Repacholi, B. (1993). Disorganized infant attachment classification and maternal psychosocial problems as predictors of hostile–aggressive behavior in the preschool classroom. *Child Development, 64*(2): 572–585.

MacLean, P. D. (1990). *The Triune Brain in Evolution: Role of Paleocerebral Functions*. New York: Plenum Press.

Maddison, S. (2010). Online obscenity and myths of freedom: dangerous images, child porn, and neoliberalism. In: F. Attwood (Ed.), *Porn.Com. Making Sense of Online Pornography* (pp. 17–33). New York: Peter Lang.

Magai, C. (2001). Emotion over the lifecourse. In: J. Birren & K. W. Schaie (Eds.), *Handbook of the Psychology of Aging* (pp. 399–426). San Diego, CA: Academic Press.

Magai, C., & Cohen, C. (1998). Attachment style and emotional regulation in dementia patients and their relation to caregiver burden. *Journals of Gerontology Series B: Psychological Sciences and Social Sciences, 53*(3): 147–154.

Mahler, M., Pine, F., & Bergman, A. (1975). *The Psychological Birth of the Human Infant*. New York: Basic Books.

Mahoney, A., Donnelly, W., Boxer, P., & Lewis, T. (2003). Marital and severe parent-to-adolescent physical aggression in clinic-referred families: mother and adolescent reports on co-occurrence and links to child behaviour problems. *Journal of Family Psychology, 17*(1): 3–19.

Main, M. (1991). Metacognitive knowledge, metacognitive monitoring, and singular (coherent) vs multiple (incoherent) model of attachment: findings and directions for future research. In: C. Parkes, J. Stevenson-Hinde, & P. Maris (Eds.), *Attachment Across the Life-Cycle* (pp. 127–160). London: Routledge.

Main, M. (1995). Recent studies in attachment with selected implication for clinical work. In: S. Goldberg, R. Muir, & J. Kerr (Eds.), *Attachment Theory: Social Development & Clinical Perspectives*. Hillsdale, NJ: Analytic Press.

Main, M., & Cassidy, J. (1988). Categories of response reunion with the parent at age six: predicted from infant attachment classifications and stable over a one-month period. *Developmental Psychology, 24*(3): 415–426.

Main, M., & Hesse, E. (1990). Parents' unresolved traumatic experiences are related to infant disorganized attachment status: is frightened and/or frightening parental behavior the linking mechanism? In: M. Greenberg, D. Cicchetti, & E. M. Cummings (Eds.), *Attachment in the Pre-School Years: Theory, Research and Intervention* (pp. 161–182). Chicago, IL: University of Chicago Press.

Main, M., & Weston, D. R. (1981). The quality of the toddler's relationship to mother and to father. *Child Development, 52*(3): 932–940.

Main, M., Kaplan, N., & Cassidy, J. (1985). Security in infancy, childhood, and adulthood. A move to the level of representation. In: I. Bretherton & E. Waters (Eds.), *Growing Points of Attachment Theory and Research, 50*(1–2), No. 209 (pp. 66–107). Monographs for the Society for Research in Child Development.

Makinen, J. A. (2006). Resolving attachment injuries in couples using emotionally focused therapy: steps towards forgiveness and reconciliation. *Journal of Consulting and Clinical Psychology, 74*(6): 1055–1064.

Malamuth, N. M. (1981). Rape proclivity among males. *Journal of Social Issues, 37*(4): 138–157.

Malamuth, N. M., & Donnerstein, E. (1982). The effects of aggressive and pornographic mass media stimuli. In: L. Berkowitz (Ed.), *Advances in Experimental Social Psychology*, Vol. 15 (pp. 103–136). New York: Academic Press.

Maltz, W., & Maltz, L. (2006). *The Pornography Trap*. New York: HarperCollins.

Manley, R. S., Rickson, H., & Standeven, B. (2000). Children and adolescents with eating disorders: strategies for teachers and school counselors. *Intervention in School & Clinic, 35*(4): 228–231.

Mann, R. E., & Hollin, C. R. (2007). Sexual offenders' explanations for their offending. *Journal of Sexual Aggression, 13*(1): 3–10.

Manning, J. C. (2006). The impact of internet pornography on marriage and the family: a review of the research. *Sexual Addiction & Compulsivity, 13*(2–3): 131–165.

Margolin, G., & Gordis, E. (2003). Co-occurrence between marital aggression and parents' child abuse potential: the impact of cumulative stress. *Violence and Victims, 18*(3): 243–258.

Marshall, L. E., & Moulden, H. M. (2006). Preparatory programs for sexual offenders. In: W. L. Marshall, Y. M. Fernandez, L. E. Marshall

& G. A. Serran (Eds.), *Sexual Offender Treatment. Controversial Issues* (pp. 200–210). Chichester: Wiley.

Marshall, W. L. (2000). Revisiting the use of pornography by sexual offenders: implications for theory and practice. *The Journal of Sexual Aggression*, 6(1/2): 67–77.

Marshall, W. L. (2006). Diagnostic problems with sexual offenders. In: W. L. Marshall, Y. M. Fernandez, L. E. Marshall, & G. A. Serran (Eds.), *Sexual Offender Treatment. Controversial Issues* (pp. 33–44). London: Wiley.

Marshall, W. L., & Barbaree, H. E. (1988). An outpatient treatment program for child molesters. In: R. A. Prentky & V. L. Quinsey (Eds.), *Human Sexual Aggression: Current Perspectives*, Vol. 528 (pp. 205–214). New York: New York Academy of Science.

Marshall, W. L., Anderson, D., & Fernandez, Y. M. (1999). *Cognitive Behavioural Treatment of Sexual Offenders*. Chichester: Wiley.

Marshall, W. L., Serann, G., Fernandez, Y. M., Mulloy, R., Thornton, D., Mann, R. E., & Anderson, D. (2003). Therapist characteristics in the treatment of sexual offenders: tentative data on their relationship with indices of behaviour change. *Journal of Sexual Aggression*, 9(1): 25–30.

Marshall, W. L., Serran, G. A., Moulden, H. M., Mulloy, R., Fernandez, Y. M., & Mann, R. E. (2002). Therapist features in sexual offender treatment: their reliable identification and influence on behaviour change. *Clinical Psychology and Psychotherapy*, 9(6): 395–405.

Maruna, S. (2001). *Making Good: How Ex-Convicts Reform and Build their Lives*. Washington, DC: American Psychological Society.

Maruna, S., & Mann, R. E. (2006). A fundamental attribution error? Rethinking cognitive distortions. *Legal and Criminological Psychology*, 11(2): 155–177.

Masterson, J. F. (1981). *The Narcissistic and Borderline Disorders*. New York: Brunner-Mazel.

Mathews, R., Mathews, J. K., & Speltz, K. (1989). *Female Sexual Offenders: An Exploratory Study*. Orwell, VT: Safer Society Press.

Matravers, A. (2003). Setting some boundaries: rethinking responses to sex offenders. In: A. Matravers (Ed.), *Sex Offenders in the Community. Managing and Reducing the Risks* (pp. 1–28). Cullompton, Devon: Willan.

McBride, C., Atkinson, L., Quilty, L. C., & Bagby, R. M. (2006). Attachment as a moderator of treatment outcome in major depression: a randomized control trial of interpersonal therapy versus cognitive behavior therapy. *Journal of Consulting and Clinical Psychology*, 74(6): 1041–1054.

McCarthy-Hoffbauer, I., Leach, C., & McKenzie, I. (2006). Deliberate self harm in children and adolescents. *Mental Health and Learning Disabilities Research and Practice*, 3(2): 107–126.

McClintock, M., & Herdt, G. (1996). Rethinking puberty: the development of sexual attraction. *Current Directions in Psychological Science*, 5(6): 178–183.

McClusky, U. (2005). *To Be Met as a Person. The Dynamics of Attachment in Professional Encounters*. London: Karnac.

McElwain, N. L., Booth LaForce, C., Lansford, J. E., Wu, X., & Dyer, W. J. (2008). A process model of attachment-friend linkages. Hostile attribution biases, language ability and mother-child affective mutuality as intervening mechanisms. *Child Development*, 76(6): 1891–1906.

McGilchrist, I. (2009). *The Master and his Emissary. The Divided Brain and the Western World*. London: Yale University Press.

McKenna, C. (1994). Malignant transference: a neurobiologic model. *Journal of the American Academy of Psychoanalysis*, 22(1): 111–127.

McKibbin, W. F., Goetz, A. T., Shackelford, T. K., Schipper, L. D., Starratt, V. G., & Stewart-Williams, S. (2007). Why do men insult their intimate partners? *Personality and Individual Differences*, 43(2): 231–241.

Megargee, E. I. (1966). *Undercontrolled and Overcontrolled Personality Types in Extreme Antisocial Aggression. Psychological Monographs*, 80(3): No. 611.

Mellody, P., Miller, A. W., & Miller, J. K. (1989). *Facing Codependence: What it is, Where it Comes From, How it Sabotages our Lives*. New York: Harper Collins.

Meloy, J. R. (1996). Stalking (obsessional following): a review of some preliminary studies. *Aggression & Violent Behavior*, 1: 147–162.

Meloy, J. R. (1998). *The Psychology of Stalking. Clinical & Forensic Perspectives*. San Diego, CA: Academic Press.

Meloy, J. R., & Gothard, R. S. (1995). A demographic and clinical comparison of obsessional followers and offenders with mental disorders. *American Journal of Psychiatry*, 152(2): 258–263.

Meltzoff, A. N., & Moore, M. K. (1995). Infants' understanding of people and things: from body imitation to folk psychology. In: J. Bermudez, A. J. Marcel & N. Eilan (Eds.), *Body and the Self* (pp. 43–69). Cambridge, MA: MIT Press.

Mental Health Foundation (2004). *Lifetime Impacts — Childhood and Adolescent Mental Health: Understanding the Lifetime Impacts*. Foundation for People with Learning Disabilities.

Miczek, K. A., Thompson, M. L., & Tornatzky, W. (1990). Subordinate animals: behavioral and physiological adaptations and opioid tolerance. In: M. R. Brown, G. F. Koob, & C. Rivier (Eds.), *Stress: Neurobiology and Neuroendocrinology* (pp. 323–357). New York: Marcel Darker.

Middleton, D., Beech, A., & Mandeville-Norden, R. (2005). What sort of person could do that? Psychological profiles of internet pornography users. In: E. Quayle & M. Taylor (Eds.), *Viewing Child Pornography on the Internet* (pp. 99–107). Lyme Regis: Russell House Publishing.

Migliorelli, R., Starkstein, S. E., Teson, A., de Quiros, G., Vazquez, S., Leiguarda, R., & Robinson, R. G. (1993). SPECT findings in patients with primary mania. *Journal of Neuropsychiatry and Clinical Neuroscience*, 5(4): 379–383.

Miklowitz, D. J., Otto, M. W., Frank, E., Reilly-Harrington, N. A., Wisneiwski, S. R., Kogan, J. N., Nierenberg, A. A., Calabrese, J. R., Marangell, L. B., Gyulai, L., Araga, M., Gonzalez, J. M., Shirley, E. R., Thase, M. E., & Sachs, G. S. (2007). Psychosocial treatments for bipolar depression: a 1-year randomized trial from the Systematic Treatment Enhancement Program. *Archives of General Psychiatry*, 64(4): 419–426.

Miklowitz, D. J., Wisneiwski, S. R., Miyahara, S., Otto, M. W., & Sachs, G. S. (2005). Perceived criticism from family members as a predictor of the one-year course of bipolar disorder. *Psychiatry Research*, 136(2–3): 101–111.

Mikulincer, M., & Shaver, P. (2003). The attachment behavioral system in adulthood: activation, psychodynamics, and interpersonal processes. In: M. P. Zenna (Ed.), *Advances in Experimental Social Psychology*, Volume 35 (pp. 53–152). San Diego, CA: Academic Press.

Milgram, S. (1974). *Obedience to Authority*. London: Tavistock.

Miller, A. (1990). *The Drama of Being a Child*. London: Virago Press.

Miller, B. C., Norton, M. C., Curtis, T., & Hill, E. J. (1997). The timing of sexual intercourse among adolescents. *Youth and Society*, 29(1): 54–83.

Milner, R. J., & Webster, S. D. (2005). Identifying schemas in child molesters, rapists, and violent offenders. *Sexual Abuse: A Journal of Research and Treatment*, 17(4): 425–439.

Miner, M. H., & Munns, R. (2005). Isolation and normlessness: attitudinal comparisons of adolescent sex offenders, juvenile offenders, and nondelinquents. *International Journal of Offender Therapy and Comparative Criminology, 49*(5): 491–504.

Minty, B. (1987). *Child Care and Adult Crime*. Manchester: Manchester University Press.

Mirrlees-Black, C. (1999). *Estimating the Extent of Domestic Violence: Findings from the 1992 British Crime Survey* (Home Office Research Bulletin no 37). London: Home Office Research and Statistics Department.

Monahan, J., & Steadman, H. (1994). *Violence and Mental Disorder: Developments in Risk Assessment*. Chicago, IL: University of Chicago Press.

Money, J. (1986). *Lovemaps: Clinical Concepts of Sexual/Erotic Health & Pathology, Paraphilia, and Gender Transposition in Childhood, Adolescence, and Maturity*. Amherst, NY: Prometheus Books.

Money, J., & Ehrhardt, A. A. (1972). *Man and Woman, Boy and Girl*. Baltimore, MD: Johns Hopkins University Press.

Moretti, M. M., & Higgins, E. T. (1999). Own versus other standpoints in self-regulations: a new look at a classic issue. *Social Cognition, 17*(22): 186–208.

Moretti, M. M., & Holland, R. (2003). The journey of adolescence. Transitions in self within the context of attachment relationships. In: S. M. Johnson & W. E. Whiffen (Eds.), *Attachment Processes in Couple and Family Therapy* (pp. 234–257). New York: Guilford Press.

Moretti, M. M., Obsuth, I., Odgers, C. L., & Reebye, P. (2006). Exposure to maternal vs. paternal partner violence, PTSD, and aggression in adolescent girls and boys. *Aggressive Behavior, 32*(4): 385–395.

Morris, J. S., Ohman, A., & Dolan, R. J. (1999). A subcortical pathway of the right amygdala mediating "unseen" fear. *Proceedings of the National Academy of Sciences of the United States, 96*(4): 1680–1685.

Morrison, A. P. (1983). Shame, ideal self and narcissism. *Contemporary Psychoanalysis, 19*(2): 295–318.

Morton, B. E., & Rafto, S. E. (2006). Corpus callosum size is linked to dichotic deafness and hemisphericity, not sex or handedness. *Brain and Cognition, 62*(1): 1–8.

Morton, J., & Johnson, M. H. (1991). CONSPEC and CONLEARN: a two-process theory of infant face recognition. *Psychological Review, 98*(2): 164–181.

Mosner, C. (1992). A response to Aviel Goodman's "Sexual addiction: designation and treatment". *Journal of Sex & Marital Therapy, 19*(3): 220–224.

Moultrie, D. (2006). Adolescents convicted of possession of abuse images of children: a new type of adolescent sex offender? *Journal of Sexual Aggression, 12*(2): 165–174.

Mullen, P. E., Pathé, M., & Purcell, R. (2000a). *Stalkers and Their Victims.* Cambridge: Cambridge University Press.

Mullen, P. E., Pathé, M., & Purcell, R. (2000b). Stalking. *The Psychologist, 13*(9): 454–459.

Murphy, W. D., & Page, I. J. (2008). Exhibitionism. Psychopathology and theory. In: D. R. Laws & W. T. O'Donohue (Eds.), *Sexual Deviance. Theory, Assessment and Treatment* (pp. 61–75). New York: Guilford Press.

Nebes, R. D., & Sperry, R. (1971). Hemispheric deconnection syndrome with cerebral birth injury in dominant arm area. *Neuropsychologia, 9*: 247–259.

Neisser, U., & Fivush, R. (1994). *The Remembering Self.* New York: Cambridge University Press.

Neufeld Bailey, H., Moran, G. S., & Penderson, D. R. (2007). Childhood maltreatment, complex trauma symptoms, and unresolved attachment in an at-risk sample of adolescent mothers. *Attachment & Human Development, 9*(2): 139–161.

Neugebauer, R., Hoek, H. W., & Susser, E. (1999). Prenatal exposure to wartime famine and development of antisocial personality disorder in early adulthood. *Journal of the American Medical Association, 282*(5): 455–462.

Nijenhuis, E. R. S., Vanderlinden, J., & Spinhoven, P. (1998). Animal defensive reactions as a model for trauma-induced dissociative reactions. *Journal of Traumatic Stress, 11*(4): 242–260.

Novaco, R. W. (1975). *Anger Control.* London: Lexington Books.

Nunes, K. L., Firestone, P., Bradsford, J. M., Greenberg, D. M., & Broom, I. (2002). A comparison of modified versions of the Static-99 and sex offender risk appraisal guide. *Sexual Abuse: A Journal of Research and Treatment, 14*(3): 253–269.

Nutt, D. (1999). Alcohol and the brain: pharmacological insights for psychiatrists. *British Journal of Psychiatry, 175*: 114–119.

O'Connor, A. A. (1987). Female sexual offenders. *British Journal of Psychiatry, 150*(5): 615–620.

O'Connor, T. G., Bredenkamp, D., Rutter, M., & English and Romanian Adoptees (ERA) Study Team (1999). Attachment disturbances and disorders in children exposed to early severe deprivation. *Infant Mental Health Journal, 20*(1): 10–29.

O'Donnell, I., & Milner, C. (2007). *Child Pornography. Crime, Computers and Society.* Cullompton, Devon: Willan.

Ogawa, J. R., Sroufe, L. A., Weinfield, N. A., Carlson, E. A., & Egeland, B. (1997). Development and the fragmented self: longitudinal study of dissociative symptomology in a nonclinical sample. *Development and Psychopathology, 9*(4): 855–879.

Okami, P., & Goldberg, A. (1992). Personality correlates of pedophilia: are they reliable indicators? *Journal of Sex Research, 29*(3): 297–328.

Orzolek-Kronner, C. (2002). The effect of attachment theory in the development of eating disorders. *Child & Adolescent Social Work Journal, 19*(6): 421–435.

O'Toole, L. (1998). *Pornocopia: Porn, Sex, Technology and Desire.* London: Serpents Tail.

Otway, L. J., & Vignoles, V. L. (2006). Narcissism and childhood recollections: a quantitative test of psychoanalytic predictions. *Personality & Social Psychology Bulletin, 32*(1): 104–116.

Pacey, S. (2004). Couples and the first baby: responding to new parents' sexual and relationship problems. *Sexual & Marital Therapy, 19*(3): 223–246.

Padesky, C. (2003). Personal communication.

Panskepp, J. (1985). Mood changes. In: P. Vinken, G. Bruyn & H. Klawans (Eds.), *Handbook of Clinical Neurology*, Vol. 45 (pp. 271–285). Amsterdam: Elsevier.

Panskepp, J. (1998). *Affective Neuroscience: The Foundations of Human and Animal Emotions.* New York: Oxford University Press.

Panskepp, J. (2004). *Textbook of Biological Psychiatry.* Hoboken, NJ: Wiley-Liss.

Pao, P. (1968). On manic–depressive psychosis. *Journal of the American Psychoanalytic Association, 16*(4): 809–832.

Papousek, H., & Papousek, M. (1979). Early ontogeny of human social interaction: its biological roots and social dimensions. In: M. von Cranach, K. Foppa, W. Lepenies, & D. Ploog (Eds.), *Human Ethology. Claims and Limits of a New Discipline. Contributions to the Colloquium Sponsored by Reimers–Stiflung* (pp. 456–478). Cambridge: Cambridge University Press.

Pathé, M., & Mullen, P. E. (1997). The impact of stalkers on their victims. *British Journal of Psychiatry, 170*: 12–17.

Perkins, D. (1989). The case for treating sex offenders. *Criminal Justice, 7*(2): 9.

Perren, S., Schmid, R., Herrmann, S., & Wettstein, A. (2007). The impact of attachment on dementia-related problem behavior and spousal caregivers' well-being. *Attachment & Human Development, 9*(2): 163–178.

Perry, B. D. (2001). The neurodevelopmental impact of violence in childhood. In: D. Schetky & E. Benedek (Eds.), *Textbook of Child and Adolescent Forensic Psychiatry* (pp. 221–238). Washington, DC: American Psychiatric Press.

Perry, B. D. (2002). Childhood experience and the expression of genetic potential: what childhood neglect tells us about nature and nurture. *Brain and Mind, 3*(1): 79–100.

Perry, B. D., Pollard, R. A., Blakley, T. L., Baker, W. L., & Vigilante, D. (1995). Childhood trauma, the neurobiology of adaptation, and "use-dependent" development of the brain. How states become traits. *Infant Mental Health Journal, 16*(4): 271–291.

Peter, T. (2006). Mad, bad or victim? Making sense of mother–daughter sexual abuse. *Feminist Criminology, 1*(4): 283–302.

Petersen, K., & Thomasius, R. (2007). *Consequences of Cannabis Use and Abuse.* Lengerich, Germany: Pabst Science.

Petersson, M., Hulting, A.-L., & Uvnas-Moberg, K. (1999). Oxytocin causes a sustained decrease in plasma levels of corticosterone in rats. *Neuroscience Letters, 264*(1–3): 41–44.

Peto, A. (1969). Terrifying eyes. A visual superego forerunner. *Psychoanalytic Study of the Child, 24*: 197–212.

Phelps, J. (2006). *Why Am I Still Depressed? Recognizing and Managing the Ups and Downs of Bipolar II and Soft Bipolar Disorder.* New York: McGraw-Hill.

Piquero, A., & Tibbetts, S. (1999). The impact of pre/perinatal disturbances and disadvantaged familial environment in predicting criminal offending. *Studies on Crime and Crime Prevention, 8*(1): 52–70.

Pithers, W. D., Marques, J. K., Gibat, C. C., & Marlatt, G. A. (1983). Relapse prevention of sexual aggressives: a self control model of treatment and maintenance of change. In: J. G. Greer & I. R. Stuart (Eds.), *The Sexual Aggressor: Current Perspectives on Treatment* (pp. 241–259). New York: Van Nostrand Reinhold.

Popovic, M. (2007). Establishing new breeds of (sex) offenders: science or political control. *Sexual & Relationship Therapy, 22*(2): 255–271.

Post, R. M., Rubinow, D. R., & Ballenger, J. C. (1986). Conditioning and sensitization in the longitudinal course of affective illness. *British Journal of Psychiatry, 149*: 191–201.

Powell, A. (2007). *Paedophiles, Child Abuse and the Internet*. Oxford: Radcliffe.

Power, A. (2007). Discussion of trauma at the threshold: the impact of boarding school on attachment in young children. *Attachment: New Directions in Psychotherapy and Relational Psychoanalysis, 1*(3): 313–320.

Power, H. (2003). Disclosing information on sex offenders: the human rights implications. In: A. Matravers (Ed.), *Sex Offenders in the Community. Managing and Reducing the Risks* (pp. 72–101). Cullompton, Devon: Willan.

Prendergast, W. E. (1993). *The Merry-Go-Round of Sexual Abuse: Identifying and Treating Survivors*. New York: Guilford Press.

Prescott, J. W. (1996). The origins of human love and violence. *Journal of Prenatal & Perinatal Psychology & Health, 10*(3): 143–188.

Proeve, M., & Howells, K. (2006). Shame and guilt in child molesters. In: W. L. Marshall, Y. M. Fernandez, L. E. Marshall, & G. A. Serran (Eds.), *Sexual Offender Treatment. Controversial Issues* (pp. 125–139). Chichester: Wiley.

Putnam, F. (2003). Ten-year research update review: child sexual abuse. *Journal of the American Academy of Child and Adolescent Psychiatry, 42*(3): 269–278.

Putnam, F. W. (1995). Development of dissociative disorders. In: D. Cicchetti & D. J. Cohen (Eds.), *Developmental Psychopathology, Vol. 2: Risk, Disorder & Adaptation* (pp. 581–608). New York: Wiley.

Quayle, E. (2005). The internet as a therapeutic medium? In: E. Quayle & M. Taylor (Eds.), *Viewing Child Pornography on the Internet* (pp. 127–144). Lyme Regis: Russell House Publishing.

Quayle, E., Erooga, M., Wright, L., Taylor, M., & Harbinson, D. (2006). *Only Pictures? Therapeutic Work with Internet Sex Offenders*. Lyme Regis: Russell House Publishing.

Quinsey, V. L. (1983). Prediction of recidivism and the evaluation of treatment programs for sex offenders. In: S. N. Verdun-Jones & A. A. Keltner (Eds.), *Sexual Aggression and the Law* (pp. 27–40). Vancouver, Canada: Simon Fraser University Criminology Research Centre.

Quinsey, V. L., Chaplin, T., C., & Varney, G. A. (1981). A comparison of rapists and non-sex offenders' sexual preferences for mutually consenting sex, rape and physical abuse of women. *Behavioral Assessment*, 3(2): 127–135.

Radzinowicz, L. (1957). *Sexual Offences: A Report of the Cambridge Department of Criminal Science*. Toronto: Macmillan.

Raine, A., Brennan, P., & Mednick, S. A. (1994). Birth complications combined with maternal rejection at age 1 year predisposes to violent crime at age 18 years. *Archives of General Psychiatry*, 51(12): 984–988.

Raine, A., Ishikawa, S. S., Arce, E., Lencz, T., Knuth, K. H., Birhie, S., LaCasse, L., & Colletti, P. (2004). Hippocampal structural asymmetry in unsuccessful psychopaths. *Biological Psychiatry*, 55(2): 185–191.

Raine, A., Lencz, T., Birhie, S., LaCasse, L., & Colletti, P. (2000). Reduced prefrontal grey matter volume and reduced autonomic activity in anti-social personality disorder. *Archives of General Psychiatry*, 57(2): 119–127.

Ramachandran, V. S. (1994). Phantom limbs, neglect syndromes and Freudian psychology. *International Review of Neurobiology*, 37: 291–333.

Rauh, H., Ziegenhain, U., Müller, B., & Wignroks, L. (2000). Stability and change in infant-mother attachment in the second year of life: relations to parenting quality and varying degrees of day-care experience. In: P. Crittenden (Ed.), *The Organization of Attachment Relationships: Maturation, Culture, and Context* (pp. 251–276). Cambridge: Cambridge University Press.

Ray, S. L. (2004). Eating disorders in adolescent males. *Professional School Counseling*, 8(1): 98–101.

Raymond, N. C., Coleman, E., Ohlerking, F., Christensen, G. A., & Miner, M. H. (1999). Psychiatric comorbidity in pedophilic sex offenders. *American Journal of Psychiatry*, 156(5): 786–788.

Renn, P. (2007). Stop thief! But what has been stolen and by whom? *Attachment: New Directions in Psychotherapy and Relational Psychoanalysis*, 1(1): 71–77.

Reynolds, P., & Kaplan, G. A. (1990). Social connections and risk for cancer: prospective evidence from the Alameda County Study. *Behavioral Medicine*, 16(3): 101–110.

Rich, P. (2006). *Attachment and Sexual Offending. Understanding and Applying Attachment Theory to the Treatment of Juvenile Sexual Offenders*. Chichester: John Wiley.

Ridgway, R., & House, S. H. (2006). *The Unborn Child.* London: Karnac.

Risin, L. I., & Koss, M. P. (1987). The sexual abuse of boys: prevalence and descriptive characteristics of childhood victimizations. *Journal of Interpersonal Violence, 2*(3): 309–323.

Rizzolatti, G., Fadiga, L., Fogassi, L., & Gallese, V. (1999). Resonance behaviours and mirror neurons. *Archives of Italian Biology, 137*(2–3): 85–100.

Roe, K. V., & Drivas, A. (1993). Planned conception and infant functioning at age three months. *American Journal of Orthopsychiatry, 63*: 120–125.

Roffman, J. L., Marci, C. D., Glick, D. M., Dougherty, D. D., & Rauch, S. L. (2005). Neuroimaging and the functional neuroanatomy of psychotherapy. *Psychological Medicine, 35*(10): 1385–1398.

Rosenfeld, H. (1971). A clinical approach to the psychoanalytic theory of the life and death instincts: an investigation into the aggressive aspects of narcissism. *International Journal of Psycho-Analysis, 52*: 169–178.

Rosenfeld, H. (1987). *Impasse and Interpretation.* London: Tavistock.

Rosenthal, P.-A., & Rosenthal, S. (1984). Suicidal behavior by pre-school children. *American Journal of Psychiatry, 141*: 520–525.

Ross, C. A. (2004). *Schizophrenia. Innovations in Diagnosis and Treatment.* New York: Haworth Maltreatment and Trauma Press.

Ross, E. D., Homan, R. W., & Buck, R. (1994). Differential hemispheric lateralization of primary and social emotions: implications for developing a comprehensive neurology for emotions, repression, and the subconscious. *Neuropsychiatry, Neuropsychology, and Behavioral Neurology, 7*(1): 1–19.

Ross, R. R., & Fabiano, E. (1985). *Time to Think: A Cognitive Model of Delinquency Prevention and Offender Rehabilitation.* Johnson City, TN: Institute of Social Sciences and Arts.

Rossi, C., Angelucci, A., Costantin, L., Braschi, C., Mazzantini, M., Babbini, F., Fabbri, M. E., Tessarollo, L., Maffei, L., Berardi, N., Caleo, M. (2006). Brain-derived neurotrophic factor (BDNF) is required for the enhancement of hippocampal neurogenesis following environmental enrichment. *European Journal of Neuroscience, 24*(7):1850-1856.

Rossi, E. (2002). *The Psychobiology of Gene Expression: Neuroscience and Neurogenesis in Therapeutic Hypnosis and the Healing Arts.* New York: W. W. Norton.

Rowe, D. (1991). *Wanting Everything: The Art of Happiness.* London: Harper Collins.

Russek, L. G., & Schwartz, G. E. (1997). Feelings of parental caring predict health status in midlife: a 35-year follow-up of the Harvard Mastery of Stress Study. *Journal of Behavioral Medicine, 20*(1): 1–13.

Rutter, M. (2000). The adoption of children from Romania. *The Social and Intellectual Development of Children Adopted into England from Romania,* The Research Findings Register 55. London: Department of Health.

Rutter, M., Andersen-Wood, L., Beckett, R., Bredenkamp, D., Castle, J., Grootheus, C., Keppner, J., Keaveny, L., Lord, C. G., O'Connor, T. G., & English and Romanian Adoptees (ERA) Study Team (1999). Quasi-autistic patterns following severe early global privation. *Journal of Child Psychology and Psychiatry, 40*(4): 537–549.

Sachs, A. (2007). Infanticidal attachment: symbolic and concrete. *Attachment: New Directions in Psychotherapy and Relational Psychoanalysis, 1*(3): 297–304.

Sagi, A., Koren-Karie, N., Gini, M., Ziv, Y., & Joels, T. (2002). Shedding further light on the effects of various types and quality of early child care on infant–mother attachment relationship: the Haifa study of early child care. *Child Development, 73*(4): 1166–1186.

Sajaniemi, N., Mäkelä, J., Salokorpi, T., von Wendt, L., Hämäläinen, T., & Hakamies-Blomqvist, L. (2001). Cognitive performance and attachment patterns at four years of age in extremely low birth weight infants after early intervention. *European Child and Adolescent Psychiatry, 10*(2): 122–129.

Saltaris, C. (2002). Psychopathy in juvenile offenders: can temperament and attachment be considered robust developmental precursors? *Clinical Psychology Review, 22*(5): 729–752.

Salter, A. C. (1988). *Treating Child Sex Offenders and Victims: A Practical Guide.* Newbury Park, CA: Sage.

Sandnabba, N., Santtila, P., Wannäs, M., & Krook, K. (2003). Age and gender specific sexual behaviors in children. *Child Abuse & Neglect, 27*(6): 579–605.

Sarkar, M., & Andreas, M. (2004). Acceptance of and engagement in risky driving behaviors by teenagers. *Adolescence, 39*(156): 687–700.

Saugstad, L. F. (1994). The maturational theory of brain development and cerebral excitability in the multifactorially inherited manic-depressive psychosis and schizophrenia. *International Journal of Psychophysiology, 18*(3): 189–203.

Scaer, R. C. (2001). *The Body Bears the Burden. Trauma, Disassociation and Disease*. New York: Haworth Medical Press.

Schaffer, H. R., & Emerson, P. E. (1964). The development of social attachments in infancy. *Monographs of the Society for Research in Child Development, 29*(3): No. 94.

Scharfe, E. (2003). Stability and change of attachment representations from cradle to grave. In: S. M. Johnson & W. E. Whiffen (Eds.), *Attachment Processes in Couple and Family Therapy* (pp. 64–84). New York: Guilford Press.

Schiffer, B., Peschel, T., Paul, T., Gizewski, E., Forsting, M., Leygraf, N., Schedlowski, M., & Krueger, T. H. C. (2006). Structural brain abnormalities in the frontostriatal system and cerebellum in pedophilia. *Journal of Psychiatric Research, 41*(9): 725–763.

Schiffer, F. (2000). Can the different cerebral hemispheres have distinct personalities? Evidence and its implications for theory and treatment of PTSD and other disorders. *Journal of Trauma and Dissociation, 1*(2): 83–104.

Schindler, A., Thomasius, R., Petersen, K., & Sack, P-M. (2009). Heroin as an attachment substitute? Differences in attachment representations between opioid, ecstacy and cannabis abusers. *Attachment and Human Development, 11*(3): 307–330.

Schindler, A., Thomasius, R., Sack, P-M., Gemeinhardt, B., & Küstner, U. (2007). Insecure family bases and adolescent drug abuse: a new approach to family patterns of attachment. *Attachment & Human Development, 9*(2): 111–126.

Schneider, J. (2000a). Effects of cybersex addiction on the family: results of a survey. *Sexual Addiction & Compulsivity, 7*(1): 31–57.

Schneider, J. (2000b). A qualitative study of cybersex participants: gender differences, recovery issues, and implications for therapists. *Sexual Addiction and Compulsivity, 7*(4): 249–278.

Schneider, J. P. (2003). The impact of compulsive cybersex behaviours on the family. *Sexual & Relationship Therapy, 18*(3): 329–354.

Schneider, J. P., & Irons, R. R. (2001). Assessment and treatment of addictive sexual disorders: relevance for chemical dependency relapse. *Substance Use and Misuse, 36*(13): 1795–1820.

Schneider, J., & Weiss, R. (2001). *Cybersex Exposed: Simple Fantasy or Obsession?* Center City, MN: Hazelton.

Schore, A. (1994). *Affect Regulation and the Origin of the Self*. Hillsdale, NJ: Lawrence Erlbaum.

Schore, A. (2001). Minds in the making: attachment, the self-organizing brain, and developmentally oriented psychoanalytic psychotherapy. *British Journal of Psychotherapy, 17*(3): 299–328.

Schore, A. (2003a). *Affect Regulation and the Repair of the Self.* New York: Norton.

Schore, A. (2003b). *Affect Dysregulation and Disorders of the Self.* New York: Norton.

Schore, A. (2003c). The seventh annual John Bowlby memorial lecture. Minds in the making: attachment, the self-organizing brain, and developmentally-orientated psychoanalytic psychotherapy. In: J. Corrigall & H. Wilkinson (Eds.), *Revolutionary Connections. Psychotherapy and Neuroscience* (pp. 7–51). London: Karnac.

Schore, A. (2003d). Early relational trauma, disorganized attachment, and the development of a predisposition to violence. In: M. F. Solomon & D. J. Siegel (Eds.), *Healing Trauma. Attachment, Mind, Body and Brain* (pp. 107–167). New York: W. W. Norton.

Schultz, N. W. (1980). A cognitive–developmental study of the grand-child–grandparent bond. *Child Study Journal, 10*(1): 7–26.

Scott, J.-P. (1979). Critical periods in organizational processes. In: F. Faulkener & J. M. Tanner (Eds.), *Human Growth, Vol 3. Neuro-biology and Nutrition* (pp. 223–241). New York: Plenum Press.

Sentencing Advisory Panel (2002). *Sentencing Advisory Panel's Advice to the Court of Appeal on Sentences Involving Child Pornography.* London: HMSO.

Serran, G. A., & Marshall, L. E. (2006). Coping and mood in sexual offending. In: W. L. Marshall, Y. M. Fernandez, L. E. Marshall, & G. A. Serran (Eds.), *Sexual Offender Treatment. Controversial Issues* (pp. 109–124). Chichester: Wiley.

Seto, M. C., & Eke, A. W. (2005). The criminal histories and later offending of child pornography offenders. *Sexual Abuse: A Journal of Research and Treatment, 17*(2): 201–210.

Seto, M. C., Cantor, J. M., & Blanchard, R. (2006). Child pornography offences are a valid diagnostic indicator of pedophilia. *Journal of Abnormal Psychology, 115*(3): 610–615.

Shapiro, F., & Maxfield, L. (2003). EMDR and information processing in psychotherapy treatment: personal development and global implications. In: M. F. Solomon & D. J. Siegel (Eds.), *Healing Trauma. Attachment, Mind, Body and Brain* (pp. 196–220). New York: W. W. Norton.

Sharron, H., & Coulter, M. (1994). *Changing Children's Minds. Feuerstein's Revolution in the Teaching of Intelligence*. Birmingham: Souvenir Press.

Shaver, P. R., & Clark, C. L. (1994). The psychodynamics of adult romantic attachment. In: J. M. Masling & R. F. Bornstein (Eds.), *Empirical Perspectives on Object Relations Theory*, Vol. 5 (pp. 105–156). Washington, DC: American Psychological Association.

Shaw, P., Greenstein, D., Lerch, J., Clasen, L., Lenroot, R., Gogtay, N., Evans, A., Rapoport, J., & Giedd, J. (2006). Intellectual ability and cortical developments in children and adolescents. *Nature*, 440(7084): 676–679.

Shaw, R. (2003). *The Embodied Psychotherapist: The Therapist's Body Story*. London: Brunner-Routledge.

Shaw, S. M. (1999). Men's leisure and women's lives: the impact of pornography on women. *Leisure Studies*, 18(3): 197–212.

Shaywitz, B. A., Shaywitz, S. E., Pugh, K. R., Constable, R. T., Skudlarski, P., Fulbright, R. K., Bronen, R. A., Fletcher, J. M., Shankweller, D. P., Katz, I., & Gore, J. C. (1995). Sex differences in the functional organization of the brain for language. *Nature*, 373(6515): 607–609.

Sheath, M. (1990). Confrontative work with sex offenders: legitimized nonce bashing. *Probation Journal*, 37(4): 159–162.

Sheldon, K., & Howitt, D. (2007). *Sex Offenders and the Internet*. Chichester: Wiley.

Sheline, Y. I., Gado, M. H., & Kraemer, H. C. (2003). Untreated depression and hippocampal volume loss. *American Journal of Psychiatry*, 160(6): 1516–1518.

Shingler, J., & Mann, R. E. (2006). Collaboration in clinical work with sexual offenders: treatment and risk assessment. In: W. L. Marshall, Y. M. Fernandez, L. E. Marshall, & G. A. Serran (Eds.), *Sexual Offender Treatment. Controversial Issues* (pp. 225–239). Chichester: Wiley.

Shorey, H., & Snyder, C. R. (2006). The role of adult attachment styles in psychopathology and psychotherapy outcomes. *Review of General Psychology*, 10(1): 1–20.

Short, R. V. (1980). The origins of human sexuality. In: C. R. Austin & R. V. Short (Eds.), *Reproduction in Mammals, Vol. 8: Human Sexuality* (pp. 1–33). Cambridge: Cambridge University Press.

Shupe, L. M. (1954). Alcohol and crime: a study of the urine alcohol concentration found in 882 persons arrested during 8 hours immediately after commission of a felony. *Journal of Criminal Law, Criminology and Police Science*, 44(5): 661–664.

Siegel, D. (1999). *The Developing Mind: Towards a Neurobiology of Inter-personal Experience*. New York: Guilford Press.

Siegel, D. (2003). An interpersonal neurobiology of psychotherapy: the developing mind and the resolution of trauma. In: M. E. Solomon & D. J. Siegel (Eds.), *Healing Trauma: Attachment, Mind, Body and Brain* (pp. 1–56). New York: Norton.

Siegle, G. J., Carter, C., & Thase, M. E. (2006). Use of fMRI to predict recovery from unipolar depression with Cognitive Behavior Therapy. *American Journal of Psychiatry, 163*(4): 735–738.

Silverman, J., & Wilson, D. (2002). *Innocence Betrayed. Paedophilia, The Media and Society*. Oxford: Blackwell.

Skuse, D. H., & Gallagher, L. (2009). Dopaminergic–neuropeptide interactions in the social brain. *Trends in Cognitive Sciences, 13*(1): 27–35.

Slaby, R. G., & Guerra, N. G. (1988). Cognitive mediators of aggression in adolescent offenders: 1. Assessment. *Developmental Psychology, 24*(4): 580–588.

Slade, A. (1999). Attachment theory and research. implications for the theory and practice of individual psychotherapy with adults. In: J. Cassidy & P. R. Shaver (Eds.), *Handbook of Attachment. Theory, Research, and Clinical Applications* (pp. 575–594). New York: Guilford Press.

Smallbone, S. W. (2005). Attachment insecurity as a predisposing and precipitating factor for young people who sexually abuse. In: M. C. Calder (Ed.), *Children and Young People who Sexually Abuse: New Theory, Research, and Practice Developments* (pp. 4–16). Lyme Regis: Russell House Publishing.

Smallbone, S. W. (2006). An attachment–theoretical revision of Marshall and Barbaree's integrated theory of the etiology of sexual offending. In: W. L. Marshall, Y. M. Fernandez, L. E. Marshall, & G. A. Serran (Eds.), *Sexual Offender Treatment. Controversial issues* (pp. 93–107). Chichester: Wiley.

Sobal, J. (1995). Social influences on body weight. In: K. D. Brownell & C. G. Fairburn (Eds.), *Eating Disorders and Obesity*. New York: Guilford Press.

Solms, M. (1996). Towards an anatomy of the unconscious. *Journal of Clinical Psychoanalysis, 5*(3): 331–367.

Solms, M., & Turnbull, O. (2002). *The Brain and the Inner World*. New York: Other Press.

Solomon, M. F. (2003). Connection, disruption, repair: treating the effects of attachment trauma on intimate relationships. In: M. F. Solomon & D. J. Siegel (Eds.), *Healing Trauma. Attachment, Mind, Body and Brain* (pp. 322–346). New York: W. W. Norton.

Solomon, R. (1980). The opponent process of acquired emotion. *American Psychologist, 35*(8): 691–712.

Sorensen, J. (2005). *Relapse Prevention in Bipolar Disorder. A Treatment Manual and Workbook for Therapist and Client.* Hatfield: University of Hertfordshire Press.

Spear, L. P. (2000). The adolescent brain and age-related behavioral manifestations. *Neuroscience and Biobehavioral Reviews, 24*(4): 417–463.

Sperry, R. W. (1966). Brain bisection and mechanisms of consciousness. In: J. Eccles (Ed.), *Brain and Conscious Experience* (pp. 217–237). New York: Springer-Verlag.

Sperry, R. W. (1982). Some effects of disconnecting the cerebral hemispheres. *Science, 217*(4566): 1223–1226.

Spitzberg, B., & Rhea, J. (1999). Obsessive relational intrusion and sexual coercion victimization. *Journal of Interpersonal Violence, 14*(1): 3–20.

Sroufe, L. A. (1977). Attachment as an organizational construct. *Child Development, 48*(4): 1189–1199.

Sroufe, L. A. (1979). Socioemotional development. In: J. D. Osofsky (Ed.), *Handbook of Infant Development* (pp. 462–516). New York: Wiley.

Sroufe, L. A. (1983a). Individual patterns of adaptation from infancy to preschool. In: M. Perlmutter (Ed.), *Minnesota Symposium on Child Psychology* (pp. 41–84). Hillsdale, NJ: Lawrence Erlbaum.

Sroufe, L. A. (1983b). Infant–caregiver attachment and patterns of adaptation in preschool: the roots of maladaptation and competence. In: M. Perlmutter (Ed.), *Minnesota Symposium in Child Psychology*, Vol. 16 (pp. 41–81).

Sroufe, L. A., Egeland, B., Carlson, E., & Collins, W. A. (2005). *The Development of the Person: The Minnesota Study of Risk and Adaptation from Birth to Adulthood.* New York: Guilford Press.

Stapleton, A. (2010). Child pornography. Classifications and conceptualizations. In: F. Attwood (Ed.), *Porn.Com. Making Sense of Online Pornography* (pp. 34–53). New York: Peter Lang.

Stein, P. T., & Kendall, J. C. (2004). *Psychological Trauma and the Developing Brain. Neurologically Based Interventions for Troubled*

Children. Binghamton, NY: Haworth Maltreatment and Trauma Press.

Strathearn, L. (2003). Long-term cognitive function in very low-birth-weight infants. *Journal of the American Medical Association, 289*(17): 2209.

Strathearn, L., Fonagy, P., Amico, J., & Montague, R. (2009). Adult attachment predicts maternal brain and oxytocin response to infant cues. *Neuropsychopharmacology, 34*(1–2): 2655–2666.

Strathearn, L., Gray, P. H., O'Callaghan, M. J., & Wood, D. O. (2001). Childhood neglect and cognitive development in extremely low birth weight infants: a prospective study. *Pediatrics in Review, 108*(1): 142–151.

Straube, T., Glauer, M., Dilger, S., Mentzel, H.-J., & Miltner, W. H. R. (2006). Effects of Cognitive Behavioral Therapy on brain activation in specific phobia. *Neuroimage, 29*(1): 125–135.

Stuss, D. T., & Alexander, M. P. (1999). Affectively burnt in: a proposed role of the right frontal lobe. In: E. Tulving (Ed.), *Memory, Consciousness and the Brain: The Talin Conference* (pp. 215–227). Philadelphia, PA: Psychology Press.

Subby, R., & Friel, J. (1984). Co-dependency: a paradoxical dependency. In: Health Communications (Ed.), *Codependency: An Emerging Issue* (pp. 31–44). Florida: Health Communications.

Sunderland, M. (2006). *The Science of Parenting*. London: Dorling Kindersley.

Symington, N. (1993). *Narcissism. A New Theory*. London: Karnac.

Tabin, J. K. (1985). *On the Way to the Self: Ego and Early Oedipal Development*. New York: Columbia University Press.

Tagney, J. P., & Dearing, R. L. (2002). *Shame and Guilt*. New York: Guilford Press.

Tagney, J. P., Wagner, P., Fletcher, C., & Gramzow, R. (1992). Proneness to shame, proneness to guilt, and psychopathology. *Journal of Abnormal Psychology, 101*(3): 469–478.

Tantum, D., & Whitaker, J. (1992). Personality disorder and self-wounding. *British Journal of Psychiatry, 161*: 451–464.

Tapert, S. F., & Schweinsburg, A. (2006). The human adolescent brain and alcohol use disorders. In: M. Galanter (Ed.), *Alcohol Problems in Adolescents and Young Adults* (pp. 177–197). New York: Springer.

Target, M., & Fonagy, P. (1996). Playing with reality: II. The development of psychic reality from a theoretical perspective. *International Journal of Psychoanalysis, 77*: 459–479.

Tarry, H., & Emler, N. (2007). Attitudes, values and moral reasoning. *British Journal of Developmental Psychology*, 25(2): 169–183.

Taylor, C. (1997). Management and treatment. In: E. V. Welldon & C. V. Velsen (Eds.), *A Practical Guide to Forensic Psychotherapy* (pp. 20–32). London: Jessica Kingsley.

Taylor, M., & Quayle, E. (2003). *Child Pornography: An Internet Crime.* Hove: Brunner Routledge.

Taylor, M., Quayle, E., & Holland, G. (2001). Child pornography, the internet, and offending. *Isuma Canadian Journal of Policy Research*, 2(2): 94–100.

Teasdale, J. D., Howard, R. J., Cox, S. G., Ha, Y., Brammer, M. J., Williams, S. C. R., & Checkley, S. A. (1999). Functional MRI study of cognitive generation of affect. *American Journal of Psychiatry*, 156(2): 209–215.

Teicher, M. H. (2000). Wounds that time won't heal: the neurobiology of child abuse. *Cerebrum*, 2(4): 50–67.

Teicher, M. H. (2002). Scars that will not heal. The neurobiology of child abuse. *Scientific American*, 286(1): 54–61.

Thatcher, R. W. (1994). Cyclical cortical reorganization: origins of human cognitive development. In: G. Dawson & K. W. Fischer (Eds.), *Human Behavior and the Developing Brain* (pp. 232–266). New York: Guilford Press.

Thomas, D. G., Whitaker, E., Crow, C. D., Little, V., Love, L., Lykins, M. S., & Lettermman, M. (1997). Event-related potential variability as a measure of information storage in infant development. *Developmental Neuropsychology*, 13(2): 205–232.

Tizard, B., & Hodges, J. (1978). The effect of early institutional rearing on the development of eight-year-old children. *Journal of Child Psychology and Psychiatry*, 19(2): 99–118.

Tjaden, P., & Theonnes, N. (1998). *Stalking in America: Findings from the National Violence Against Women Survey.* Washington, DC: National Institute of Justice and Centre for Disease Control & Prevention.

Tomak, S., Weschler, F. S., Ghahramanlou-Holloway, M., Virden, T., & Nademin, M. E. (2009). An empirical study of the personality characteristics of internet sex offenders. *Journal of Sexual Aggression*, 15(2): 139–148.

Tomkins, S. S. (1963). *Affect/Imagery/Consciousness, Vol. 2. The Negative Effects.* New York: Springer.

Trevarthen, C. (2001). The neurobiology of early communication: intersubjective regulations in human brain development. In: A. F. Klaverboer & A. Gramsbergen (Eds.), *Handbook on Brain and Behaviour in Human Development*. Dordrecht: Kluwer.

Trevarthen, C., & Aitken, K. J. (1994). Brain development, infant communication, and empathy disorders: intrinsic factors in child mental health. *Development and Psychopathology, 6*: 597–633.

Turnbull, O. (2003). Emotion, false beliefs, and the neurobiology of intuition. In: J. Corrigall & H. Wilkinson (Eds.), *Revolutionary Connections* (pp. 135–162). London: Karnac.

Tyman, H., & Worthington, R. (2009). Female sex offending: what do we actually know? *Forensic Update, 99*: 13–18.

Tyrer, P. (2000). *Personality Disorders. Diagnosis, Management & Course* (2nd edn). Oxford: Butterworth-Heinemann.

Van Balen, R. (1990). The therapeutic relationship according to Carl Rogers: only a climate? A dialogue? Or both? In: G. Lietaer, J. Rombants, & R. van Balen (Eds.), *Client-Centered and Experiential Psychotherapy in the Nineties* (pp. 65–86). Leuven: Leuven University Press.

Van der Kolk, B. A. (1988). The trauma spectrum: the interaction of biological and social events in the genesis of the trauma response. *Journal of Traumatic Stress, 1*(3): 273–290.

Van der Kolk, B. A. (1989). The compulsion to repeat the trauma. *Psychiatric Clinics of North America, 12*(2): 389–411.

Van der Kolk, B. A. (2003). Posttraumatic stress disorder and the nature of trauma. In: M. F. Solomon & D. J. Siegel (Eds.), *Healing Trauma. Attachment, Mind, Body and Brain* (pp. 168–195). New York: W. W. Norton.

Van der Kolk, B. A., Perry, J. C., & Herman, J. L. (1991). Childhood origins of self-destructive behavior. *American Journal of Psychiatry, 148*: 1665–1671.

Van IJzendoorn, M. H., & Bakermens-Kraneburg, M. J. (1999). Attachment representations in mothers, fathers, adolescents, and clinical groups: a meta-analytic search for normative data. *Journal of Consulting and Clinical Psychology, 64*(1): 8–21.

Van IJzendoorn, M. H., & Sagi, A. (1999). Cross-cultural patterns of attachment: universal and contextual dimensions. In: J. Cassidy & P. Shaver (Eds.), *Handbook of Attachment: Theory, Research, and Clinical Application* (pp. 713–734). New York: Guilford Press.

Vandiver, D. M. (2006). A prospective analysis of juvenile male sex offenders: characteristics and recidivism rates as adults. *Journal of Interpersonal Violence*, 21(5): 673–688.

Vandiver, D. M., & Kercher, G. (2004). Offender and victim characteristics or registered female sexual offenders in Texas: a proposed typology of female sexual offenders. *Sexual Abuse*, 16(2): 121–137.

Vas Dias, S. (2000). Inner silence: one of the impacts of emotional abuse on the developing self. In: U. McClusky & C. A. Hooper (Eds.), *Psychodynamic Perspectives on Abuse: The Cost of Fear* (pp. 159–171). London: Jessica Kingsley.

Venga, R. (2005). *Brain, Personality & Addictive Behaviours*. Leicester: Matador.

Verny, T., & Kelly, J. (1981). *The Secret Life of the Unborn Child*. London: Warner.

Verrier, N. N. (1993). *The Primal Wound. Understanding the Adopted Child*. Baltimore, MD: Gateway.

Veríssimo, M., & Salvaterra, F. (2006). Maternal secure-base scripts and children's attachment security in an adopted sample. *Attachment & Human Development*, 8(3): 261–273.

Vianna, D. M. L., Graeff, F. G., Brandao, M. L., & Landeira-Fernandez, J. (2001). Defensive freezing evoked by electrical stimulation of the periaqueductal gray: comparison between dorsolateral and ventrolateral regions. *Neuroreport*, 12(18): 4109–4112.

Virkkunen, M. (1985). Urinary free cortisol secretion in habitually violent offenders. *Acta Psychiatrica Scandinavia*, 72(1): 40–44.

Vizard, E. (2006). Sexually abusive behaviour by children and adolescents. *Child and Adolescent Mental Health*, 11(1): 2–8.

Vosmer, S., Hackett, S., & Callanan, M. (2009). "Normal" and "inappropriate" childhood sexual behaviours: findings from a Delphi study of professionals in the United Kingdom. *Journal of Sexual Aggression*, 15(3): 275–288.

Vyas, A., Mitra, R., Shankaranaryana Rao, B. S., & Chattarji, S. (2002). Chronic stress induces contrasting patterns of dendritic remodeling in hippocampal and amygdaloid neurons. *Journal of Neuroscience*, 22(15): 6810–6818.

Wakeling, H. C., Webster, S. D., Moulden, H. M., & Marshall, W. L. (2007). Decisions to offend in men who sexually abuse their daughters. *Journal of Sexual Aggression*, 13(2): 81–100.

Walker, A., Kershaw, C., & Nicholas, S. (2007). *Crime in England and Wales 2005/2006*. London: Home Office.

Walker, L. E. (1979). *The Battered Woman*. New York: Harper & Row.

Walsh, A. (1995). Parental attachment, drug use and facultative sexual strategies. *Social Biology, 42*(1–2): 95–107.

Walzer, S., Gerald, P. S., & Shah, S. A. (1978). The XYY genotype. *Annual Review of Medicine, 29*(1): 563–570.

Ward, E. (1988). *Father–Daughter Rape*. London: The Women's Press.

Ward, T., & Connolly, M. (2008). A human-rights based practice framework for sexual offenders. *Journal of Sexual Aggression, 14*(2): 87–98.

Ward, T., & Marshall, W. L. (2004). Good lives, etiology and the rehabilitation of sex offenders: a bridging theory. *Journal of Sexual Aggression, 10*(2): 153–169.

Ward, T., Hudson, S. M., & Marshall, W. L. (1996). Attachment style in sex offenders. A preliminary study. *Journal of Sex Research, 33*(1): 17–26.

Waters, E., Merrick, S., Treboux, D., Crowell, J., & Albersham, L. (2000). Attachment security in infancy and early adulthood: a twenty-year longitudinal study. *Child Development, 71*(3): 684–689.

Waters, E., Wippman, J., & Sroufe, L. A. (1979). Attachment, positive affect, and competence in the peer group: two studies in construct validation. *Child Development, 50*(3): 821–829.

Watt, D. F. (1990). Higher cortical functions and the ego: explorations of the boundary between behavioral neurology, neuropsychology, and psychoanalysis. *Psychoanalytic Psychology, 7*(4): 487–527.

Watters, S. O. (2001). *Real Solutions for Overcoming Internet Addictions*. Michigan, MS: Real Solutions.

Watts, S., Bush, R., & Wilson, P. (1994). Partners of problem drinkers: moving into the 1990's. *Drug and Alcohol Review, 13*(4): 401–407.

Webster, J. D. (1997). Attachment style and wellbeing in elderly adults: a preliminary investigation. *Canadian Journal on Aging, 16*(1): 101–111.

Weinstock, M. (1997). Does prenatal stress impair coping and regulation of hypothalamic–pituitary–adrenal axis? *Neuroscience and Biobehavioral Reviews, 21*(1): 1–10.

Welldon, E. V. (1997). The practical approach. In: E. V. Welldon & C. van Velsen (Eds.), *A Practical Guide to Forensic Psychotherapy* (pp. 13–19). London: Jessica Kingsley.

Welldon, E. V., & van Velsen, C. (1997). *A Practical Guide to Forensic Psychotherapy*. London: Jessica Kingsley.

West, D. J. (1980). *Treatment in Theory and Practice, Sex Offenders in the Criminal Justice System* (pp. 141–149). Cambridge: University of Cambridge Institute of Criminology.

West, M. L., & Sheldon-Keller, A. E. (1994). *Patterns of Relating: An Adult Attachment Perspective*. New York: Guilford Press.

Westen, D., Nakash, O., Thomas, C., & Bradley, R. (2006). Clinical assessment of attachment patterns and personality disorder in adolescents and adults. *Journal of Consulting and Clinical Psychology, 74*(6): 1065–1085.

Whittle, N., Bailey, S., & Kurtz, Z. (2006). *The Needs and Effective Treatment of Young People Who Sexually Abuse: Current Evidence*. London: Home Office: Department of Health, National Institute for Mental Health in England.

Wilkinson, M. (2006). *Coming to Mind. The Mind–Brain Relationship: a Jungian Clinical Perspective*. London: Routledge.

Williams Committee Report (1979). *Obscenity and Film Censorship* (Cmnd: 7772). London: HMSO.

Williams, L. M., & Finkelhor, D. (1990). The characteristics of incestuous fathers: a review of recent studies. In: W. L. Marshall, D. R. Laws, & H. E. Barbaree (Eds.), *Handbook of Sexual Assault: Issues, Theories, and Treatment* (pp. 231–255). New York: Plenum Press.

Wilson, C., Gardener, F., Burton, J., & Leung, S. (2006). Maternal attributions and young children's conduct problems. *Infant and Child Development, 15*(2): 109–121.

Wilson, J., & Hernstein, R. (1985). *Crime and Human Nature*. New York: Simon & Schuster.

Wilson, J. S., Ermshar, A. L., & Welsh, R. K. (2006). Stalking as paranoid attachment: a typological and dynamic model. *Attachment & Human Development, 8*(2): 139–157.

Winnicott, D. W. (1960). The theory of parent–infant relationship. *International Journal of Psychoanalysis, 41*: 585–595.

Winnicott, D. W. (1971). *Playing and Reality*. New York: Basic Books.

Wismer Fries, A. B., Ziegler, T. E., Kurian, J. R., Jacoris, S., & Pollak, S. D. (2005). Early experiences in humans is associated with changes in neuropeptides critical for regulating social behavior. *Proceedings of the National Academy of Sciences of the United States, 102*(47): 17237–17240.

Wittling, W. (1995). Brain asymmetry in the control of autonomic–physiologic activity. In: R. Davidson & K. Hugdahl (Eds.), *Brain Asymmetry* (pp. 305–358). Cambridge, MA: MIT Press.

Wortley, R., & Smallbone, S. W. (2006). Applying situational principles to sexual offences against children. *Situational Prevention of Child Sexual Abuse. Crime Prevention Studies, 19*: 7–36. New York: Willan.

Wyre, R. (1987). *Working with Sex Abuse*. London: Perry.

Wyre, R. (2003). Personal communication.

Yamada, H., Sadato, N., Konishi, Y., Muramoto, S., Kimura, K., Tanak, M., Yonekura, Y., Ishii, Y., & Itoh, H. (2000). A milestone for normal development of the infantile brain detected by functional MRI. *Neurology, 55*(2): 218–223.

Yates, A., Beutler, L. E., & Crago, M. (1983). Characteristics of young violent offenders. *Journal of Psychiatry and Law, 11*: 137–149.

Young, K. (1998). *Caught in the Net. How to Recognize the Signs of Internet Addiction and a Winning Strategy for Recovery*. New York: Wiley.

Young, K., Cooper, A., Griffin-Shelley, E., O'Mara, J., & Buchanan, J. (2000). Cybersex and infidelity online: implications for evaluation and treatment. *Sexual Addictions & Compulsivity, 7*(1): 59–74.

Young, K., Griffin Shelley, E., Cooper, A., O'Mara, J., & Buchanan, J. (2000). Online infidelity: a new dimension in couple relationships with implications for evaluation and treatment. *Journal of Sexual Addiction & Compulsivity, Special Issue: Cybersex: The Dark Side of the Force*, Chap 3: 62–63.

Young, K., O'Mara, J., & Buchanan, J. (2001). Cybersex and infidelity online: implications for evaluation and treatment. *Sexual Addiction and Compulsivity, 7*(7): 50–74.

Yurgelun-Todd, D. A., & Killgore, W. D. (2006). Fear-related activity in the prefrontal cortex increases with age during adolescence: a preliminary fMRI study. *Neuroscience Letters, 406*(3): 194–199.

Zahn-Waxler, C., McKnew, D. H., Cummings, M., Davenport, W. B., & Radke-Yarrow, M. (1984). Problem behaviors and peer interaction of young children with a manic–depressive parent. *American Journal of Psychiatry, 141*(2): 236–240.

Zeanah, C. H. (1996). Beyond insecurity: a reconceptualization of attachment disorders in infancy. *Journal of Consulting and Clinical Psychology, 64*(1): 42–52.

Zeanah, C. H., Mammen, O., & Lieberman, A. (1993). Disorders of attachment. In: C. H. Zeanah (Ed.), *Handbook of Infant Mental Health* (pp. 332–349). New York: Guilford Press.

Zillman, D. (1979). *Hostility and Aggression*. Hillsdale, NJ: Lawrence Erlbaum.

Zitzman, S., & Butler, M. (2005). Attachment, addiction, and recovery: conjoint marital therapy for recovery from sexual addiction. *Sexual Addiction & Compulsivity*, 12(4): 311–337.

Zona, M., Sharma, L., & Lane, J. (1993). A comparative study of erotomanic and obsessional subjects in a forensic sample. *Journal of Forensic Sciences*, 38(4): 894–903.

INDEX

Abel, G. G., 189, 211, 244, 251, 259, 305
Abelin, E., 37, 305
Abrams, J. L., 153, 305
Abrams, K. Y., 56, 62–63, 328
Abrams, L. S., 87, 305
abuse, xvii, 56, 59, 62–63, 66, 69–70, 77, 86, 97–98, 111, 136, 139, 142–143, 146–147, 159–163, 187, 190, 197, 204, 207, 211–212, 217, 239–240, 243, 245, 250, 252, 261, 263–264, 292, 295, 300–301
    see also: alcohol, drugs, substance
child(hood), xi, xvii, xx, 9, 56, 58–63, 68–69, 80–82, 94, 97–98, 109, 132–135, 137–138, 142, 147, 160, 163–164, 184, 197, 203–215, 217, 230, 239–241, 243–246, 252–253, 255, 260, 263–267
emotional, 56, 69, 78–79, 81, 122, 159, 227
intrafamilial, 246
maternal, 131
parental, 79, 97, 163
physical, 9, 56, 61, 69, 78, 80–81, 94–95, 122, 133, 138, 142, 205, 234
self, 139
sexual, xx, 56, 60–61, 63, 77–78, 80–81, 95, 109, 138, 142, 160, 164, 187, 190, 206–207, 213, 240, 245–246, 252–253, 266
abusive care-giver/parent, xv, xix, 57, 62–63, 97, 126, 133, 135
Adams, M. J., 306
addiction, xx, 53, 60, 78, 90–93, 106, 111, 114, 127, 136, 138, 146, 153, 155, 162, 176–180, 184, 188–194, 201–203, 209, 215, 218, 236, 292, 296–298 see also: alcohol, drugs, Internet
cigarettes/nicotine, 91, 127, 192, 233
food, 91, 179
gambling, 179
religion, 91, 179

sexual, xix, 91, 155, 174–179,
181–182, 184, 188, 191–193,
199, 201, 203, 208–209, 216,
219, 233
shopping, 91, 179, 215
work, 91, 127, 179
Adelson, E., 69, 322
Adkerson, D. L., 299, 312
adolescent, xiv, xix, xx, 3–4, 64, 67,
71, 76–77, 81–93, 95–100, 115,
121, 130, 138, 150, 187, 189–190,
202, 239, 242, 247–249, 252–253,
293, 298
Adolphs, R., 44, 306
adoption/adoptive
children, xiii–xiv, 46, 65–70, 246,
292
mother, 66–67, 69–70
parents, xiv, 65–67, 69–70
adrenaline, 1, 13, 27, 46–48, 65, 91,
128, 145, 155, 162, 178, 246, 286
nor-, 20, 179
Adult Attachment Interview, 114,
290
affection, x, 3, 26, 36, 76, 82, 108,
156, 224
aggression, 8, 10, 13, 38, 54, 64, 67,
69, 78–81, 86, 94–99, 113, 121,
135, 144–145, 161–163, 166–167,
169, 173, 189, 193, 212, 226,
230–231, 250–251, 257, 263, 283,
294–296
passive–, 52, 90
Ahmad, S., 142, 306
Ainsworth, M. D. S., 3–4, 50, 306
Aitken, K. J., 28, 355
Akdeniz, Y., 203, 207, 306
Akiskal, H. S., 92, 99, 124, 166–170,
306, 309, 332–333
Akiskal, K., 92, 99, 124, 166–168,
170, 333
Albersham, L., 104, 357
alcohol/alcoholics, 53, 60, 83, 89,
91–92, 127, 135–136, 138,
153–154, 175, 179, 216, 231–232,
267–268, 271, 286, 293

abuse, 136, 232, 268 see also:
substance abuse
addiction, 53, 91, 127, 132, 179,
192, 233
Alexander, M. P., 27, 353
Alexander, P. C., 160, 306
Allen, J. G., 197, 306
Almergi, J. B., 29, 327
Alpern, L., 56, 335
Ames, E. W., 67, 306
Amico, J., 54, 353
Anda, R. F., 60, 321
Andersen-Wood, L., 68, 347
Anderson, B., 91–92, 309
Anderson, C. A., 230, 306
Anderson, D., 300, 337
Andreas, M., 84, 347
Andreason, N. C., 171, 306
Andrews, B., 283–284, 329
Angelucci, A., 287, 346
anger, 4, 13, 15–16, 37–38, 47, 50, 52,
54–55, 57, 85, 88, 90, 99,
109–110, 121–123, 125, 127,
133–135, 145, 152–154, 157–158,
160–161, 164, 167–168, 170, 181,
199, 219, 224, 231, 235, 245,
250–251, 257, 274, 283, 294–295,
297
anxiety, x, 10, 13, 20, 25, 46, 50–51,
64, 81, 93, 107, 109–110, 113,
127, 130–132, 140–142, 151,
155–156, 167, 188, 198–199, 224,
230, 246, 254, 277–278, 293, 299
disorder, 93, 131, 168, 244
separation, 10, 24, 27, 30, 38, 47,
63, 239
Aou, S., 179, 306
Appleby, L., 137, 307
Araga, M., 170–171, 339
Araji, S., 300, 321
Arce, E., 145, 345
assault, 13, 78, 96, 136, 159, 162, 206,
224, 248, 250–251, 253
Asuan-O'Brien, A., 160, 334
Atkinson, B. J., 13, 45, 58, 153, 307
Atkinson, L., 281–282, 337

attachment
  adult, 4, 104–105, 186
  ambivalent, 55, 90, 111, 113, 138,
    169–170, 248
  avoidant, 51, 71, 100, 112–113,
    115, 118, 123, 127, 131, 133,
    159, 196, 218, 227, 237, 251,
    282, 284, 286
  bond, 4, 132, 162, 179, 225, 245,
    281
  childhood, 4, 104, 107, 112–114, 152
  development, 28, 35, 37
  disorganized, xv, 56, 64, 114, 133,
    283
  dysfunction, 132–133, 138, 233
  figure(s), xii, xvii, 3–4, 23, 31–32,
    50, 55, 63, 88, 100, 109,
    113–114, 126, 163, 226, 253,
    276, 280, 283–284, 300
  infant, 34, 104, 278, 281
  infanticidal, 142–143
  injury, xix, 10, 66, 86, 157, 215,
    292–294, 297
  insecure, x, xix, 4, 9–10, 41, 48, 52,
    58, 68, 71, 76, 78, 81, 85, 87,
    107–108, 111, 113, 115, 122,
    136, 140, 142, 144, 146, 151,
    156, 160–161, 168–169, 176,
    178–180, 186–188, 197, 202,
    225–227, 231–232, 238–239,
    253, 278, 285, 294
  multiple, xi, xiii
  paranoid, 226
  preoccupied, 50–51, 89, 108, 133,
    138, 160–161, 232
  reactive, 68–69
  secure, xiii, xix, 5–6, 10, 28, 35,
    65–66, 69, 76, 78, 85, 91, 93,
    105, 127, 156, 161, 179,
    186–187, 219, 277–279, 302
  theory, x, xix, 104–105
  trauma, 112, 156–157, 298
attention deficit and hyperactivity
    disorder (ADHD), xiv, 68,
    95–96, 168
Attwood, F., 200, 214, 307

autism, 68, 144
autonomy, 5, 71, 82, 85–86, 120, 162,
    186, 189, 284
Awad, G., 190, 307
axons, 18–19, 32, 83

Babbini, F., 287, 346
Babchishin, K., 269, 331
Bach-y-Rita, G., 146, 307
BAD-ME, 57, 61–62
Bagby, R. M., 281–282, 337
Bagley, C., 63, 97, 307
Bailey, A. J., 62, 311
Bailey, S., 81, 358
Bak, M., 142, 307
Baker, W. L., 59, 343
Bakermens-Kraneburg, M. J., 154,
    355
Ballenger, J. C., 166, 344
Bancroft, J., 79, 81, 198, 240, 251,
    259, 299, 307, 330
Bandura, A., 145, 307
Barbaree, H. E., 240, 243, 254, 308,
    310, 337
Barbas, H., 276, 308
Barlow, D. H., 251, 259, 305
Barnett, D., 56, 313
Barnett, L., 285, 319
Barone, L., 87–88, 308
Barron, M., 208, 308
Bartels, A., 109, 308
Bartholomew, K., 51, 63, 107, 161,
    163, 308
Bartosh, D. L., 263, 308
Basch, M. F., 280, 308
Bateman, A. W., 126, 141, 308
Bates, A., 260, 266, 308, 320
Bayart, D., 169, 332
Baylis, G. C., 186, 324
Beaudoin, G., 195, 331
Beauregard, M., 195, 331
Bechara, A., 144, 308
Beck, A. T., 131, 150, 295, 308–309
Beckett, R., 68, 260, 309, 347
Beech, A., 210, 212, 254, 259–261,
    268–269, 309, 316, 322, 339

behaviour
  antisocial, 6, 95, 98, 124
  criminal, 97, 131, 255
  disorders, 58, 131, 166
  sexual, 76, 79–82, 109, 174–175,
    177–178, 185, 189–190, 192,
    194, 210, 241, 243–244,
    298–299
  violent, 9, 63, 69, 96, 131, 146, 162,
    230–231
Behen, M., 46, 314
Belsky, J., 10, 76–77, 309
Benazzi, F., 168, 309
Bench, C. J., 20, 309
Beniart, S., 91–92, 309
Benkelfat, C., 134, 330
Bennett, A., 65, 333
Benoit, D., 70, 309
Bentall, R., 167, 309
Berardi, N., 287, 346
Bergman, A., 35, 37, 120, 335
Bergner, R., 199, 296, 311
Berkowitz, L., 231, 309
Berlin, F. S., 191–192, 199, 215, 323
Berne, E., 109, 309
Beutler, L. E., 145, 359
Beyko, M., 267, 310
bipolar disorder, xix, 140, 166–171
Birhie, S., 145, 345
Birnbaum, G. E., 109, 310
birth trauma, 7-9
Black, D. A., 246, 310
Blackburn, R., 229, 259, 310
Blackshaw, L., 262, 323
Blak, T., 243–244, 310, 312
Blakley, T. L., 59, 343
Blanchard, E. B., 251, 259, 305
Blanchard, R., 210–211, 228,
    243–244, 310, 312, 349
Blehar, M. C., 3–4, 306
Bloomberg, D., 229, 311
Blos, P., 38, 310
Blumberg, H. P., 134, 318
Boardman, M., 63, 142, 310
Bocij, P., 227, 310
Bogaert, A. F., 240, 243, 308, 310

Bohus, M., 138, 310
Boies, S., 185, 192–193, 199, 315
Bond, A., 137, 327
Boon, J. C. W., 224, 310
Booth LaForce, C., 6, 338
Boring, A., 59, 317
Borysenko, J., 25, 310
Borysenko, M., 25, 310
Boucher, R., 213, 313
Boulet, J. R., 229, 311
Bourbeau, L. S., 112, 318
Bourgouin, P., 195, 331
Bow, J., 159, 311
Bowlby, J., x–xii, xix, 4, 10–11, 39,
    104, 118–119, 144, 158, 275, 311
Boxer, P., 159, 190, 311, 335
Bradbury, T. N., 150, 152, 314, 321
Bradford, J. M. W., 229, 269, 311,
    331
Bradley, R., 133, 282, 358
Bradsford, J. M., 268, 341
Braeutigam, S., 62, 311
brain
  amygdala, 13, 20, 24–25, 28,
    31–33, 39, 44–46, 50–51,
    57–62, 77–78, 83–84, 86, 93,
    108, 120, 134, 158, 180,
    186–187, 189–190, 193–194,
    197, 203, 209, 214, 250, 277
  cerebellum, 243, 289
  child's/infant's, xiii, xix, 23,
    28–29, 32, 39, 51, 58–60, 64,
    66, 69, 71, 135, 186, 243
  cingulate, 20, 28, 32, 39, 47, 59,
    145, 195, 277
  corpus callosum, 17, 21–23, 45,
    58–59, 280, 288
  cortex, 16–17, 20, 24–25, 27–28,
    32–33, 36–38, 45, 47, 51, 54,
    58–59, 83–84, 86, 92, 134, 137,
    145, 158, 179, 193, 195, 197,
    241, 243, 276–278, 280, 282,
    289–290
  damage, 132, 231
  development, xix, 20, 29, 66, 69,
    75, 188, 202, 239, 290

hemisphere(s), 17, 19–23, 28, 32–33, 36, 39–40, 44–47, 65, 77, 84, 86, 98, 133, 158, 187, 194, 197, 203, 219, 225, 276, 279–281, 288–289, 291

hippocampus, 13, 24, 27–28, 33, 44, 46, 48, 58–61, 92, 134, 277, 287, 291, 294

hypothalamus, 25, 29, 37, 54, 194–195, 250

hypothalamus–pituitary–adrenal pathway (HPA axis), 23–24, 44, 46, 50, 58–59, 64–65, 78, 84, 158, 180, 198, 219, 294

left, 20–22, 28–29, 44–46, 54, 59, 75, 134, 158, 197–198, 279–280, 282, 287, 290, 298

limbic system, 16, 20, 24, 28, 31, 33, 35–36, 44–45, 47, 108, 277, 280, 283

neurone(s), 17–19, 23, 26, 28, 30, 32–33, 59, 83, 276

prefrontal lobe, 29, 46

right, xix, xx, 20–22, 28–29, 32–33, 40–41, 46–47, 59–62, 69, 75, 87, 98, 100, 124–125, 134, 158, 180, 187–189, 194, 197–198, 202, 219, 239, 278–281, 286–287, 289–290, 297–298

stem, 16, 51, 58, 137

Brammer, M. J., 44, 354

Brandao, M. L., 64, 356

Braschi, C., 287, 346

Braunwald, K. G., 56, 313

Brazelton, T. B., 25, 311

Bredenkamp, D., 66–68, 342, 347

Bremner, J. D., 60, 65, 311, 333

Brennan, K. A., 111, 311

Brennan, P., 9, 345

Bridges, A., 199, 296, 311

Brisch, K. H., xvi, 113, 133, 311

British Crime Survey, 158, 223, 233

Bronen, R. A., 21, 350

Broom, I., 268, 341

Broucek, F. J., 121–123, 311–312

Brown, N. W., 125, 312

Brown, R., 28, 312

Browne, C. J., 112, 312

Browne, K. D., 159, 163, 265, 269, 316, 318

Brownmiller, S., 251, 312

Buchanan, J., 185, 201, 359

Buck, R., 21–22, 28, 312, 346

Budd, T., 223, 228, 312

Bumby Cognitive Distortions Scale, 299

Bunclark, J., 139, 316

Burkart, B. R., 253, 323

burnout, 197–198, 289 see also: stress

Burns, N., 252, 321

Burton, J., 49, 358

Bush, R., 154, 357

Bussière, M. T., 210, 266–267, 326

Butler, M., 297, 360

Byng-Hall, J., 58, 312

Cahn, B. R., 290, 312

Calabrese, J. R., 170–171, 339

Caleo, M., 287, 346

Callanan, M., 79, 81, 356

Cantor, J. M., 210–211, 228, 243–244, 310, 312, 349

Carden, S. W., 92, 312

Cardoner, N., 59, 326

CARE, 23–24, 27–30, 35–36, 40, 44–45, 47, 49–50, 61, 64, 77, 88, 99, 105–106, 143, 150–151, 157–158, 187, 254, 278, 281, 297

circuit, 25, 27, 35, 49, 51, 91, 178, 289, 294

Careaga, A., 192–193, 196, 199, 216, 312

Carich, M. S., 299, 312

Carich–Adkerson Victim Empathy and Self Report Inventory, 299

Carlson, E. A., 6, 11, 63–64, 93–95, 119, 312, 342, 352

Carlson, V. J., 56, 119, 312–313

Carmen, E. H., 98, 160, 313

Carmona, J., 160, 334

Carnes, L., 198, 299, 307

Carnes, P., 174–175, 177–178, 192–193, 203, 216–217, 266, 313, 317
Carr, J., 204, 212, 313
Carroll, R., 278, 313
Carter, C., 276, 351
Carter, D., 213, 313
case study
   Conner, xviii, xix, 221–222, 235, 303
   Gordon, xviii–xx, 2, 11–16, 40–41, 43–44, 60, 71, 73–75, 100–101, 103–104, 115, 117–118, 127–130, 147–150, 164–165, 172, 181–183, 219–222, 233, 235–236, 270–271, 273–275, 303
   Jenny, 11–13, 15–16, 40–41, 43–44, 71, 220
   Joe, 11–13, 41, 71, 220
   John, 103
   Rachel, xix, 150, 164–165, 172–173, 181–184, 219–222, 233, 235–236, 270, 303
Casey, B., 59, 317
Cassidy, J., 50, 70, 108, 187, 313, 335–336
Castle, J., 68, 347
Cavanagh Johnson, T., 80, 313
Ceballos-Baumann, A. O., 59, 326
Chamberlain, D., xi, 12, 25–26, 313
Chaplin, T., C., 259, 345
Charlton, B., 27, 313
Charney, D., 65, 333
Chattarji, S., 59, 356
Checkley, S. A., 44, 354
child and adolescent mental health services (CAMHS), 100
child(ren) see also:
   adoption/adoptive
   biological, 66, 246
   foster, 69, 246
   step-, 69, 246
Chin, D., 160, 334
Chiron, C., 32, 44, 187, 313
Chisholm, K. A., 66, 314

Cho, E., 13, 78, 320
Choy, A., 244, 310
Christensen, B. K., 243, 310
Christensen, G. A., 244, 345
Christian, R., 257, 326
Christie, M. M., 250, 314
Chugani, D., 46, 314
Chugani, H., 46, 314
Cicchetti, D., 56, 313
Clark, C. L., 132, 350
Clark, D., 59, 317
Clasen, L., 86, 350
Clulow, C., 51, 55, 153, 160, 314
Cobb, R. J., 150, 314
Cobbs, G., 86, 327
co-dependency, xix, 119, 126, 149, 151, 153–156, 159, 161, 163, 170, 296
cognitive behavioural therapy (CBT), xviii, 170, 216, 255, 261, 277, 282, 291, 297
Cohen, C., 113, 335
Cohen, L. E., 270, 314
Cohen, L. J., 243, 314
Cole-Detke, H., 87–88, 314
Coleman, E., 244, 345
Coley, R. L., 99, 314
Colletti, P., 145, 345
Collins, W. A., 6, 11, 93–94, 97, 119, 352
Combating Paedophile Information Networks in Europe (COPINE), 206
comorbidity, 136, 140, 167, 179, 244
conduct disorder, 59, 78, 130, 168
Connolly, M., 259, 357
Constable, R. T., 21, 350
Constantine, L., 79, 314
Cookston, J. T., 77, 314
Cooper, A., 184–185, 192–193, 195–196, 199, 201, 213, 215, 219, 266, 314–315, 359
Cooper, P. J., 87, 315
Corley, M., 297, 315
Corodimas, K. P., 87, 189, 315
Corter, C., 9, 325

Cortoni, F., 267, 315
Cosford, P., 106, 315
Costantin, L., 287, 346
Coulter, M., 26, 50, 350
Cowan, C. P., 161, 315
Cowan, P., 161, 315
Cowburn, M., 256, 315
Cox, S. G., 44, 354
Coyne, B. J., 251, 305
Coyne, L., 197, 306
Cozolino, L., xvi, 93, 134, 279, 316
Crago, M., 145, 359
Craig, L. A., 260–261, 265, 268–269, 316
Cramer, B. G., 25, 311
Crandell, L., 52, 321
criminal justice systems, 68, 139, 247, 268
Crittenden, P. M., 37, 48, 53, 55, 62, 76, 139, 316
Crow, C. D., 35, 354
Crowder, J. D., 232, 318
Crowe, M., 139, 316
Crowell, J., 104, 150, 316, 357
Crown Prosecution Service (CPS), 205
Csikszentmihalyi, M., 203, 316
Cudmore, L., 105, 316
Cue, K., 285, 319
Cullen, K., 243, 314
Cummings, E. M., 58, 317
Cummings, M., 169, 359
Curtis, T., 77, 339
cyclothymia, 56, 83, 165–169
Cytryn, L., 169, 323

Dabbs, J. M. J., 96, 316
Damasio, A., 18, 29, 34, 44, 49, 144, 195, 285, 306, 308, 316–317
Daneback, K., 185, 315
Davenport, R., xvii, 263, 299–300, 317
Davenport, W. B., 169, 359
Davies, M., 63, 142, 310
Davies, P. T., 58, 317
Davies, W., 81, 323

Davila, J., 106, 156–157, 275, 317
Davin, P. A., 252, 317
Davis, K. E., 152, 332
Davis, K. L., 137, 323
Davis, R. A., 191, 317
day care, 10, 252
de Graaf, R., 142, 307
de Quiros, G., 20, 339
de Zulueta, F., 146–147, 231, 318
Deakin, J. F., 44, 318
Dear, G. E., 153, 163, 317
Dearing, R. L., 284, 353
DeBellis, M. D., 59–60, 78, 188, 317
delinquency, 92–97, 99, 135, 190, 249
Delmonico, D. L., 177–178, 188, 203, 217, 266, 227, 317
DeLuca, R. V., 252, 326
delusions, 137, 143–144, 167, 232
DeMaria, R., 110, 123, 292, 318
dementia, 112–113, 179
dendrites, 13, 18, 58, 83, 219, 276, 294
Dennis, W., 67–68, 318
depression, x, xii, 13, 17, 20, 30, 32, 38, 47–48, 52, 55, 57, 60–61, 71, 83, 113, 120, 124, 131–132, 134, 137, 140–141, 151, 156–157, 160, 165–168, 170–172, 181, 186, 198–199, 222, 224, 227, 230, 236, 244, 246, 253–254, 271, 276, 283, 287, 291, 293, 299, 303
    manic, 165–166, 169
Deus, J., 59, 326
development(al) see also:
    attachment, brain
    child, 34–35, 37, 39, 52, 54, 63, 71, 79, 81, 119, 119, 135, 140, 186–187
    neural, 23, 25, 33, 47, 65, 67, 76, 84, 86, 105, 107, 202, 281
Diamond, G. S., 82, 85, 318
Dickey, R., 243–244, 310
Diehl, M., 112, 318
Dietz, P. E., 232, 318
diffusion tensor imaging (DTI), 40, 277

Dilger, S., 45, 277, 353
disassociation, 111, 133, 194, 198, 283, 291
Disinhibited Attachment Disorder, 68
dissociation, 61, 63–65, 146, 240
dissociative identity disorder (DID), 63, 142–143
distress, ix, xiv, 13, 20, 24, 26–27, 30, 47, 51, 69, 78, 87–88, 92, 100, 131–132, 135, 140–141, 145, 150–153, 157–158, 177, 199–200, 211, 214, 221, 223, 277, 286, 290 see also: burnout, stress
Dittman, V., 204, 323
divorce, xii, 78, 95, 151, 226
Dixon, L., 159, 163, 318
Dobbing, J., 33, 318
Dolan, R. J., 20, 44, 108, 186, 309, 318, 324, 340
Donegan, N. H., 134, 318
Donnelly, W., 189, 335
Donnerstein, E., 259, 336
Doren, D. M., 265–266, 268, 319
Dougherty, D. D., 276, 346
Dozier, M., 285, 319
Drake, C. R., 249, 319
Drake, R. E., 142, 325
Draper, P., 76–77, 309
dreaming, 29, 144
Drivas, A., 11, 346
Driver, J., 186, 324
drugs, 83, 87, 89, 92–93, 96, 99, 136–138, 141, 144, 179, 267, 286, 293 see also: opiates, opiods
  abuse, 60, 136, 268 see also: substance abuse
  addiction, 53, 91–92, 132, 175, 179, 192
  amphetamines (speed), 92, 136
  cannabis, 92–93, 136, 286
  cocaine, 93, 136–137, 216
  ecstasy, 93
  heroin, 92–93
Dubowitz, H., 231, 319

Dulac, O., 32, 44, 187, 313
Dutton, D. G., 51, 63, 159, 161–163, 308, 319, 333
Dyer, W. J., 6, 338
dysregulation, 67, 100, 113, 121, 124, 169, 189 see also: regulation

earned security, xviii, 65, 284
eating disorders, 87–89, 140
  anorexia, 55, 87, 89–90, 138, 168
  binge, 55, 138
  bulimia, 87, 90, 169
  compulsive, 51, 138
Ebner, U., 138, 310
Edwards, P., 154, 319
Edwards, V., 60, 321
Eells, T. D., 279, 319
Effective Thinking Skills Course (ETS), 258
Egeland, B., 6, 11, 64, 93–94, 97, 119, 319, 342, 352
Ehrhardt, A. A., 239, 340
Eke, A. W., 210, 349
Ellis, D. P., 231, 319
Elnick, A. B., 112, 318
Emerson, P. E., xi, 3, 37, 348
Emler, N., 95, 354
Emmelkamp, P. M. G., 224, 331
emotional intelligence, 6, 47, 61, 87
emotional memories, 7, 36, 44
empathy, 6, 54, 56, 108, 124–126, 128, 135, 144–145, 147, 186, 198, 253, 270, 282, 295, 297, 300
  blocked, 123
  spontaneous, 122
  victim, 213, 219, 244, 255, 257, 263–264
English and Romanian Adoptees (ERA) Study Team, 66–68, 342, 347
ephebophilia, 242, 244, 247, 263
Epstein, R. S., 285, 319
Erenay, N., 204, 323
Erikson, E., 120, 319
Ermshar, A. L., 223–224, 226, 358
Eron, L. D., 78, 319

Erooga, M., 208–209, 214, 216, 344
erotomania, 227, 232
Essex, M., 13, 78, 320
Etherington, K., 246, 253, 320
Etkin, A., 291, 320
Evans, A., 86, 350
Everhart, E., 86, 332
exhibitionism, 111, 175, 238, 244,
    248–249, 251
eye movement desensitization and
    reprocessing (EMDR), 280

Fabbri, M. E., 287, 346
Fabiano, E., 255, 346
Fadiga, L., 26, 346
Fagg, J., 137, 327
Falke, R., 144, 327
Faller, K. C., 253, 320
Falshaw, L., 260, 320
fantasy, 77, 124, 177, 193, 204, 208,
    233, 238, 257 see also:
    narcissism / narcissistic, sexual
Farley, P., 287, 320
Farrington, D. P., 94, 320
Favazza, A. R., 137, 320
FEAR, xvi, 24–25, 29–30, 34, 36, 41,
    44, 47–48, 52, 55–57, 61, 64–65,
    77, 87, 89–90, 98, 113, 123–124,
    146, 150, 154, 161, 168–170, 187,
    226, 231, 240, 243, 246, 271, 277,
    290, 294, 302
  circuit, 41, 44, 46, 50, 52, 56, 62,
    91, 106, 131, 138, 178, 232,
    240, 249
Federici, R. S., 69, 320
Feelgood, S., 243, 320
Feeney, J., 39, 150, 320
Feher, E., 81, 323
Feldman, L. B., 123, 321
Felitti, V. L., 60, 321
Felson, M., 270, 314
Ferenz-Gillies, R., 86, 332
Fernandez, W. I., 85, 330
Fernandez, Y. M., 262, 265, 300, 321,
    337
Ferrari, P., 169, 332

Ferree, M., 196, 321
Ferren, D. J., 244, 310
fetish, 82, 185, 213, 237–240, 248
Few, A. L., 160, 321
Field, T., 35, 321
Fields, R. D., 17, 321
Fincham, F. D., 152, 321
Fink, G., 186, 324
Finkelhor, D., 61, 246, 252, 254, 300,
    321, 358
Finn, P., 240, 330
Firestone, P., 268–269, 331, 341
Fischer, K. W., 75, 321
Fisher, D., xvii, 259–260, 263,
    299–300, 309, 317, 321–322
Fisher, J., 52, 321
Fitzherbert, C., 262, 322
Fivush, R., 28, 341
Flak, V., 259–260, 322
Fletcher, C., 256, 353
Fletcher, J. M., 21, 96, 322, 350
Fletcher, P., 44, 318
Fogassi, L., 26, 346
Foley, T. P., 266, 322
Fonagy, P., xv, 36, 54, 114, 126, 133,
    281–282, 291, 308, 322, 353
Ford, H., 253, 322
Fordham, A. S., 260, 309
Forsting, M., 22, 243, 348
Frackowiak, R. S., 20, 309
Fraiberg, S., 69, 322
Fraley, R. C., 150, 322
Frank, E., 170–171, 339
Freeman, A., 131, 140, 309, 333
freeze response, 24, 44, 48, 53, 56,
    64–65, 87, 127, 198, 291
Frei, A., 204, 323
Freud, S., 39, 79, 119, 175, 245, 280,
    323
Friedman, A., 20, 323
Friedman, J. I., 137, 323
Friedrich, W., 81, 323
Friel, J., 154, 353
Friendship, C., 260, 320
Frith, C. D., 44, 318
Fritz, G., 253, 323

Fromuth, M. E., 253, 323
frottage / frotteurism, 175, 238, 244, 248
Frustaci, K., 59, 317
Fulbright, R. K., 21, 134, 318, 350
Furby, L., 262, 323

Gado, M. H., 60, 350
Gaensbauer, T. J., 169, 323
Gage, P., 231
Galbreath, N. W., 191–192, 199, 215, 323
Gallagher, B., 205, 323
Gallagher, L., 25, 351
Gallese, V., 26, 346
Galynker, I., 243, 314
Gannon, T. A., 251, 323
Gans, S., 243, 314
Garby, T., 263, 308
Gardener, F., 49, 358
Gargaro, S., 257, 328
Garrett, J., 200, 296, 333
Garrison, K., 254–255, 257, 324
gay see: sexuality, homo-
Gazzaniga, M., 22, 324
Gedo, J., 277, 324
Gemeinhardt, B., 93, 348
gender difference, 21, 64, 84, 106, 195, 228, 293
George, C., 114, 290, 324
George, N., 186, 324
Gerald, P. S., 97, 357
Gerber, A., 133, 282, 322
Gergely, G., 29, 324
Gerhardt, S., xiii, 47, 134, 324
Ghaemi, S. N., 167, 324
Ghahramanlou-Holloway, M., 212, 354
Gibat, C. C., 250, 343
Giedd, J., 59, 86, 317, 350
Gilby, R., 257, 324
Gillespie, A. A., 207, 247–248, 257, 324
Gilligan, J., 96, 147, 230–231, 324
Gini, M., 10, 347
Gizewski, E., 22, 243, 348

Gizzarelli, R., 299, 327
Glaser, D., 47, 324
Glauer, M., 45, 277, 353
glia cells, 17, 219
Glick, B., 136, 325
Glick, D. M., 276, 346
Glick, I. D., 171, 306
Glocker, F. X., 138, 310
Glueck, E. T., 135, 324
Glueck, S., 135, 324
Godsi, E., 147, 158, 230–231, 324
Goetz, A. T., 156, 338
Goffman, E., 209, 325
Gogtay, N., 86, 350
Gold, P. W., 87, 189, 315
Goldberg, A., 243, 342
Goldberg, B., 257, 324
Goldberg, S., 9, 325
Goldberger, L., 120, 325
Golden, G., 213, 219, 266, 315
Goldstein, A. P., 136, 325
Goleman, D., 6, 33–34, 47, 325
Gonzalez, J. M., 170–171, 339
Goodman, A., 174, 325
Goodman, L. A., 142, 325
Goodwin, F. K., 167, 324
Gordis, E., 159, 336
Gordon, H. W., 60, 325
Gore, J. C., 21, 134, 318, 350
Gothard, R. S., 223, 226, 338
Gottman, J., 152, 294, 325
Gracewell Clinic, 262
Graeff, F. G., 64, 356
Graf, M., 204, 323
Graham-Kevan, N., 159, 161, 325
Gramzow, R., 256, 353
grandiosity, 119, 121–124, 126–127, 136, 166, 170–171, 226
Gray, P. H., xi, 353
Gray, S., 263, 308
Green, A. H., 138, 325
Green, R. G., 230, 325
Greenall, P. V., 249, 251, 257, 325
Greenberg, D. M., 268, 341
Greenberger, D., 141, 214, 325
Greenfield, D., 198–199, 315, 325

Greenspan, S. I., 6, 326
Greenstein, D., 86, 350
Gregory, E., 34, 326
Greyston, A. D., 252, 326
grief, xiv, xvi, 4, 48–49, 63, 69
Griffin, E., 177–178, 203, 217, 227, 266, 313, 317
Griffin-Shelley, E., 185, 201, 326, 359
Griffiths, D., 257, 326
Grootheus, C., 68, 347
Groth, A. N., 250, 326
Grubin, D., 260, 268, 326
Guerra, N. G., 145, 351
Guiducci, V., 87–88, 308
Guild, D., 251, 259, 305
guilt, xii, 10, 54, 140, 147, 178, 192, 213, 231, 252
Gundel, H., 59, 326
Gyulai, L., 170–171, 339

Ha, Y., 44, 354
Hackett, S., 79, 81, 356
Hagan, L. K., 38, 326
Hakamies-Blomqvist, L., 9, 347
Hall, Richard C. W., 97, 242–244, 253, 267, 326
Hall, Ryan C. W., 97, 242–244, 253, 267, 326
Halliday, R., 257, 326
Hämäläinen, T., 9, 347
Hanson, R. K., 210, 260, 266–269, 299, 326–327
Hantouche, E. G., 169, 332
Harbinson, D., 208–209, 214, 216, 344
Hargrove, M. F., 96, 316
Harlow, N., 211, 244, 305
Harmon, R. J., 169, 323
Harper, G. W., 85, 330
Harrington, A., 20, 327
Harris, A. J. R., 260, 269, 326–327
Harris, L. J., 29, 327
Harter, S., 86, 327
Hartmann, E., 144, 327
Harvey, C., 154, 319
Harwood, R. L., 119, 312

Haw, C., 138, 327
Hawton, K., 137–138, 327
Hazan, C., xviii, 104–105, 158, 327, 332
healing, xvi, 219, 276, 280, 287, 289, 294, 297–298, 301
Heard, D. H., 105, 327
Heath, L., 79, 327
Hebb, D. O., 30, 328
hebephilia, 242, 244, 263
Heilbrun, A. B., 145, 328
Heinz, J. W., 257, 328
hemispheric lateralization, 20–21
Henderson, A., 51, 63, 161, 163, 308
Henderson, M., 229, 328
Hennessy, M., 244, 328
Herdt, G., 76, 338
Herman, B. A., 91, 328
Herman, J. L., 57, 60, 62–63, 65, 135, 137–138, 245–246, 328, 355
Hernstein, R., 232, 358
Herpertz, S. C., 134, 330
Herrmann, S., 113, 343
Herzog, J. M., 37, 328
Hess, E. H., 28, 186, 328
Hesse, E., 56, 62–63, 328, 336
Hesson-McInnis, M., 199, 296, 311
Heyman, R. E., 246, 310
Hicks, D., 79, 328
Higgins, E. T., 88, 340
Higgitt, A., 291, 322
Hildyard, K. L., 131, 328
Hill, E. J., 77, 339
Hiller, J., 194, 328
Hinde, R., 35, 328
Hindley, M., 252
Hingsburger, D., 257, 326
Hodges, J., 68, 354
Hoek, H. W., xvi, 341
Hof, L., 110, 123, 292, 318
Hofer, M. A., 48, 92, 312, 329
Hogue, T. E., 265, 316
Holland, G., 206, 354
Holland, R., 86, 95, 161, 340
Hollin, C. R., 250, 336

Holmes, J., 5, 106, 111, 132, 142, 225, 250, 276, 329
Holtzworth-Munroe, A., 159, 329
Homan, R. W., 21–22, 346
Home Office, 96, 252, 329
homophobia, 156, 293 *see also*: sexual, homo-
Hook, A., 283–284, 329
Hook, E. B., 97, 329
hormones *see also*: adrenaline, opiod
acetylcholine, 91, 178
androgen, 96, 230, 254
cortisol, 1, 13, 27, 29, 46–48, 53, 58, 65, 69, 78, 91, 178
dopamine, 20, 25–26, 32, 44, 46, 53–54, 91–92, 124, 134, 137, 144, 178–179, 186, 192, 195, 214
endorphins, 29, 92, 178, 286, 295
enkephalin, 64, 178, 286
glutamate, 91, 178
neuropeptides, xx, 25, 27, 29, 67, 254
oestrogen, 96, 230
oxytocin, 25, 27, 29–30, 38, 53–54, 67, 91, 97, 143–144, 178, 186, 190, 241, 253–254
peptides, 19, 24, 138, 179, 191
progesterone, 96, 230
serotonin, 32, 96, 132, 230, 254
testosterone, 38, 96–97, 194, 230, 250, 253
vasopressin, 29, 67, 91, 143, 178, 194, 254
House, S. H., xiii, 7, 25, 27, 230, 346
Houston, K., 138, 327
Howard, J., 98, 329
Howard, R. J., 44, 354
Howells, K., 284, 344
Howitt, D., 207, 210, 212, 244, 255, 259–260, 262, 264, 266, 329, 350
Hoyer, J., 243, 320
Hrouda, D. R., 232, 318
Hudson, D., 191
Hudson, K., 246, 329

Hudson, S. M., 241, 244–245, 255, 329, 333, 357
Hudson-Allez, G., 228, 329
Hulting, A.-L., 29, 343
Huntoon, J., 197, 306
Hurley, R. A., 134, 330
Hutton, L., 81, 329
hyperactivity, 13, 27, 36, 51, 53, 56–60, 64, 68, 96, 107, 135, 197–198, 219, 286 *see also*: attention deficit hyperactivity disorder
hyperarousal, 36, 52, 59, 276
hypervigilance, 13, 52, 56, 59, 119, 122, 126–127, 157, 224, 282

ICD-10, 242–243, 247, 330
imprinting, 27–28, 35, 39, 120, 239–240
incest, 241–242, 246, 252, 263–264, 266
infantophile, 242, 263
Inokuchi, A., 179, 306
Insel, T. R., 144, 330
intelligence quotient (IQ), 67, 86, 94, 97, 145, 190, 244, 266
internal working model, 11, 27, 77, 275–276, 290
Internet, xix, 103, 111, 115, 148, 177, 181, 184–185, 189–190, 193–194, 196–199, 202–203, 205–207, 211, 214–216, 227–228, 245, 248, 263, 294, 297, 299
addiction, xix, 184, 189, 191–196, 198–199, 201, 208–210, 215–218, 296–298
offenders, 190, 203, 205, 207, 209, 212–213, 216–217, 241, 258, 266, 270, 299
pornography, xix, 175, 184–185, 192, 195–196, 199–201, 203, 208, 214–217, 219, 228, 237, 248, 263, 265, 296
viewing, 192–193, 199, 203, 206, 210, 219, 245, 263, 267, 269, 298

intervention
  clinical, 251, 281
  cognitive, 217, 256, 290
  medical, 7, 63, 139
  physical, 139
  psychological, 284
  therapeutic, 219, 280
  treatment, 141, 257
Irons, R. R., 179, 348
Irwin, M. J., 136, 325
Ishii, Y., 28, 359
Ishikawa, S. S., 145, 345
Itoh, H., 28, 359
Izard, C. E., 40, 110, 330

Jack, C., 257, 334
Jacobvitz, D., 56, 60, 133, 335
Jacoris, S., 67, 358
Jambaque, I., 32, 44, 187, 313
Jamil, O. B., 85, 330
Janssen, E., 198, 240, 299, 307, 330
Janssen, I., 142, 307
jealousy, 12, 41, 51, 109, 154, 156,
  161, 181, 199
Jellicoe-Jones, L., 257, 325
Jenkins, A., 250, 255, 263, 284, 301,
  330
Jenkins, P., 184, 203, 212, 330
Joels, T., 10, 347
Johnson, M. H., 28, 340
Johnson, P. A., 134, 330
Johnson, S. M., 123, 153, 156, 157,
  330
Jones, S., 214, 330,
Josephson, G. J., 156, 331
Joubert, S., 195, 331
Judd, D., 105, 316
Juhasz, C., 46, 314

Kabat-Zinn, J., 290, 331
Kahr, B., 142–143, 331
Kalin, N. H., 13, 53, 64, 78, 320, 331
Kalishian, M. M., 154, 331
Kamphuis, J. H., 224, 331
Kandel, E. R., 291, 320
Kaplan, G. A., 108, 345

Kaplan, N., 70, 114, 290, 324, 336
Kapur, N., 44, 137, 307, 318
Karama, S., 195, 331
Karpman, S., xvi, 13, 146, 161–162,
  331
Karpman triangle, xvi, 146, 161–162
Katz, I., 21, 350
Kaufman, J., xvii, 97, 245, 331
Keaveny, L., 68, 347
Kelly, J., 7–9, 13, 33, 109, 142, 356
Kelly, K. F., 257, 328
Kendall, J. C., 59, 352
Kennedy, R., 133, 282, 322
Keppner, J., 68, 347
Kercher, G., 253, 356
Kernberg, O., 132, 180, 197, 331
Kershaw, C., 159, 230, 357
Keshavan, M., 59, 317
Kienlen, K. K., 232, 331
Killgore, W. D., 83–84, 331, 359
Kimmel, M., 208, 308
Kimura, K., 28, 359
King, E. G., 243, 314
Kingston, D. A., 269, 331
Kinzl, J. F., 109, 331
Kirkpatrick, L. A., 152, 332
Kirsch, E. A., 29, 327
Klassen, P. E., 243–244, 310, 312
Klein, M., 13, 57, 78, 123, 320, 332
Knight, R. A., 213, 251, 313, 332
Knuth, K. H., 145, 345
Ko, J. Y., 167, 324
Kobak, R., 47, 86–88, 158, 314, 332
Kochman, F. J., 169, 332
Kogan, J. N., 170–171, 339
Kohut, H., 122, 332
Kolb, L. C., 65, 332
Konishi, Y., 28, 359
Koren-Karie, N., 10, 347
Koss, M. P., 60, 253, 321, 346
Koukkou, M., 29, 332
Krabbendam, L., 142, 307
Kraemer, H. C., 60, 350
Krone, T., 204, 207–208, 212, 332
Krook, K., 80, 347
Krueger, T. H. C., 22, 243, 348

Kruttschnitt, C., 79, 327
Krystal, H., 75, 333
Krystal, J., 65, 333
Kuban, M. E., 243–244, 310, 312
Kuebli, J., 38, 326
Kulik, J., 28, 312
Kumari, V., 276, 333
Kurian, J. R., 67, 358
Kurtz, Z., 81, 358
Küstner, U., 93, 348

Labouvie-Vief, G., 112, 318
Lacadie, C., 134, 318
LaCasse, L., 145, 345
Lake, B., 105, 327
Lake, F., 231, 333
Lancker, V., 26, 333
Lancrenon, S., 169, 332
Landau, J., 200, 296, 333
Landeira-Fernandez, J., 64, 356
Landolt, M. A., 161, 333
Lane, J., 232, 360
Lanning, K. V., 82, 209, 333
Lansford, J. E., 6, 338
Lanthier, R. D., 250, 314
Lara, D. R., 92, 99, 124, 166–168, 170, 333
Laws, D. R., 255, 333
Layden, M. A., 140, 333
Lazarus, R. S., 230, 333
Leach, C., 92, 338
LeDoux, J. E., 16, 18, 33, 45, 59–60, 83–84, 87, 108, 158, 180, 189, 193–194, 209, 280, 315, 333
Lee, S., 91–92, 309
Lehmann, D., 29, 332
Leigh, T., 133, 282, 322
Leiguarda, R., 20, 339
Lencz, T., 145, 345
Lenroot, R., 86, 350
LePage, A., 231, 309
Lerch, J., 86, 350
Lerner, H., 155, 334
Leroux, J-M., 195, 331
lesbian see: sexuality, homo-
Lettermman, M., 35, 354

Leung, S., 49, 358
Levene, J., 190, 307
Levine, P., 134, 334
Levitin, D. J., 289, 334
Levy, K. N., 275, 317
Levy, T. M., 66, 68, 120–121, 334
Lewis, D., 263, 308
Lewis, T., 190, 335
Leygraf, N., 22, 243, 348
Lieb, K., 138, 310
Lieberman, A., 69, 359
Lifton, R. J., 64, 334
Lilienfeld, S. O., xviii, 256, 334
Limberger, M., 138, 310
Lindemann, E., 146, 334
Linden, D. E. J., 276, 334
Lindgren, S., 200, 334
Lindsay, W. R., 257, 334
Lingford-Hughes, A., 93, 334
Liotti, G., 57, 277, 334
Little, V., 35, 354
Loeb, T., 160, 334
Loewenstein, P., 256, 315
Lojkasek, M., 9, 325
Lolita syndrome, 263
Lopez-Sala, A., 59, 326
Lord, C. G., 68, 347
LOSS, 30, 47–49, 53, 61–62, 89, 105, 115, 146, 150, 154, 161, 168, 179, 226, 271, 280
    circuit, xiv, 9, 30–31, 47–51, 57, 65–66, 77, 187, 296
Lounes, R., 32, 44, 187, 313
Love, L., 35, 354
lovemap, 77, 187, 238
LUST, 24, 61, 91, 105–106, 150–151, 194, 240, 250
    circuit, 61–62, 76–77, 105, 115, 178, 187–188, 191, 195, 239
Lykins, M. S., 35, 354
Lyons-Ruth, K., 56, 60, 133, 335

MacLean, P. D., 16, 91, 335
Maddison, S., 212–213, 335
Maffei, L., 287, 346
Magai, C., 113, 335

Maheu, M., 199, 315
Mahler, M., 35, 37, 120, 335
Mahoney, A., 189, 335
Main, M., 37, 50, 54, 56–57, 62–63,
    70, 113–114, 276, 290, 324, 328,
    335–336
Mäkelä, J., 9, 347
Makinen, J. A., 157, 330, 336
Malamuth, N. M., 251, 259, 336
Maltz, L., 193, 336
Maltz, W., 193, 336
Mammen, O., 69, 359
Mandelbaum, T., 47, 332
Mandeville-Norden, R., 210, 212,
    339
Mangweth, B., 109, 331
Manley, R. S., 89, 336
Mann, R. E., 250, 256, 262, 300,
    336–337, 350
Manning, J. C., 199, 336
Månsson, S-A., 185, 315
Marangell, L. B., 170–171, 339
Marci, C. D., 276, 346
Margolin, G., 159, 336
Marks, J. S., 60, 321
Marlatt, G. A., 250, 343
Marold, D. B., 86, 327
Marques, J. K., 250, 343
Marshall, L. E., 198, 250, 259, 262,
    300, 336, 349
Marshall, W. L., 213, 219, 241, 246,
    250, 254, 262, 266–267, 269, 300,
    314–315, 337, 356–357
Martell, D. A., 232, 318
Martin-Mittage, B., 59, 326
Martinson, F., 79, 314
Maruna, S., 256, 284, 337
masochism, 236–237, 248
Massachusetts Treatment Centre,
    Version 3 (MTC:R3), 251
Masterson, J. F., 124, 337
masturbation, 101, 176, 195, 199,
    201, 207, 228, 247, 260
    compulsive, 138, 148, 173, 175,
        181–182, 192, 241, 298, 303
Mathews, J. K., 252, 337

Mathews, R., 252, 337
Matravers, A., xiv, xvi, 337
Matthews, D. B., 232, 318
Mattinson, J., 223, 228, 312
Mattoon, G., 133, 282, 322
Maxfield, L., 280, 349
Mazzantini, M., 287, 346
McBride, C., 281–282, 337
McCarthy-Hoffbauer, I., 92, 338
McClintock, M., 76, 338
McClusky, U., 105, 281, 327, 338
McCowan, E. J., 230, 325
McElwain, N. L., 6, 338
McGeoch, P., 243, 314
McGilchrist, I., 22, 338
McGlashan, T. H., 134, 318
McKenna, C., 280, 338
McKenzie, I., 92, 338
McKibbin, W. F., 156, 338
McKnew, D. H., 169, 323, 359
Medeiros, B. L., 99, 314
Mednick, S. A., 9, 345
Meehan, J. C., 159, 329
Megargee, E. I., 95, 338
Mellody, P., 155, 338
Meloy, J. R., 223, 226, 231–233, 338
Meltzoff, A. N., 26, 338
Mental Health Foundation, 75, 87,
    339
mentalization, 126, 276–277, 283
Mentzel, H.-J., 45, 277, 353
Merrick, S., 104, 357
Metcalf, C., 266, 308
Miczek, K. A., 49, 339
Middleton, D., 210, 212, 339
Migliorelli, R., 20, 339
Miklowitz, D. J., 170–171, 339
Mikulincer, M., 108, 198, 339
Milgram, S., 230, 339
Miller, A. W., 122, 155, 338–339
Miller, B. C., 77, 339
Miller, J. K., 155, 338
Miller, L., 231, 319
Millikin, J., 157, 330
Mills, T., 98, 160, 313
Milner, C., 204, 213–214, 342

Milner, R. J., 250, 339
Miltner, W. H. R., 45, 277, 353
mind–body link, ix, xix, 285
Minde, K., 9, 325
mindfulness, xix, 6, 71, 210, 216,
    218, 228, 270, 283, 285, 290–291,
    298
Miner, M. H., 190, 244, 249, 340, 345
Minty, B., 99, 340
Mirrlees-Black, C., 233, 340
misattunement, 5–6, 36, 278
Mitchell, I. J., 254, 309
Mitra, R., 59, 356
Miyahara, S., 171, 339
Mizuno, Y., 179, 306
Monahan, J., 232, 340
Money, J., 77, 187, 203, 237–239, 340
Montague, R., 54, 353
mood and sexuality, 198 see also:
    questionnaires
Moore, M. K., 26, 338
Moran, G. S., 64, 78, 291, 322, 341
Moretti, M. M., 86, 88, 95, 161, 340
Morris, J. S., 44, 108, 318, 340
Morrison, A. P., 54, 340
Morrison, F., 257, 334
Morse, S. B., 140, 333
Morton, B. E., 21, 340
Morton, J., 28, 340
Morton, K. E., 260, 327
Mosner, C., 174, 341
mother see also: adoption/adoptive
    biological, xi, xiii, 3, 7, 24–25,
        36–37, 65–67, 70, 186, 243,
        252
    child–/infant–, xii, 7, 25, 36, 66
    good-enough, 294
    step-, 252
    working, x, 10
Moulden, H. M., 246, 259, 262, 300,
    336–337, 356
Moultrie, D., 190, 341
Muczik, O., 46, 314
Mueser, K., 142, 325
Mullen, P. E., 222–224, 233, 341, 343
Müller, B., 10, 345

Mulloy, R., 262, 300, 337
Munns, R., 190, 249, 340
Muramoto, S., 28, 359
Murphy, W. D., 249, 341
myelin, xiv, 19, 30, 32, 83
Myhill, A., 223, 228, 312

Nabbout, R., 32, 44, 187, 313
Nademin, M. E., 212, 354
Nagy, F., 46, 314
Nakash, O., 133, 282, 358
Narayan, M., 60, 311
narcissism/narcissistic, 6, 115,
    118–119, 121–127, 136, 160–161,
    170, 186, 220, 226, 271
    classic, 122–125
    compensatory, 122–124, 126, 135,
        147, 170, 284, 303
    fantasy, 124, 126, 226, 231
    personality, 117, 122–123, 130, 244
    primary, 119, 121, 147
    rage, 121, 123, 125, 127–128, 146,
        160, 232, 251, 275
    style, xix, 121, 125–127, 159, 244,
        250
    wound, 170
Narcissus, 118–119, 126
National Institute for Clinical
    Excellence (NICE), xvii–xviii
Nebes, R. D., 20, 341
Neisser, U., 28, 341
Neufeld Bailey, H., 64, 78, 341
Neugebauer, R., xvi, 341
neural see also: development
    circuit, 23, 33, 37, 47
    connections, 11, 18, 30, 191, 219,
        276
    pathways, 18–19, 33, 36, 38, 40,
        49, 91, 180, 186–187, 190, 194,
        197, 202, 218
    pruning, 85–86, 189, 239
    template, 11, 57, 63, 105, 186, 278,
        294
neuro-
    chemistry, 90
    genesis, 59, 219, 287–288

psychology, 40, 69, 145, 231
transmitters, 18–20, 32, 46, 96, 230
  see also: hormones
neuropsychologically-based
  attachment disorder, 69
Newman, C. F., 140, 333
Nicholas, S., 159, 230, 357
Nicholls, T., 159, 319
Nierenberg, A. A., 170–171, 339
Nijenhuis, E. R. S., 108, 198, 341
Nikiforov, K., 243, 314
Nishino, H., 179, 306
Noller, P., 39, 150, 320
Nordenberg, D., 60, 321
Norton, M. C., 77, 339
Novaco, R. W., 230, 341
Nunes, K. L., 268, 341
Nutt, D., 93, 179, 334, 341

obsessive–compulsive disorder
  (OCD), 51, 130–131, 168, 174
Obsuth, I., 95, 340
O'Callaghan, M. J., xi, 353
O'Connor, A. A., 252, 341
O'Connor, T. G., 66–68, 342, 347
Odgers, C. L., 95, 340
O'Donnell, I., 204, 213–214, 342
Ogawa, J. R., 64, 342
Ohlerking, F., 244, 345
Ohman, A., 108, 340
Okami, P., 243, 342
Oki, M., 83, 331
Oldfield, M., 144, 327
Olley, S., 257, 334
Olson, I. R., 134, 318
O'Mara, J., 185, 201, 359
omnipotence, 6, 119–122, 125, 136,
  186
Oomura, Y., 179, 306
Operation
  Appal, 204
  Avalanche, 203–204
  Ore, 204, 266
  Starburst, 203
opiates, 24, 27, 29–30, 89–92, 127,
  134, 138, 178–180, 190

opioids, 48, 64, 91, 139–140, 146,
  178, 186
Orlans, M., 66, 68, 120–121, 334
orphans, x, 243
  Kosovan, 197
  Lebanese, 67
  Romanian, 46, 67–68
  Russian, 67
Orzolek-Kronner, C., 90, 342
Osborn, C., 189, 305
O'Toole, L., 201, 342
Otto, M. W., 170–171, 339
Otway, L. J., 124, 342

Pacey, S., xii, 151, 342
Padesky, C., 141, 214, 325, 342
paedophile(s)/paedophilia, xiv, xvi,
  xx, 77, 100, 184, 203, 205–207,
  210–212, 215, 218–219, 228,
  236–237, 239–244, 246–248, 258,
  260, 263–264, 266
Page, I. J., 249, 341
panic, x, 46, 65, 108, 140, 188
PANIC, 24, 29–31, 36, 41, 45, 47–48,
  51, 61–62, 64–65, 89, 105, 150,
  154, 168, 178, 187, 271, 277, 290,
  294
  circuit, 27, 30, 46–47, 50, 52, 64,
    67, 77, 91–92, 106, 150, 154,
    158, 178, 190
Panskepp, J., xiv, 23, 27, 29–30, 33,
  38, 44, 90–93, 98, 137, 144, 194,
  231, 250, 277, 328, 342
Pao, P., 170, 342
Papousek, H., 26, 342
Papousek, M., 26, 342
paranoid, 113, 130, 133, 137, 211,
  224, 226
paraphilia, xviii, 77, 82, 184,
  189–190, 215, 235–236, 238–240,
  244, 247, 251, 263, 298
parasympathetic nervous system,
  16, 48, 64, 219
parent(s) see also: abusive,
  adoption/adoptive, mother
  –child relationship, 69, 154, 281

grand-, xi, 3, 10, 32, 78, 119, 292
single, 11
Parker, K. C. H., 70, 309
Parry, C. D., 232, 318
Pask-McCartney, C., 136, 325
Pathé, M., 222–224, 233, 249, 319,
    341, 343
Paul, T., 22, 243, 348
peer group, 86, 88
Penderson, D. R., 64, 78, 341
penile plethysmograph (PPG), 210,
    213, 259–260
periaqueductal grey, 33, 250
peripheral nervous system, 16
Perkins, D., 254, 343
Perren, S., 113, 343
Perry, B. D., xiii, 50, 58–59, 64, 67,
    69, 83, 86, 343
Perry, J. C., 62, 138, 355
personality disorder see also:
    narcissism/narcissistic
    antisocial, xvi, 69, 131, 169, 226
    avoidant, 55, 133
    borderline, 51, 130, 134–135, 138,
        142, 159, 169
Peschel, T., 22, 243, 348
Peter, T., 253, 343,
Petersen, K., 93, 286, 343, 348
Petersson, M., 29, 343
Peto, A., 57, 133, 343
Phelps, J., 171, 343
Pine, F., 35, 37, 120, 335
Pinto, O., 92, 99, 124, 166–168, 170,
    333
Pipp, S. L., 75, 321
Piquero, A., 9, 343
Pithers, W. D., 250, 343
Pittenger, C., 291, 320
Planchon, L., 185, 192–193, 315
PLAY, 24, 27–29, 35–36, 61, 77, 88,
    105, 150–151, 187, 281, 289
    circuit, 35–37, 44, 49, 91, 105–106,
        178
Polan, H. J., 291, 320
Polich, J., 290, 312
Pollak, S. D., 67, 358

Pollard, R. A., 59, 343
Popovic, M., 248, 344
pornography, xix, 80, 110, 115, 160,
    175–177, 181, 185, 188–189,
    192–196, 199–201, 203–204,
    207–209, 211–216, 228, 235–236,
    238, 247, 249, 296–297 see also:
    Internet
positron emission tomography
    (PET), 40, 46, 277
Post, R. M., 166, 344
post traumatic stress disorder
    (PTSD), xvi, 58, 60, 65, 95, 131,
    136, 146, 157, 197, 217, 283, 286
Potokar, J., 93, 334
Poulson, M. C., 20, 323
Powell, A., 255, 344
Power, A., 78, 344
Power, H., 269, 344
Poznansky, O., 243, 314
practising period, xiii, 5, 37, 47,
    55–56, 71, 85, 119, 186, 239
premature babies, 7–9
Prendergast, W. E., 180, 344
Prentky, R., 213, 251, 313, 332
Prescott, J. W., xi, 26, 344
primary care, 132, 167, 228
prison system, xvii, 257
probation service(s), 215, 257–258,
    260
Proeve, M., 284, 344
promiscuity, 77, 87, 238, 240
prostitution, 115, 160, 164, 173, 175,
    177, 181, 183, 201, 237
protoconversation, 28, 37, 154, 284
psychopathology, x, xx, 4, 38, 63, 89,
    92, 95, 100, 129, 133, 139, 143,
    168–169, 189, 242, 247, 249,
    290
psychopaths, 131, 144–145, 147
psychopathy, 97–98, 131, 144, 147,
    167
puberty, xix, 62, 71, 73, 75–77, 79,
    82, 85, 90, 100, 187, 194,
    238–239, 242, 298
Pugh, K. R., 21, 350

Purcell, R., 223–224, 233, 341
Putnam, D., 185, 192–193, 315
Putnam, F. W., 63–64, 344

Quayle, E., 206, 208–209, 213–214,
216, 257, 344, 354
questionnaires, 223, 261, 299
Hanson Sex Attitude, 299
Mood and Sexuality, 199, 299
Sexual Excitation/Inhibition
(SES/SIS), 299
Quilty, L. C., 281–282, 337
Quinsey, V. L., 254, 259, 344–345

R. v. Bowden (2000), 206
R. v. Smith (2003), 206
Rabama, I., 136, 325
Radke-Yarrow, M., 169, 359
Radzinowicz, L., 263, 345
Rafto, S. E., 21, 340
rage, xii, xiv, 4, 57, 95, 108, 118, 121,
125, 128, 133–134, 162, 170, 173,
181–182, 188, 222, 226, 231, 246
see also: narcissism/narcissistic
RAGE, xvi, 24, 29–30, 36, 44, 47, 52,
54–56, 61, 65, 77, 87, 90, 92, 98,
113, 115, 124, 150, 154, 158,
168–170, 187, 226, 231, 240, 243,
246, 249–250, 271, 277, 294, 302
circuit, 41, 44, 52, 91, 99, 106, 131,
138, 158, 161, 178, 196,
231–232, 249–251, 277
Raine, A., 9, 145, 345
Ramachandran, V. S., 22, 345
rape, xv, 78, 118, 136, 147, 160, 215,
224, 227, 237, 241, 248–251, 255,
259, 268–269
rapid eye movement (REM) sleep,
29, 144
Rapoport, J., 86, 350
Rauch, S. L., 276, 346
Rauh, H., 10, 345
Ray, S. L., 89, 345
Raymond, N. C., 244, 345
Reactive Attachment Disorder,
68–69

recidivism, xvii, 210, 215, 217, 233,
249, 254, 256, 260–270
Reebye, P., 95, 340
regulation, xix, 45, 52, 121, 134, 144,
194, 202, 280–281, 291 see also:
dysregulation, self
Reiker, P. P., 98, 160, 313
Reilly-Harrington, N. A., 170–171,
339
Renn, P., 146, 345
Repacholi, B., 56, 335
resilience, 5–6, 97, 125, 286
reuptake, 19, 254
Reynolds, P., 108, 345
Rhea, J., 227, 352
Rich, P., 50, 81, 125, 132, 135, 180,
197, 244–245, 255, 345
Rickson, H., 89, 336
Ridgway, R., xiii, 7, 25, 27, 230, 346
Rifkin, A., 56, 62–63, 328
Risin, L. I., 253, 346
risk
assessment, 146, 211, 232–233,
261, 265–266, 268–270, 300
factor(s), xvi, 9, 92, 94, 133, 246,
267–270
management, 259, 265, 269
Matrix (2000), 266, 269
prediction, 269
Rivkin, I., 160, 334
Rizzolatti, G., 26, 346
Road Traffic Accidents (RTA), 78,
286, 289
Robinson, J., 137, 307
Robinson, R. G., 20, 339
Roch Lecours, A., 195, 331
Roe, K. V., 11, 346
Roffman, J. L., 276, 346
Rosen, K. H., 160, 321
Rosenberg, S. D., 142, 325
Rosenfeld, H., 119, 346
Rosenthal, P.-A., 57, 346
Rosenthal, R. J., 137, 320
Rosenthal, S., 57, 346
Ross, C. A., 143, 346
Ross, E. D., 21–22, 346

Ross, M. W., 185, 315
Ross, R. R., 255, 346
Rossi, C., 287, 346
Rossi, E., 219, 287–288, 346
Rouleau, J.-L., 251, 305
Rowe, D., 31, 347
Rubinow, D. R., 166, 344
Russ, D., 144, 327
Russek, L. G., 108, 347
Russell, C., 186, 324
Rutter, M., 66–68, 342, 347
Ryan, N., 59, 317

Sachs, A., 143, 347
Sachs, G. S., 170–171, 339
Sack, P-M., 93, 348
Sadato, N., 28, 359
sadism, 95, 145, 206, 223, 237, 242, 244, 251 see also: masochism
Sagi, A., 5, 10, 347, 355
Sajaniemi, N., 9, 347
Salokorpi, T., 9, 347
Saltaris, C., 131, 347
Salter, A. C., 255, 347
Salvaterra, F., 66, 356
Sandnabba, N., 80, 347
Sands, J., 33, 318
Sanislow, C. A., 134, 318
Santtila, P., 80, 347
Sarkar, M., 84, 347
Saugstad, L. F., 83, 347
Saunders, E., 190, 307
Sawyer, D., 191–192, 199, 215, 323
Scaer, R. C., 60, 78, 283, 286, 295, 348
Schaffer, H. R., xi, 3, 37, 348
Scharfe, E., 10, 348
Schedlowski, M., 22, 243, 348
Schiffer, B., 22, 243, 348
Schiffer, F., 22, 348
Schindler, A., 93, 348
Schipper, L. D., 156, 338
schizophrenia, 131, 137, 142–144
Schmid, R., 113, 343
Schneider, J., 297, 315
Schneider, J. P. 177, 179, 196, 199–200, 216, 296–297, 348

Schore, A., xiii, 5, 13, 24, 32, 34–36, 38–39, 53–54, 59–60, 83, 86, 98, 108, 132, 135–136, 169–170, 180, 186–187, 189–190, 194, 197–198, 277, 280, 283, 348–349
Schulkin, J., 87, 189, 315
Schultz, N. W., xi, 349
Schwartz, G. E., 108, 347
Schweinsburg, A., 92, 353
Scott, C. K., 152, 321
Scott, H., 299, 327
Scott, J.-P., 32, 349
Scott Long, J., 198, 299, 307
Scwartz, B., 138, 310
Seabrook, L., 86, 332
Second World War, x, xvi, 112
SEEKING, xiv, 23–25, 27, 29–31, 35, 40, 44, 47, 50–51, 61, 64–65, 90–91, 105–106, 144, 150, 178, 186–187, 189–191, 193, 195, 203, 250, 281, 287, 294
    circuit, 24–26, 49, 65, 88, 99, 106, 137, 144, 186, 190–191, 193–195, 203–204, 209, 214
self
    awareness, 33
    -control, 277
    -esteem, 54, 61, 81, 85, 100, 111, 120, 122–123, 160, 167, 199, 201, 297, 300
    harm, 57, 85, 87, 90, 92, 98, 131, 134, 136–140, 171, 282
    -mutilation, 139, 146
    protection, 24, 50
    reflective, 36, 291
    -regulation, 136, 291
    soothe, 6, 188, 190, 196, 199, 236, 271, 298
Seng-ts'an, C., 302
Sentencing Advisory Panel (SAP), 206, 349
sequelae, 31, 50, 55
Serran, G. A., 198, 250, 262, 300, 337, 349
Seto, M. C., 210–211, 228, 240, 308, 349

Sex Offender Need Assessment
Rating (SONAR), 269
Sex Offender Risk Appraisal Guide
(SORAG), 269
Sex Offender's Register, 206
Sex Offenders Treatment
Programme (SOTP), 216,
256–260, 262
sexual *see also*: abuse, behaviour
arousal, 24, 79–80, 101, 185, 189,
194–196, 198, 200, 203,
210–211, 237–238, 240, 249,
253–254, 259–261, 293
dysfunction(s), 109, 241, 299
experience, 80–81, 164, 253
fantasy, 212
identity, 89
relationship, 40, 90–91, 111, 154,
162, 164, 173–174, 192, 196,
201, 240, 243, 295, 298
template, 62, 75–79, 81, 100, 176,
187–188, 237–239, 244, 253,
292, 298
sexuality
adult, 8, 109
bisexual, 85, 240, 243
hetero-, 156, 161, 177, 184, 200,
238, 240, 293, 295
homo-, xiii, 77, 85, 146, 156, 161,
177, 184, 239–240, 243, 295
trans-, 85, 195, 236
Shackelford, T. K., 156, 338
Shah, S. A., 97, 357
shame, xi, 12–13, 48, 52–54, 57, 71,
73, 93, 108, 119–122, 125, 127,
132–134, 140–141, 147, 156, 175,
178, 186, 192, 199, 203, 216,
218–219, 226, 231, 240, 256, 262,
264, 274–275, 283–284, 298, 301,
303
Shankaranaryana Rao, B. S., 59, 356
Shankweller, D. P., 21, 350
Shapiro, F., 280, 349
Shapiro, V., 69, 322
Sharma, L., 232, 360
Sharron, H., 26, 50, 350

Shaver, P. R., 104, 108, 111, 132, 198,
311, 327, 339, 350
Shaw, J., 137, 307
Shaw, P., 86, 350
Shaw, R., 285, 350
Shaw, S. M., 200, 350
Shaywitz, B. A., 21, 350
Shaywitz, S. E., 21, 350
Sheath, M., 258, 350
Sheldon, K., 210, 212, 255, 266, 350
Sheldon-Keller, A. E., 132, 358
Sheline, Y. I., 60, 350
Sheridan, L., 224, 310
Shingler, J., 300, 350
Shirley, E. R., 170–171, 339
Shlosberg, E., 112, 312
Shorey, H., 51, 95, 106, 108, 133, 198,
275, 350
Short, R. V., 248, 350
Shupe, L. M., 136, 350
Siegel, D., 13, 53, 66, 197, 209–210,
280, 284, 291, 294, 301, 351
Siegle, G. J., 276, 351
Silverman, J., 204, 351
Simkin, S., 137, 327
Skoff, B., 144, 327
Skudlarski, P., 21, 134, 318, 350
Skuse, D. H., 25, 351
Slaby, R. G., 145, 351
Slade, A., 3, 118, 282–283, 351
Slep, A. M., 246, 310
Smallbone, S. W., 76–77, 180,
189–190, 244, 255, 270, 351, 359
smell, 2, 8, 24–26, 45, 65, 237
Smith, A. H. W., 257, 334
Snyder, C. R., 51, 95, 106, 108, 133,
198, 275, 350
Sobal, J., 88, 351
social intelligence, 27
social phobia, 54
sociopathic, 144, 244, 267
Solms, M., 21–22, 24, 30, 132, 144,
194, 231, 351
Solomon, M. F., 294, 352
Solomon, R., 239, 352
Sorensen, J., 171, 352

Southwick, S., 65, 333
Spear, L. P., 83, 189, 352
Special Care Baby Units (SCBU),
    7–8, 221
specific serotonin reuptake
    inhibitors (SSRIs), 254
Speltz, K., 252, 337
Sperry, R. W., 20, 288, 341, 352
Spinhoven, P., 108, 198, 341
Spitz, A. M., 60, 321
Spitzberg, B., 227, 352
splitting, 19, 64–65, 127, 135, 146,
    193, 288
Spring, M., 153, 305
Sroufe, L. A., xv, 6, 11, 14, 54, 64,
    93–94, 97, 119, 319, 342, 352, 357
stalking, xviii–xix, 162, 221–224,
    226, 228–229, 231–233, 235, 263
    cyber-, 227
Standeven, B., 89, 336
Stapleton, A., 211–212, 247, 352
Starkstein, S. E., 20, 339
Starratt, V. G., 156, 338
Static-99, 266, 268
Steadman, H., 232, 340
Steele, H., xv, 133, 282, 291, 322
Steele, M., xv, 133, 282, 291, 322
Stein, P. T., 59, 352
Steinberg, L., 76–77, 309
Stern, R., S., 82, 85, 318
Stewart, T. M., 232, 318
Stewart-Williams, S., 156, 338
Stoll, K., 253, 323
Stormer, C. C., 87, 305
Strathearn, L., xi, 8–9, 26, 53–54, 69,
    353
Straube, T., 45, 277, 353
stress, xvi–xvii, 5–6, 12–13, 25, 27,
    29, 32, 39, 46, 52–53, 55–56,
    58–60, 62, 78, 87, 91, 94–95, 99,
    108–109, 120, 125, 132, 134, 154,
    157, 163, 169, 175, 179–181, 189,
    197–199, 217, 225, 227, 230, 254,
    279, 283, 286, 289, 291–294
    see also: burnout, distress,
    post traumatic stress disorder

Stringer, I., 265, 316
Strong, D., 198, 299, 307
Strong, S. M., 243, 310
Structured Anchored Clinical
    Judgement (SACJ), 266,
    268–269
Stuart, G. L., 159, 329
Stuss, D. T., 27, 353
Subby, R., 154, 353
subjectivity, 31, 137, 261, 280, 287
    inter-, 277
substance abuse, 92, 134, 136, 138,
    140, 159, 226, 232, 253, 283
    see also: alcohol, drugs
suicide, 60, 126, 131, 137, 139, 224,
    230
Sunderland, M., xiii, 5, 353
Susser, E., xvi, 341
Swithenby, S. J., 62, 311
Symington, N., 125, 353
sympathetic arousal, 13, 48, 54–55,
    87, 120, 123, 158, 198
sympathetic nervous system, 16, 18,
    24, 44, 47, 48, 51, 64, 120, 134,
    178, 219
synaptic gap, 18–19, 32
Syrota, A., 32, 44, 187, 313
Systematic Treatment Enhancement
    Programmes for Bipolar
    Disorder (STEP-BD), 170

Taber, K. H., 134, 330
Tabin, J. K., 239, 353
Tagney, J. P., 256, 284, 353
Tanak, M., 28, 359
Tantum, D., 37, 353
Tapert, S. F., 92, 353
Target, M., 133, 281–282, 322, 353
Tarry, H., 95, 354
Taylor, C., 256, 354
Taylor, M., 206, 208–209, 213–214,
    216, 344, 354
Teasdale, J. D., 44, 354
Teicher, M. H., 58–59, 354
temporal lobe, 17, 243
    epilepsy, 243

Temporini, H., 137, 323
Teson, A., 20, 339
Tessarollo, L., 287, 346
Thames Valley Project, 260
Thase, M. E., 170–171, 276, 339, 351
Thatcher, R. W., 287, 354
Thatcherism, 316
Theonnes, N., 162, 354
Thomas, C., 133, 282, 358
Thomas, D. G., 35, 354
Thomasius, R., 93, 286, 343, 348
Thompson, M. L., 49, 339
Thornton, D., 268–269, 300, 326, 337
Tibbetts, S., 9, 343
Tikkanen, R., 185, 315
Tizard, B., 68, 354
Tjaden, P., 162, 354
Tomak, S., 212, 354
Tomkins, S. S., 119, 354
Tornatzky, W., 49, 339
torture, 78, 138, 143, 214
touch, 2, 8, 18, 26–27, 41, 43, 71, 76, 123, 137, 165, 208, 213, 237–238, 241, 289
Townsend, E., 138, 327
Tranel, D., 44, 144, 306, 308, 317
transference, 60, 141–142, 228, 281, 284
    counter-, 143, 281, 283
transgenerational transmission, xii, xv, xviii, 67, 70, 77, 94, 97, 125, 151, 231, 253, 292, 296
transvestitism, 237
trauma, xv–xvii, xix–xx, 56, 58–62, 64–65, 70, 78, 82, 86, 88, 98, 110–111, 114, 132–135, 139, 142, 146, 151, 157, 160, 163, 179–180, 188–190, 197–198, 207, 217, 231, 238, 243–244, 253, 263–264, 276–278, 280, 283, 286–287, 291–292, 298, 300–301 see also: attachment, birth trauma, post traumatic stress disorder
Treboux, D., 104, 150, 316, 357

Trevarthen, C., 28, 135, 355
Turnbull, O., 21–22, 24. 30, 137, 144, 194, 231, 351, 355
Tyman, H., 252, 355
Tyrer, P., 131, 141, 308, 355

UK Court of Appeal, 206
UK Sentencing Advisory Panel (SAP), 206
University of Minnesota, 94
US Department of Justice, 203–204
Utting, D., 91–92, 309
Uvnas-Moberg, K., 29, 343

Van Balen, R., 261, 355
Van der Kolk, B. A., 62, 136, 138–139, 146, 160, 250, 355
Van Duyne, C., 232, 318
Van IJzendoorn, M. H., 5, 154, 355
van Os, J., 142, 307
van Velsen, C., 258, 358
vandalism/vandalization, 77, 87, 98, 176, 187, 238–239, 253, 292, 298
Vanderlinden, J., 108, 198, 341
Vanderveer, P., 213, 313
Vandiver, D. M., 253, 260, 356
Varney, G. A., 259, 345
Vas Dias, S., 36, 356
Vazquez, S., 20, 339
Venga, R., 31, 356
Veríssimo, M., 66, 356
Verny, T., 7–9, 13, 33, 109, 142, 356
Verrier, N. N., 70, 356
Vess, J., 244, 328
Vianna, D. M. L., 64, 356
Vigilante, D., 59, 343
Vignoles, V. L., 124, 342
violence, xi, xv, 9, 11, 13, 58, 64, 67, 71, 78–79, 83, 94–96, 98–99, 110, 136, 144–147, 158–160, 162–163, 182, 214, 227, 229–233, 241, 250–251, 257, 262–263, 267, 269, 274, 294–296 see also: behaviour
    compulsive, 136

domestic, xix, 13, 58–60, 78,
94–95, 147, 156, 158–159, 161,
163, 186, 189–190, 226, 231,
233, 294
institutional, 147
psychopharmacological, 136
Virden, T., 212, 354
Virkkunen, M., 69, 356
Vizard, E., 81, 356
Vollebergh, W., 142, 307
von Wendt, L., 9, 347
Vorst, H., 240, 330
Vosmer, S., 79, 81, 356
voyeurism, 111, 175, 192, 207, 212,
215, 238, 241, 244, 248, 249, 251,
263
Vukadinovic, Z., 198, 299, 307
Vyas, A., 59, 356

Wagner, N., 253, 323
Wagner, P., 256, 353
Wakeling, H. C., 246, 356
Walker, A., 159, 230, 357
Walker, J., 244, 328
Walker, L. E., 162, 357
Wall, S., 3–4, 306
Waller, N. G., 150, 322
Walsh, A., 77, 357
Walzer, S., 97, 357
Wannäs, M., 80, 347
Ward, D., 79, 327
Ward, E., 252, 357
Ward, T., 241, 244–245, 251,
254–255, 259, 269, 323, 329, 333,
357
Warren, J., 232, 318
Waters, E., xv, 3–4, 104, 306, 357
Watson, J., 29, 324
Watson, M. S., 244, 310
Watt, D. F., 22, 57, 357
Watters, S. O., 216, 357
Watts, S., 154, 357
Weaver, C., 243, 314
Webb, R., 200, 296, 333
Webster, J. D., 112, 357
Webster, S. D., 246, 250, 339, 356

Weeks, G., 110, 123, 292, 318
Weiner, P., 231, 319
Weinfield, N. A., 64, 342
Weinrott, M. R., 262, 323
Weinstock, M., 198, 357
Weiss, R., 200, 216, 348
Welldon, E. V., 258, 358
Welsh, R. K., 223–224, 226, 358
Wernz, M., 138, 310
Weschler, F. S., 212, 354
West, A. G., 249, 251, 325
West, D. J., 264, 358
West, F., 231
West, M. L., 132, 358
West, R., 252
Westen, D., 133, 282, 358
Weston, D. R., 37, 336
Wettstein, A., 113, 343
Wexler, B. E., 134, 318
Whitaker, E., 35, 354
Whitaker, J., 37, 353
Whitehead, P. C., 154, 319
Whitesell, N. R., 86, 327
Whittle, N., 81, 358
Whyte, B., 81, 329
Wignroks, L., 10, 345
Wilkinson, M., 284, 358
Williams, J., 160, 334
Williams, L. M., 246, 358
Williams, S. C. R., 44, 354
Williams Committee Report, 205,
358
Williamson, D. F., 60, 321
Willimans, L. M., 252, 321
Wilson, C., 49, 256, 315, 358
Wilson, D., 204, 351
Wilson, J. S., 223–224, 226, 232, 358
Wilson, P., 154, 357
Winnicott, D. W., 39, 358
Wippman, J., xv, 357
Wismer Fries, A. B., 67, 358
Wisneiwski, S. R., 170–171, 339
Wittling, W., 22, 359
Wolf, L., 257, 324
Wolfe, D., 131, 328
Wong, S., 267, 310

Wood, D. O., xi, 353
Wood, M., 63, 307
Woolfe, R., 96, 322
Worthington, R., 252, 355
Wortley, R., 270, 359
Wright, J., 81, 323
Wright, L., 208–209, 214, 216, 344
Wu, X., 6, 338
Wyatt, G., 160, 334
Wyre, R., 262, 359

Yamada, H., 28, 359
Yates, A., 145, 359
Yates, P. M., 269, 331
Yonekura, Y., 28, 359
Young, K., 185, 199, 201, 359

Young, L., 63, 307
Yurgelun-Todd, D. A., 83–84, 331, 359

Zahn-Waxler, C., 169, 359
Zeanah, C. H., xiv, 68–69, 359
Zeifman, D., 105, 327
Zeki, S., 109, 308
Ziegenhain, U., 10, 345
Ziegler, T. E., 67, 358
Zigler, E., xvii, 97, 245, 331
Zillman, D., 145, 230, 360
Zitzman, S., 297, 360
Ziv, Y., 10, 347
Zona, M., 232, 360
Zucker, K. J., 243, 310